ELSEVIER
MOSBY

Vice President, Global Medical Reference: Mary Gatsch
Editor: Kerry Holland
Developmental Editor: Barbara Cohen-Kligerman
Production Supervisor, Electronic Year Books: Donna M. Skelton
Electronic Article Manager: Mike Sheets
Illustrations and Permissions Coordinator: Dawn Vohsen

2014 EDITION

Composition by TNQ Books and Journals Pvt Ltd, India

Editorial Office:
Elsevier
Suite 1800
1600 John F. Kennedy Blvd.
Philadelphia, PA 19106-3399

International Standard Serial Number: 8756-5005
International Standard Book Number: 978-0-323-26471-6

2

The Year Book
NEONATAL AN
PERINATA
MEDICIN

ELSEVIER
MOSBY

Editorial Board

Contributing Editors

David H. Adamkin, MD

Professor of Pediatrics; Director of Division of Neonatology; Director of Nutritional Research; Rounsavall Chair of Neonatal Medicine; Co-Director of Neonatal Fellowship, University of Louisville, Louisville, Kentucky

Varsha Bhatt-Mehta, PharmD, MS, FCCP

Clinical Professor, College of Pharmacy and Department of Pediatrics and Communicable Diseases, Medical School, University of Michigan, Ann Arbor Michigan

Monika Bhola, MD

Associate Professor of Pediatrics, Rainbow Babies and Children's Hospital, Case Western Reserve University, Cleveland, Ohio

Heather H. Burris, MD, MPH

Assistant Professor of Pediatrics, Division of Newborn Medicine, Boston Children's Hospital; Attending Neonatologist, Department of Neonatology, Beth Israel Deaconess Medical Center, Boston, Massachusetts

Christina A. Buysse, MD

Fellow in Developmental and Behavioral Pediatrics, Division of Neonatal and Developmental Medicine, Lucile Packard Children's Hospital, Stanford University, Palo Alto, California

Alexis S. Davis, MD, MS

Clinical Assistant Professor of Neonatology, Division of Neonatal and Developmental Medicine, Lucile Packard Children's Hospital, Stanford University, Palo Alto, California

Juliann M. Di Fiore, BSEE

Research Engineer, Case Western Reserve University Neonatology, Rainbow Babies & Children's Hospital, Cleveland, Ohio

Jonathan M. Fanaroff, MD, JD

Associate Professor of Pediatrics, Case Western Reserve University School of Medicine; Director, Rainbow Center for Pediatric Ethics; Co-Director, Neonatal Intensive Care Unit, Rainbow Babies & Children's Hospital, Cleveland, Ohio

Samir Gupta, DM, MD, FRCPCH, FRCPI

Professor of Neonatology, Durham University; Deputy Director, Research and Development; Consultant Neonatologist, University Hospital of North Tees, Stockton, United Kingdom

Naomi Laventhal, MD, MA

Assistant Professor, Department of Pediatrics and Communicable Diseases, Division of Neonatal-Perinatal Medicine, University of Michigan, C.S. Mott Children's Hospital, Ann Arbor, Michigan

M. Jeffrey Maisels MD, DSc

Chair Emeritus and Professor; Director, Academic Affairs, Department of Pediatrics, Oakland University William Beaumont School of Medicine, Royal Oak, Michigan

Richard J. Martin, MD
Drusinsky-Fanaroff Chair in Neonatology, Rainbow Babies & Children's Hospital; Professor of Pediatrics, Case Western Reserve University, Cleveland, Ohio

Christopher C. McPherson, PharmD
Departments of Pharmacy and Pediatric Newborn Medicine, Brigham and Women's Hospital, Boston, Massachusetts

Pak Cheung Ng, MD, FRCPCH, FRCP (Lond,Edin)
Professor of Pediatrics and Chairman, Department of Pediatrics, Chinese University of Hong Kong, Hong Kong, China

Kenneth Pituch, MD
Professor of Pediatrics and Communicable Diseases; Medical Director, Pediatric Palliative Care Program, C.S. Mott Children's Hospital, University of Michigan, Ann Arbor, Michigan

Karen M. Puopolo, MD, PhD
Chief, Section on Newborn Pediatrics, Pennsylvania Hospital; Associate Professor of Clinical Pediatrics, University of Pennsylvania Perelman School of Medicine, Children's Hospital of Philadelphia Newborn Care at Pennsylvania Hospital, Philadelphia, Pennsylvania

Martha Sola-Visner, MD
Attending Neonatologist, Boston Children's Hospital; Assistant Professor of Pediatrics, Harvard Medical School, Boston, Massachusetts

Rebecca J. Vartanian, MD
Clinical Assistant Professor, Department of Pediatrics, University of Michigan Health System, Ann Arbor, Michigan

Nicole K. Yamada, MD
Fellow in Neonatal-Perinatal Medicine; Division of Neonatal and Developmental Medicine, Lucile Packard Children's Hospital, Stanford University, Palo Alto, California

Table of Contents

Journals Represented ix

Introduction xi

1. The Fetus 1
2. Epidemiology and Pregnancy Complications 5
3. Genetics and Teratology 19
4. Labor and Delivery 31
5. Infectious Disease and Immunology 55
6. Cardiovascular System 73
7. Respiratory Disorders 89
8. Central Nervous System and Special Senses 125
9. Gastrointestinal Health and Nutrition 153
10. Hematology and Bilirubin 205
11. Renal, Metabolism, and Endocrine Disorders 221
12. Miscellaneous 229
13. Pharmacology 245
14. Postnatal Growth and Development/Follow-Up 255
15. Ethics 279

Article Index 293

Author Index 303

Journals Represented

Journals represented in this YEAR BOOK are listed below.

Acta Obstetricia et Gynecologica Scandinavica
Acta Paediatrica
American Journal of Clinical Nutrition
American Journal of Epidemiology
American Journal of Obstetrics and Gynecology
American Journal of Perinatology
Antimicrobial Agents and Chemotherapy
Archives of Disease in Childhood
Archives of Disease in Childhood Fetal and Neonatal Edition
Australia & New Zealand Journal of Obstetrics and Gynaecology
BioMedical Central Pediatrics
British Journal of Obstetrics and Gynaecology
Clinical Chemistry
Developmental Medicine and Child Neurology
Diabetes Care
Early Human Development
European Journal of Obstetrics, Gynecology and Reproductive Biology
Fertility and Sterility
Frontiersin Cellular and Infection Microbiology
Genome Medicine
International Journal of Gynaecology and Obstetrics
Journal of Dental Research
Journal of Infectious Diseases
Journal of Neurosurgery Pediatrics
Journal of Parenteral and Enteral Nutrition
Journal of Pediatric Gastroenterology and Nutrition
Journal of Pediatric Surgery
Journal of Pediatrics
Journal of Perinatology
Journal of the American College of Surgeons
Journal of the American Medical Association
Journal of the American Medical Association Ophthalmology
Journal of the American Medical Association Pediatrics
Journal of Ultrasound in Medicine
Lancet
Nature Medicine
Neonatology
Neuroradiology
New England Journal of Medicine
Nutrients
Obstetrics and Gynecology
Paediatric and Perinatal Epidemiology
Pediatric Infectious Disease Journal
Pediatric Neurology
Pediatric Radiology
Pediatric Research
Pediatrics

Proceedings of the National Academy of Sciences of the United States of America
Public Library of Science One
Radiology
Seizures
Transfusion
Ultrasound in Obstetrics & Gynecology

Standard Abbreviations

The following terms are abbreviated in this edition: acquired immunodeficiency syndrome (AIDS), cardiopulmonary resuscitation (CPR), central nervous system (CNS), cerebrospinal fluid (CSF), computed tomography (CT), deoxyribonucleic acid (DNA), electrocardiography (ECG), health maintenance organization (HMO), human immunodeficiency virus (HIV), intensive care unit (ICU), intramuscular (IM), intravenous (IV), magnetic resonance (MR) imaging (MRI), ribonucleic acid (RNA), and ultrasound (US).

Note

To facilitate the use of the Year Book of Neonatal and Perinatal Medicine® as a reference tool, all illustrations and tables included in this publication are now identified as they appear in the original article. This change is meant to help the reader recognize that any illustration or table appearing in the Year Book of Neonatal and Perinatal Medicine® may be only one of many in the original article. For this reason, figure and table numbers will often appear to be out of sequence within the Year Book of Neonatal and Perinatal Medicine®.

Introduction

It is with a real sense of accomplishment and excitement that the editors present the 2014 edition of the YEAR BOOK OF NEONATAL AND PERINATAL MEDICINE. It is a labor of love and a continuing challenge to find suitable articles to review, but it is also a great learning experience. Each editor has a focus area, but we also range beyond our comfort zones and enlist the assistance of our talented colleagues so that the reader has exposure to a broad range of topics and opinions. We are grateful to our colleagues who so willingly and substantially contribute to each edition.

We are pleased to present our opinions on many randomized controlled trials as well as other important scientific endeavors that move the field forward. Genetics and fetal evaluation for genetic disorders from cell free maternal plasma feature prominently, as do the controversial outcomes in trials to determine optimal saturations in very low birth weight infants. There is copious information on nutrition and the ever-present necrotizing enterocolitis together with much information on therapeutic hypothermia. Long-term neuro-developmental outcomes and a variety of ethical dilemmas are also included.

Attention to quality improvement (QI) programs and safety is essential to providing good patient care. The Institute of Medicine has six specific aims for improvement. The headlines are safety, effectiveness, patient-centered, timely, efficient, and equitable. A key element for the success of quality initiatives is an enthusiastic staff that undergoes rigorous education and training to develop a culture of communication and teamwork. The benefits of QI programs are exemplified in the current YEAR BOOK in a number of reports ranging from preventing moderate hypothermia in preterm babies by warming the resuscitation area, delayed clamping or milking of the umbilical cord, a standardized investigation to determine the etiology of severe hyperbilirubinemia, and the treatment of hypoglycemia, to highlight a few examples. Not only do these interventions save lives and reduce morbidity, they are also extremely cost effective. We wholeheartedly endorse the comments of McAdams, "The failure to more broadly implement delayed cord clamping in neonates ignores published benefits of increased placental blood transfusion at birth and may represent an unnecessary harm for vulnerable neonates."[1] As participation in QI programs is an integral component of recertification in Neonatology, I anticipate that we will witness many more examples.

We are grateful to Elsevier for their continued support and confidence in the editorial staff and thank in particular Barbara Cohen-Kligerman, who has been of inestimable value in keeping us on time and on track so that she could assemble this book. We hope that the readers enjoy the book as much as we have enjoyed assembling these manuscripts and commentaries.

Avroy A. Fanaroff
William E. Benitz
Steven M. Donn
Josef Neu
Lu-Ann Papile
Linda J. Van Marter

Reference

1. McAdams RM. Time to implement delayed cord clamping. *Obstet Gynecol.* 2014; 123:549-552.

1 The Fetus

Conservative management of antenatally diagnosed cystic lung malformations

Ng C, Stanwell J, Burge DM, et al (Univ Hosp Southampton NHS Foundation Trust, UK)

Arch Dis Child 99:432-437, 2014

Aim.—To review the outcome of all antenatally diagnosed conservatively managed congenital lung malformations (CLMs) managed at our centre.

Methods.—All patients diagnosed antenatally with cystic lung malformations from 2001 to 2011, at a tertiary referral paediatric surgical centre practising a policy of conservative management of asymptomatic cases, were retrospectively reviewed. Data were collected from medical case notes and radiology reports. Ethical approval was obtained from our institutional research and development department.

Results.—The complete records of 74 fetuses antenatally diagnosed with CLM were reviewed. There were 72 live births, at a median gestation of 39.6 weeks. Emergency lobectomy was performed in one symptomatic neonate. Elective lobectomies were performed at parental request in three asymptomatic infants, one of whom had a family history of synovial sarcoma. Two patients developed pneumonia in the affected lobe during early childhood and proceeded to lobectomy at the age of 3 years. One patient with a bronchopulmonary sequestration required embolisation for cyanotic episodes. The remaining 65 patients have been conservatively managed to date, and none have required hospital admission. Less than a quarter report mild respiratory symptoms such as cough or wheeze. Median follow-up is 5 years.

Conclusions.—This retrospective cohort study of 74 consecutive CLMs diagnosed antenatally over a 10-year period demonstrates that most of these lesions will remain asymptomatic throughout childhood. Although the natural history of CLMs in later years remains to be elucidated, we hope that this report on medium-term outcomes will be useful to clinicians who undertake antenatal counselling and may inform the discussion on how best to manage these children.

► The most common fetal lung cysts are due to congenital cystic adenomatoid malformations (CCAM) and pulmonary sequestration. Lima et al,[1] reporting on prenatal and perinatal aspects of CCAMs, noted an incidence of 1:1980 with the diagnosis at mean gestational age of 24 ± 3.7 weeks. In their series, progression of the lesions occurred in 11 cases (44%), stability in 6 (24%), and regression in 8 (32%). Radiographic abnormalities were found in 22 of 23 patients studied. Three patients with polyhydramnios and hydrops, which are bad prognostic signs, died. Tsai et al[2] reported a series of 58 patients with CCAM and noted that with the advent of 3-dimensional ultrasound capability, more lesions were now being recognized in the second trimester. Taking the technology to the next level, Pacharn et al[3] reported that "Prenatal MRI is highly accurate in defining congenital lung anomalies. When fetal MRI findings suggest a specific diagnosis, postnatal findings confirmed the prenatal MRI diagnosis in 98% of cases." This is impressive because their series at the Cincinnati referral center included more than 50 cases. The commonest lesion encountered was CCAM followed by sequestration and a few cases of bronchogenic cysts, which are extremely rare and arise from abnormal buds from the primitive esophagus and tracheobronchial tree. They are typically unilocular arising from the posterior wall of the airway and may be readily recognized by ultrasound as a unilocular cystic lesion in the fetal thorax. If the heart is being compressed and there is evidence of hydrops, the cyst may be aspirated.

It is reassuring to learn from the Ng et al study that the trend toward less invasive surgery on the fetus was not hazardous for the babies. Indeed, few of the 74 patients with fetal lung lesions needed surgery through childhood. Fetuses with large CCAMs associated with hydrops are predisposed to perinatal mortality, and therefore prenatal intervention is required.

A. A. Fanaroff, MD, FRCPE

References

1. Lima JS, Camargos PA, Aguiar RA, Campos AS, Aguiar MJ. Pre and perinatal aspects of congenital cystic adenomatoid malformation of the lung. *J Matern Fetal Neonatal Med.* 2014;27:228-232.
2. Tsai HF, Cheng YC, Ko HC, et al. Prenatal diagnosis of fetal congenital cystic adenomatoid malformation of the lung using three-dimensional ultrasound: comparison between the 20th and 21st centuries. *Taiwan J Obstet Gynecol.* 2013;52: 90-96.
3. Pacharn P, Kline-Fath B, Calvo-Garcia M, et al. Congenital lung lesions: prenatal MRI and postnatal findings. *Pediatr Radiol.* 2013;43:1136-1143.

Absent Fetal Nasal Bone: What Does it Mean for the Euploid Fetus?

Dukhovny S, Wilkins-Haug L, Shipp TD, et al (Brigham and Women's Hosp, Boston, MA; et al)

J Ultrasound Med 32:2131-2134, 2013

Objectives.—Our purpose was to review the outcomes of singleton pregnancies in which an absent nasal bone was noted on first- or second-trimester sonography and aneuploidy was not present.

Methods.—We identified singleton pregnancies from 2005 to 2011 in which an absent nasal bone was noted on sonography, aneuploidy was excluded, and newborn examinations were available for review. Sonographic reports were reviewed for anomalies, growth, and amniotic fluid volume. Newborn records were reviewed for physical examinations, complications, and radiologic or genetic tests.

Results.—We identified 142 fetuses with a sonographic appearance of an absent nasal bone. We excluded 52 cases with aneuploidy and 33 in which newborn examination information was unavailable. Fifty-seven cases met inclusion criteria. For 3 euploid fetuses with an absent nasal bone on sonography, the presence of additional anomalies on second-trimester sonography ultimately signaled an adverse outcome: the presence of multiple congenital anomalies, a microdeletion syndrome, and a specific genetic diagnosis.

Conclusions.—All cases with adverse outcomes had additional prenatal sonographic findings. For the remainder, normal newborn examination findings provide some reassurance, especially in the setting of otherwise normal second-trimester sonographic findings. A microarray as a test for microdeletion and duplication syndromes in this situation could be considered.

▶ Langdon Down first reported a small nasal bone in Trisomy 21, frequently referred to as *Down syndrome.*[1] Subsequently, with careful ultrasound surveillance, it has been reported that absence of the fetal nasal bone in the first trimester yields a likelihood ratio for Down syndrome of 27.8, and in the second trimester, the likelihood ratio is 83.[2,3] A recent systematic review and meta-analysis[4] reported the pooled estimates of positive and negative likelihood ratios (for Trisomy 21) were 40.08 (95% confidence interval [CI], 18.10–88.76) and 0.71 (95% CI, 0.64–0.79), respectively, for absent nasal bone and 15.15 (95% CI, 8.15–28.16) and 0.47 (95% CI, 0.34–0.64), respectively, for hypoplastic nasal bones. No relevant differences were found between the various means of defining nasal hypoplasia. They concluded that absence or hypoplasia of the nasal bones show high specificity and low but acceptable sensitivity in identifying fetuses with Down syndrome.

It has been estimated that between 0.5% and 2.8% of euploid fetuses on either first- or second-trimester ultrasound scan will have images consistent with delayed ossification of the nasal bone.

To the authors' knowledge, this study is the first to evaluate newborn outcomes from women with an absent nasal bone in euploid fetuses. This data gap presents a dilemma for the health care team with regard to counseling parents when this situation arises. Three of the 57 eligible patients with a normal karyotype, all with additional abnormalities to the absent nasal bones, had major problems and genetic abnormalities. They concluded that in the absence of other malformations, the families can be reassured. However, they recommended detailed fetal anatomic survey in the second trimester and cautiously advised microarray studies, "given the subtleties of presentation of microdeletion and duplication syndromes." They correctly identified the lack of uniform identification and recording of the fetal nasal bones as a limitation of the study and most authors called for "a prospective cohort with long-term follow-up of euploid fetuses with an absent nasal bone and normal postnatal examination findings is needed to determine how often an absent nasal bone is a normal variant vs a marker for subtle syndromes or developmental delays."

A. A. Fanaroff, MD, FRCPE

References

1. Down JL. Observations on an ethnic classification of idiots. *Lond Hosp Rep.* 1866;3:259-262.
2. Cicero S, Curcio P, Papageorghiou A, Sonek J, Nicolaides K. Absence of nasal bone in fetuses with trisomy 21 at 11–14 weeks of gestation: an observational study. *Lancet.* 2001;358:1665-1667.
3. Bromley B, Lieberman E, Shipp TD, Benacerraf BR. Fetal nose bone length: a marker for Down syndrome in the second trimester. *J Ultrasound Med.* 2002; 21:1387-1394.
4. Moreno-Cid M, Rubio-Lorente A, Rodríguez MJ, et al. Systematic review and meta-analysis of performance of second-trimester nasal bone assessment in detection of fetuses with Down syndrome. *Ultrasound Obstet Gynecol.* 2014;43: 247-253.

2 Epidemiology and Pregnancy Complications

The Effect of Real-Time Continuous Glucose Monitoring in Pregnant Women With Diabetes: A randomized controlled trial

Secher AL, Ringholm L, Andersen HU, et al (Rigshospitalet, Copenhagen, Denmark; et al)

Diabetes Care 36:1877-1883, 2013

Objective.—To assess whether intermittent real-time continuous glucose monitoring (CGM) improves glycemic control and pregnancy outcome in unselected women with pregestational diabetes.

Research Design and Methods.—A total of 123 women with type 1 diabetes and 31 women with type 2 diabetes were randomized to use real-time CGM for 6 days at 8, 12, 21, 27, and 33 weeks in addition to routine care, including self-monitored plasma glucose seven times daily, or routine care only. To optimize glycemic control, real-time CGM readings were evaluated by a diabetes caregiver. HbA_{1c}, self-monitored plasma glucose, severe hypoglycemia, and pregnancy outcomes were recorded, with large-for-gestational-age infants as the primary outcome.

Results.—Women assigned to real-time CGM ($n = 79$) had baseline HbA_{1c} similar to that of women in the control arm ($n = 75$) (median 6.6 [range 5.3–10.0] vs. 6.8% [5.3–10.7]; $P = 0.67$) (49 [34–86] vs. 51 mmol/mol [34–93]). Forty-nine (64%) women used real-time CGM per protocol. At 33 weeks, HbA_{1c} (6.1 [5.1–7.8] vs. 6.1% [4.8–8.2]; $P = 0.39$) (43 [32–62] vs. 43 mmol/mol [29–66]) and self-monitored plasma glucose (6.2 [4.7–7.9] vs. 6.2 mmol/L [4.9–7.9]; $P = 0.64$) were comparable regardless of real-time CGM use, and a similar fraction of women had experienced severe hypoglycemia (16 vs. 16%; $P = 0.91$). The prevalence of large-for-gestational-age infants (45 vs. 34%; $P = 0.19$) and other perinatal outcomes were omparable between the arms.

Conclusions.—In this randomized trial, intermittent use of real-time CGM in pregnancy, in addition to self-monitored plasma glucose seven

times daily, did not improve glycemic control or pregnancy outcome in women with pregestational diabetes.

▶ Current treatment of diabetes in pregnancy relies on intermittent self-monitoring of blood glucoses using finger sticks to monitor capillary blood glucoses.

Continuous glucose monitoring (CGM) systems are a relatively new technology that allow frequent glucose measurements (every 5 minutes) and the ability to monitor glucose trends in real time. Whereas there has been great optimism that the more liberal use of CGM systems will improve outcomes in diabetic pregnancy the evidence speaks otherwise. Voormolen,[1] after a systematic review, concluded, "Current evidence on the efficacy of CGM on improving glycemic control during pregnancy as well as on the effectiveness on pregnancy outcome is limited to two randomized controlled trials (RCTs) with contradicting results. Evidence on the cost effectiveness is lacking. Further proper RCTs on the effectiveness and cost-effectiveness of CGM in pregnancy are required before wide implementation in practice." Nonetheless many investigators believe that there is a huge potential for their use in research and clinical practice and trials. It is anticipated that CGMs will improve detection of both hyperglycemia and hypoglycemia and help stabilize glucose levels so that HbA_{1c} levels can be kept at reasonable levels.

In Secher et al's randomized trial, CGM did not improve glucose control compared with multiple glucose measurements. HbA_{1c}, self-monitored plasma glucose values, and plasma glucose profiles of biochemical hypo- or hyperglycemia were similar throughout pregnancy in women using real-time CGM versus control subjects for the entire study population Sixteen percent of women in each group experienced hypoglycemia.

The inevitable conclusion from the trial is that CGM is not ready for prime time. It may be helpful in selected cases. Intensive focus in gestational diabetes needs to be directed at diet, including carbohydrate counting and control of weight gain.

Starikov et al[2] posed the question as to whether the HbA_{1c} in the first trimester would predict adverse pregnancy outcomes. The frequencies of composite maternal adverse pregnancy outcomes (birth at <37 weeks, preeclampsia, and medically indicated birth <39 weeks), and composite fetal adverse pregnancy outcomes (shoulder dystocia, Apgar scores <7 at 5 minutes, small for gestational age [SGA], large for gestational age [LGA], and stillbirth) were compared between HbA_{1c} categories (<6.5, 6.5–7.4, 7.5–8.4, and ≥8.5%). There was an increased risk of shoulder dystocia in those women with HbA_{1c} ≥8.5% but otherwise no statistically significant correlations. However, the teaching remains that tight control of blood sugars before conception reduces the prevalence of birth defects in insulin-dependent diabetics. This practice should be continued.[3]

A. A. Fanaroff, MD, FRCPE

References

1. Voormolen DN, DeVries JH, Evers IM, Mol BW, Franx A. The efficacy and effectiveness of continuous glucose monitoring during pregnancy: a systematic review. *Obstet Gynecol Surv.* 2013;68:753-763.
2. Starikov RS, Inman K, Chien EK, et al. Can hemoglobin A1c in early pregnancy predict adverse pregnancy outcomes in diabetic patients? *J Diabetes Complications.* 2014;28:203-207.
3. Cordua S, Secher AL, Ringholm L, Damm P, Mathiesen ER. Real-time continuous glucose monitoring during labour and delivery in women with type 1 diabetes - observations from a randomized controlled trial. *Diabet Med.* 2013;30:1374-1381.

Impact of ART on pregnancies in California: an analysis of maternity outcomes and insights into the added burden of neonatal intensive care

Merritt TA, Goldstein M, Philips R, et al (Loma Linda Univ School of Medicine, CA; et al)

J Perinatol 34:345-350, 2014

Objective.—We reviewed the occurrence of prematurity, low birth weight, multiple gestations, frequency of stillbirths and maternity care-associated variables including hospital stay and hospital charges of women conceiving using assisted reproductive technology (ART) or artificial insemination (AI) compared with women with a history of infertility who conceived naturally, and all other naturally conceived pregnancies in California at non-federal hospitals between 2009 and 2011. At a single center, infants born after ART/AI were compared with infants provided care in the normal nursery.

Study Design.—Publically available inpatient data sets from the California Office of Statewide Health Planning and Development for years 2009—2011 using data from all California non-federal hospitals were used to determine the impact of ART on a variety of pregnancy-related outcomes and infant characteristics. Infant data from a single center was used to determine hospital charges for infants delivered over an 18-month period to compare the hospital and physician charges indexed to similar charges for infants admitted to the 'normal' newborn nursery.

Result.—Among ART/AI pregnancies, there was a 4—5-fold increase in stillbirths, compared with a 2—3-fold increase among women with infertility compared with other naturally conceiving women. ART/AI pregnancies underwent more cesarean sections (fourfold), and a near fourfold increase in the rate of preterm deliveries. Multiple gestations were increased 24—27-fold compared with naturally conceived pregnancies. Maternal hospital stay and hospital charges were increased among those undergoing ART/AI. Infant charges were increased multi-fold for singletons, twins and triplets delivered after ART/AI compared with naturally conceived infants.

Conclusion.—Multiple births, preterm births and a higher overall rate of fetal anomalies were found in California after ART/AI for 2009—2011. Cesarean section rates, longer length of maternal stay and hospital charges among women receiving ART/AI could be lowered if emphasis on elective single embryo transfers was a higher priority among providers. Charges for the care of infants delivered after ART/AI are substantially higher than among naturally conceived infants born late preterm or at term. Families seeking ART/AI need to be informed of the impact of these adverse pregnancy outcomes, including neonatal outcomes and charges for medical care for their infant(s), when considering ART/AI.

▶ This article opens a large can of worms, from "It's not nice to fool mother nature" to "Always read the fine print" to "In the interests of full disclosure ...." Yet these are important data in the age of assisted reproductive technology (ART). In this ambitious study, Merritt and colleagues looked at the outcomes of infants born after ART or artificial insemination (AI) and compared them with infants delivered to women with a history of infertility who conceived naturally and to all infants born from naturally conceived pregnancies in (nonfederal hospitals) in California between 2009 and 2011. A single center was used to determine differences in both physician and facility charges. Not surprisingly, ART/AI infants had higher rates of stillbirth (4- to 5-fold higher) compared with infants born after maternal infertility without ART/AI (2- to 3-fold higher) or naturally conceived infants. There was a higher rate of cesarean delivery and a 4-fold increase in preterm birth. Multifetal gestation increased 24- to 27-fold with ART/AI compared with natural conception. The rate of fetal anomalies also increased. Hospital and physician charges were found to be significantly higher, as was maternal length of stay, in pregnancies conceived with ART/AI.

As the authors suggest, this information needs to be provided to women seeking to become pregnant through either ART or AI. Because the charges escalate dramatically for multifetal gestation, this also needs to be communicated not only to patients but to infertility specialists, and counseling needs to include a discussion about the increased risks and costs of carrying twins or higher-order multiples in ART/AI pregnancies, which may be superimposed on prematurity and its attendant complications.

S. M. Donn, MD

Amnioinfusion in very early preterm prelabor rupture of membranes (AMIPROM): pregnancy, neonatal and maternal outcomes in a randomized controlled pilot study

Roberts D, Vause S, Martin W, et al (Liverpool Women's NHS Foundation Trust, UK; St Mary's Hosp, Manchester, UK; Birmingham Women's NHS Foundation Trust, Edgbaston, UK; et al)

Ultrasound Obstet Gynecol 43:490-499, 2014

Objective.—To assess short- and long-term outcomes of pregnant women with very early rupture of membranes randomized to serial amnioinfusion or expectant management, and to collect data to inform a larger, more definitive clinical trial.

Methods.—This was a prospective non-blinded randomized controlled trial with randomization stratified for pregnancies in which the membranes ruptured between 16 + 0 and 19 + 6 weeks' gestation and 20 + 0 and 23 + 6 weeks' gestation to minimize the risk of random imbalance in gestational age distribution between randomized groups. Intention-to-treat analysis was used. The study was conducted in four UK hospital-based fetal medicine units (Liverpool Women's NHS Trust, St Mary's Hospital Manchester, Birmingham Women's NHS Foundation Trust and Wirral University Hospitals Trust). The participants were women with confirmed preterm prelabor rupture of membranes at 16 + 0 to 24 + 0 weeks' gestation. Women with multiple pregnancy, fetal abnormality or obstetric indication for immediate delivery were excluded. Participants were randomly allocated to either serial weekly transabdominal amnioinfusions if the deepest pool of amniotic fluid was < 2 cm or expectant management until 37 weeks' gestation. Short-term maternal, pregnancy and neonatal and long-term outcomes for the child were studied. Long-term respiratory morbidity was assessed using validated respiratory questionnaires at 6, 12 and 18 months of age and infant lung function test at around 12 months of age. Neurodevelopment was assessed using the Bayley Scales of Infant Development, second edition (BSID-II) at corrected age of 2 years.

Results.—Fifty-eight women were randomized to the study. Two babies were excluded from the analysis because of termination of pregnancy for lethal anomaly, leaving 56 participants (28 assigned to serial amnioinfusion and 28 to expectant management) recruited between 2002 and 2009. There was no significant difference in perinatal mortality (19/28 vs 19/28; relative risk (RR) 1.0 (95% CI, 0.70-1.43)) and maternal or neonatal morbidity. The overall chance of surviving without long-term respiratory or neurodevelopmental disability was 4/56 (7.1%); 4/28 (14.3%) in the amnioinfusion group and 0/28 in the expectant group (RR 9.0 (95% CI, 0.51-159.70)).

Conclusions.—This pilot study found no major differences in maternal, perinatal or pregnancy outcomes. The study was not designed to show a difference between the groups and the number of survivors was too small to draw any conclusions about long-term outcomes. It does, however, signal that a larger definitive study to evaluate amnioinfusion for improvement in healthy survival is needed. The pilot suggests that, with appropriate funding, such a study is feasible.

▶ When membranes rupture during the second trimester, it is an uphill battle to salvage the fetus and newborn. Evidence from observational studies support the notion that transabdominal amnioinfusion can significantly improve outcomes in which preterm premature rupture of membranes (PPROM) occurs between 16 and 26 weeks' gestation.[1] However, van Teeffelen found no controlled trials in their Cochrane review and stated: "There is currently no evidence to evaluate the use of transabdominal amnioinfusion in women with oligohydramnios secondary to rupture of fetal membranes before 26 weeks for improving perinatal outcome. Further research examining the effects of this intervention is needed."[2]

They were thus in agreement with Hofmeyr's earlier Cochrane review, which concluded: "These results are encouraging but are limited by the sparse data and unclear methodological robustness, therefore further evidence is required before amnioinfusion for PPROM can be recommended for routine clinical practice."[3]

Absence of amniotic fluid before 23 weeks' gestation makes pulmonary hypoplasia with respiratory insufficiency extremely likely, and despite heroic efforts, survivors free of respiratory or neurodevelopmental problems are few and far between. Furthermore, preterm delivery is inevitable, and there are high rates of chorioamnionitis and neonatal infections. Efforts to restore fluid with transabdominal amnioinfusion have, for all intents and purposes, proved to be futile; nonetheless, this line of therapy continues to be explored.[1,2]

The Roberts AMIPROM study is reported above. This is the first randomized trial to address respiratory and neurodevelopmental outcomes after transabdominal amnioinfusion. No infants in the control group survived without respiratory or neurologic problems compared with 7% and 14% without respiratory and neurodevelopmental outcomes, respectively, in the transabdominal amnioinfusion group. Admittedly, this is a small sample size, so the investigators are encouraged by the feasibility of doing a large trial. I personally would not fund such a study and believe newer approaches are needed.

A. A. Fanaroff, MD, FRCPE

References

1. Porat S, Amsalem H, Shah PS, Murphy KE. Transabdominal amnioinfusion for preterm premature rupture of membranes: a systematic review and metaanalysis of randomized and observational studies. *Am J Obstet Gynecol.* 2012;207: 393.e1-393.e11.
2. Van Teeffelen S, Pajkrt E, Willekes C, Van Kuijk SM, Mol BW. Transabdominal amnioinfusion for improving fetal outcomes after oligohydramnios secondary to preterm prelabour rupture of membranes before 26 weeks. *Cochrane Database Syst Rev.* 2013;(8):CD009952.
3. Hofmeyr GJ, Essilfie-Appiah G, Lawrie TA. Amnioinfusion for preterm premature rupture of membranes. *Cochrane Database Syst Rev.* 2011;(12):CD000942.

EXPRESS study shows significant regional differences in 1-year outcome of extremely preterm infants in Sweden

Serenius F, For the EXPRESS study group (Uppsala Univ, Sweden; Karolinska Univ Hosp, Huddinge, Stockholm, Sweden; et al)

Acta Paediatr 103:27-37, 2014

Aim.—The aim of this study was to investigate differences in mortality up to 1 year of age in extremely preterm infants (before 27 weeks) born in seven Swedish healthcare regions.

Methods.—National prospective observational study of consecutively born, extremely preterm infants in Sweden 2004–2007. Mortality was compared between regions. Crude and adjusted odds ratios and 95% CI were calculated.

Results.—Among 844 foetuses alive at mother's admission for delivery, regional differences were identified in perinatal mortality for the total group (22–26 weeks) and in the stillbirth and perinatal and 365-day mortality rates for the subgroup born at 22–24 weeks. Among 707 infants born alive, regional differences were found both in mortality before 12 h and in the 365-day mortality rate for the subgroup (22–24 weeks) and for the total group (22–26 weeks). The mortality rates were consistently lower in two healthcare regions. There were no differences in the 365-day mortality rate for infants alive at 12 h or for infants born at 25 weeks. Neonatal morbidity rates among survivors were not higher in regions with better survival rates. Perinatal practices varied between regions.

Conclusion.—Mortality rates in extremely preterm infants varied considerably between Swedish healthcare regions in the first year after birth, particularly between the most immature infants.

▶ It has become fashionable to have catchy nomenclature for the large multicenter trials and national cohorts. Hence we have become familiar with the EXPRESS, EPICURE, MOSAIC, SUPPORT, BOOST, NOPAIN, STOP-ROP, and CAP trials to mention a few.[1-4] Without a program, it is difficult to recognize players on the sports field, and so one constantly needs to expand and refresh one's memory regarding these various trials. A characteristic of every large trial—whether it is a randomized intervention or a national cohort—has been the center and regional variation in outcomes and practice. A disconcerting feature of this is the inability to pinpoint the different practices responsible for the variability.

This report from Sweden is no exception. I am, however, encouraged that whatever is accounting for the differences appear to be present within the first 12 hours of life, so perhaps further probing of this extensive database will yield some answers.

Serenius et al note that in fetuses alive at mother's admission for delivery and delivered at 22 to 26 weeks, the stillbirth rate ranged from 8.2% to 22% ($P = .06$), perinatal mortality rate ranged from 22% to 46% ($P < .01$), and 365-day mortality ranged from 31% to 54% ($P = .12$). Huge swings. For the 22- to 24-week group, regional variations in mortality were wide, and all outcomes differed ($P < .001$). Strikingly, there were no regional mortality differences in the 25- to 26-week group.

In infants born alive at 22–26 weeks (Table 4 in the original article), the 365-day mortality rate ranged from 18% to 43% ($P = .02$), with wider and highly significant regional differences at 22 to 24 weeks' gestation.

There were large regional differences in the rate of death before 12 hours after birth in both the total cohort ($P < .01$) and the 22- to 24-week group ($P < .001$) but only trivial and nonsignificant differences in 365-day mortality between infants alive at 12 hours. The rate of major neonatal morbidities between survivors at 1 year did not differ between the regions.

The take-home message is that there remain huge regional differences in outcome, mainly at the borders of viability (22–24 weeks). There are differences in perinatal care highlighted by the lack of administration of antenatal corticosteroids to many of these infants.[5] The encouraging news is that the infants who survive, even at the youngest gestational ages, do not have increased disabilities.

A. A. Fanaroff, MD, FRCPE

References

1. EXPRESS Group. Incidence of and risk factors for neonatal morbidity after active perinatal care: extremely preterm infants study in Sweden (EXPRESS). *Acta Paediatr.* 2010;99:978-992.
2. Costeloe KL, Hennessy EM, Haider S, Stacey F, Marlow N, Draper ES. Short term outcomes after extreme preterm birth in England: comparison of two birth cohorts in 1995 and 2006 (the EPICure studies). *BMJ.* 2012;345:e7976.
3. EXPRESS Group, Fellman V, Hellström-Westas L, Norman M. One-year survival of extremely preterm infants after active perinatal care in Sweden. *JAMA.* 2009; 301:2225-2233.
4. Stoll BJ, Hansen NI, Bell EF, et al. Neonatal outcomes of extremely preterm infants from the NICHD Neonatal Research Network. *Pediatrics.* 2010;126:443-456.
5. Carlo WA, McDonald SA, Fanaroff AA, et al. Association of antenatal corticosteroids with mortality and neurodevelopmental outcomes among infants born at 22 to 25 weeks' gestation. *JAMA.* 2011;306:2348-2358.

Outcomes of Infants Born at 22 and 23 Weeks' Gestation

Ishii N, for the Neonatal Research Network (Aiiku Hosp, Minato, Tokyo, Japan; et al)
Pediatrics 132:62-71, 2013

Objective.—To provide instructive information on death and neurodevelopmental outcomes of infants born at 22 and 23 weeks' gestational age.

Methods.—The study cohort consisted of 1057 infants born at 22 to 25 weeks in the Neonatal Research Network, Japan. Neurodevelopmental impairment (NDI) at 36 to 42 months' chronological age was defined as any of the following: cerebral palsy, hearing impairment, visual impairment, and a developmental quotient <70. A systematic review was performed by using databases of publications of cohort studies with neonatal and neurodevelopmental outcomes at 22 and 23 weeks.

Results.—Numbers and incidences (%) of infants with death or NDI were 60 (80%) at 22 weeks and 156 (64%) at 23 weeks. In logistic regression analysis, gestational ages of 22 weeks (odds ratio [OR]: 5.40; 95% confidence interval [CI]: 2.48–11.76) and 23 weeks (OR: 2.14; 95% CI: 1.38–3.32) were associated with increased risk of death or NDI compared with 24 weeks, but a gestational age of 25 weeks (OR: 0.65; 95% CI: 0.45–0.95) was associated with decreased risk of death or NDI. In the systematic review, the medians (range) of the incidence of death or NDI in 8 cohorts were 99% (90%–100%) at 22 weeks and 98% (67%–100%) at 23 weeks.

Conclusions.—Infants born at 22 and 23 weeks' gestation were at higher risk of death or NDI than infants at born at 24 weeks. However, outcomes were improved compared with those in previous studies. There is a need for additional discussions on interventions for infants born at 22 or 23 weeks' gestation.

▶ Counseling parents in anticipation of delivery of preterm infants at the margins of viability remains one of the most difficult tasks required of perinatal health care providers. The emotional intensity of an impending pregnancy loss is compounded by uncertainty about and, too often, inconsistency in the empiric data available to inform the discussion. This report from the Japanese Neonatal Research Network attempts to address that need. The authors highlight the observation of improving survival rates among infants born at 22 to 23 weeks of gestation, but even that muted enthusiasm should be tempered by a careful examination of their data:

	Gestational Age (n [% of total])			
	22 Weeks	23 Weeks	24 Weeks	25 Weeks
n	75	245	332	405
Died	48 (64)	91 (38)	76 (22)	60 (13)
Lost	4 (5)	35 (14)	76 (22)	95 (23)
Profound NDI	7 (9)	45 (18)	23 (7)	36 (9)
Moderate NDI	7 (9)	25 (10)	68 (20)	80 (20)
No/minimal NDI	9 (12)	49 (20)	89 (27)	134 (33)

First, it is notable that far fewer infants were born at 22 weeks than during each subsequent week of gestation, even though the trial design ensured capture of live-born infants who died in the delivery room as well as those admitted to the neonatal intensive care unit, and rates of transfer from outside facilities were similar (8 to 10%) across groups. The cesarean delivery rate increased from 24% at 22 to 42%, 67%, and 73% at 23, 24, and 25 weeks, respectively, suggesting a much more aggressive approach to obstetric intervention as gestation advanced. Data gathered from those who survive delivery at 22 or 23 weeks despite a hands-off approach to obstetric intervention should not be used to guide decisions about management of all fetuses or infants at that early stage. Second, among infants born at 22 or 23 weeks, the probability of survival with profound neurodevelopmental impairment (NDI) is nearly the same as that of survival with no or minimal impairment, but among those surviving infants born at 24 or 25 weeks, no or minimal impairment is nearly 4 times as likely as profound NDI. Clearly, supportive treatment is a much better gamble after 23 weeks. Finally, loss of nearly 30% of survivors from follow-up evaluation raises concern about the reliability of the estimates of NDI rates. Although it is important to advise prospective parents of infants at risk for birth at 22 to 23 weeks that the probability of survival with no or minimal impairment is not zero, they also need to be aware that the risk of profound impairment is comparable and may be higher if obstetric interventions lead to survival of less robust members of these high-risk cohorts.

W. E. Benitz, MD

Antecedents of Cerebral Palsy and Perinatal Death in Term and Late Preterm Singletons

McIntyre S, Blair E, Badawi N, et al (Univ of Sydney, New South Wales, Australia; Children's Natl Med Centre, Washington, DC; Natl Insts of Health, Bethesda, MD)
Obstet Gynecol 122:869-877, 2013

Objective.—To examine the antecedents of cerebral palsy and of perinatal death in singletons born at or after 35 weeks of gestation.

Methods.—From a total population of singletons born at or after 35 weeks of gestation, we identified 494 with cerebral palsy and 508 neonates in a matched control group, 100 neonatal deaths, and 73 intrapartum stillbirths (all deaths in selected birth years). Neonatal death and cerebral palsy were categorized as without encephalopathy, after neonatal encephalopathy, or after neonatal encephalopathy considered hypoxic–ischemic. We examined the contribution of potentially asphyxial birth events, inflammation, fetal growth restriction, and birth defects recognized by age 6 years to each of these outcomes and to intrapartum stillbirths.

Results.—The odds of total cerebral palsy after potentially asphyxial birth events or inflammation were modestly increased (odds ratio [OR] 1.9, 95% confidence interval [CI] 1.1–3.2 and OR 2.2, 95% CI 1.0–4.2, respectively). However, potentially asphyxial birth events occurred in 34% of intrapartum stillbirths and 21.6% of cerebral palsy after hypoxic–ischemic encephalopathy. Inflammatory markers occurred in 13.9% and 11.9% of these outcomes, respectively. Growth restriction contributed significantly to all poor outcome groups. Birth defects were recognized in 5.5% of neonates in the control group compared with 60% of neonatal deaths and more than half of cases of cerebral palsy without hypoxic–ischemic encephalopathy. In children with cerebral palsy, a potentially asphyxial birth event, inflammation, or both were experienced by 12.6%, whereas growth restriction, a birth defect, or both were experienced by 48.6% ($P < .001$).

Conclusion.—Fetal growth restriction and birth defects recognized by age 6 years were more substantial contributors to cerebral palsy and neonatal death than potentially asphyxial birth events and inflammation.

Level of Evidence.—II.

▶ In this total population case-control study the authors' objective was to gain more specific information concerning pathways to perinatal death or cerebral palsy in term and late-preterm singletons. In an attempt to identify etiologically more homogenous groups of cerebral palsy and neonatal death, study subjects were stratified according to newborn neurologic status, then the contribution of 4 major risk factors (potentially asphyxial birth events, indicators of inflammation, fetal growth restriction and birth defects) alone or in combination was quantified for each of the outcomes.

Eligible cases of cerebral palsy comprised all registrants of the Western Australia Cerebral Palsy Register born in Western Australia between January 1, 1980, and December 31, 1995, excluding those whose cerebral palsy was acquired postnatally. Control subjects and intrapartum stillbirth and neonatal death data were obtained from the Maternal Child Health Research Database, which includes 99.5% of all registered births.

The authors used population-attributable fractions to estimate the proportion of cerebral palsy risk that could be attributed to each of the 4 major risk factors. When estimated relative risk is used to calculate population-attributable fractions, as was done in this study, there invariably is an overestimation regarding the impact of the risk factor. In addition, one of the assumptions underlying valid population-attributable fraction estimation is that there is a causal relationship between the risk factor and the disease. For these reasons, the percentages reported in the abstract most likely are biased and do not indicate that there is a causal relationship between cerebral palsy and neonatal death and any of the risk factors. Thus, the authors' conclusion that fetal growth restriction and birth defects are more substantial contributors to cerebral palsy and neonatal death than potentially asphyxial birth events and inflammation needs to be validated by additional studies.

L. A. Papile, MD

Claims for compensation after alleged birth asphyxia: a nationwide study covering 15 years

Andreasen S, Backe B, Øian P (Nordland Hosp, Bodø, Norway; Norwegian Univ of Technology and Science, Trondheim, Norway; Univ of Tromsø, Norway)

Acta Obstet Gynecol Scand 93:152-158, 2014

Objective.—To analyze compensation claims with neurological sequela or death following alleged birth asphyxia.

Design.—A cohort study.

Setting.—A nationwide study in Norway.

Sample.—All claims made to The Norwegian System of Compensation to Patients (NPE) concerning sequela related to alleged birth asphyxia, between 1994 and 2008. A total of 315 claims of which 161 were awarded compensation.

Methods.—Examination of hospital records, experts' assessments and the decisions made by the NPE, the appeal body and courts of law.

Main Outcome Measures.—Characteristics of deliveries resulting in intrapartum asphyxia and causes of substandard care categorized in eight groups.

Results.—In the 161 compensated cases, 107 children survived (96 with neurological sequela), and 54 children died. Human error was a frequent reason of substandard care, seen as inadequate fetal monitoring (50%), lack of clinical knowledge and skills (14%), noncompliance with clinical guidelines (11%), failure in referral for senior medical help (10%) and error in drug administration (4%). System errors were registered in only 3%, seen as poor organization of the department, lack of guidelines and time conflicts. The health personnel held responsible for substandard care was an obstetrician in 49% and a midwife in 46%.

Conclusions.—Substandard care is common in birth asphyxia, and human error is the cause in most cases. Inadequate fetal monitoring and lack of clinical knowledge and skills are the most frequent reasons for compensation after birth asphyxia.

▶ This article reports the results of a study that attempted to determine the reasons for payment of compensation claims after allegations of neurologic injury from birth asphyxia in Norway. The authors compared claims made to the Norwegian system of compensation to patients with reports of suspected substandard care made to the Norwegian Board of Health Supervision. The objective was to analyze cases with neurologic complications or death to identify the most prevalent reasons for substandard care and to suggest quality improvement measures.

Although the methodology used in this study is somewhat subjective and the experts who reviewed the cases consisted only of obstetricians, not neonatologists or pediatric neurologists, some of the conclusions appear to be valid and exportable to practice in other countries in the developed world. Substandard care caused by human error was found to be a main factor in the majority of cases and included inadequate fetal monitoring, lack of clinical knowledge or skills, noncompliance with written guidelines, failure to obtain more senior help in a timely manner, and, to a much lesser degree, errors in drug administration. Substandard system errors included poor departmental organization, time conflicts in the delivery room, and lack of written guidelines, but these were involved substantially less often than human error. Far and away, the most frequent reason for compensating these claims in Norway was inadequate fetal monitoring. It will be interesting to see if the recent reclassification system in the United States will have an impact on this in our own country.

In the United States, our tort system allows for a claim to be made under virtually any circumstance. Thus, a poor outcome often results in a claim of medical negligence because the claimant must prove that there was a departure from acceptable standards of care and that this departure was causally linked to the injury. The data from the Norwegian study, however, may be quite applicable to understanding factors that lead patients or their families to litigation.

S. M. Donn, MD

Assisted reproductive technologies impair the expression and methylation of insulin-induced gene 1 and sterol regulatory element-binding factor 1 in the fetus and placenta

Lou H, Le F, Zheng Y, et al (Zhejiang Univ, People's Republic of China)
Fertil Steril 101:974-980, 2014

Objective.—To evaluate the cholesterol metabolism linked to assisted reproductive technology (ART) by analyzing the expression levels and DNA methylation patterns of the insulin-induced gene (INSIG), sterol regulatory element-binding protein (SREBP), and SREBP cleavage-activating protein in the fetus and placenta.

Design.—Experimental research study.

Setting.—An IVF center, university-affiliated teaching hospital.

Patient(s).—Four patients groups were recruited: pregnancies after IVF/intracytoplasmic sperm injection (ICSI) (n = 55), natural pregnancies (n = 40), multifetal reduction after IVF/ICSI (n = 56), and multifetal reduction after controlled ovarian hyperstimulation (COH) (n = 42).

Intervention(s).—Expression and DNA methylation of INSIG-SREBP-SREBP cleavage-activating protein in the fetus and placenta samples were determined.

Main Outcome Measure(s).—The expression and DNA methylation patterns were tested by real-time quantitative polymerase chain reaction (PCR) and pyrosequencing.

Result(s).—In the ICSI treatment group, significantly higher levels of triglycerides and apolipoprotein-B were observed in cord blood compared with controls. Meanwhile, in ICSI-conceived fetuses, the expression of *INSIG1* was significantly higher, and methylation rates were lower, than in the IVF and control groups. Furthermore, in the placenta, the *INSIG1* and *SREBF1* transcripts were also significantly higher with lower methylation rates in the ICSI group than in the IVF and control groups.

Conclusion(s).—Our results indicated that the dysregulation of *INSIG1* and *SREBF1* caused by ART were observed not only in the fetus but also in the placenta, primarily in the ICSI group. However, the long-term sequelae of this dysregulation should be closely followed.

▶ To study the associations of different modes of reproductive technology with DNA methylation and expression of insulin-induced gene (*INSIG1*) and sterol regulatory element-binding protein (*SREBF1*) in fetuses and placenta, a group of Chinese investigators analyzed cord blood and placentas from 3 groups of pregnancies: pregnancies achieved by in vitro fertilization (IVF)/intracytoplasmic sperm injection (ICSI) ($n = 55$), natural pregnancies ($n = 40$), and multifetal reduction after IVF/ICSI ($n = 56$) and multifetal reduction after ovarian hyperstimulation ($n = 42$). The investigators used pyrosequencing and real-time polymerase chain reaction to analyze DNA methylation and expression. In the ICSI treatment group, significantly higher levels of triglycerides and apolipoprotein-B were observed in cord blood compared with natural pregnancies. Expression of *INSIG1* was higher and methylation levels lower among fetuses conceived from IVF or naturally without ICSI. The investigators also noted lower methylation in ICSI of both *INSIG1* and *SREBF1* in placenta compared with non-ICSI IVF or control groups. Although the long-term sequelae of these findings was not established in this article, because the majority of IVF in the United States moves toward ICSI due to the higher success rates, epigenetic dysregulation remains a concern and investigation of subtle metabolic effects is warranted.

H. H. Burris, MD

3 Genetics and Teratology

DNA Sequencing versus Standard Prenatal Aneuploidy Screening

Bianchi DW, for the CARE Study Group (Tufts Med Ctr and Tufts Univ School of Medicine, Boston, MA)

N Engl J Med 370:799-808, 2014

Background.—In high-risk pregnant women, noninvasive prenatal testing with the use of massively parallel sequencing of maternal plasma cell-free DNA (cfDNA testing) accurately detects fetal autosomal aneuploidy. Its performance in low-risk women is unclear.

Methods.—At 21 centers in the United States, we collected blood samples from women with singleton pregnancies who were undergoing standard aneuploidy screening (serum biochemical assays with or without nuchal translucency measurement). We performed massively parallel sequencing in a blinded fashion to determine the chromosome dosage for each sample. The primary end point was a comparison of the false positive rates of detection of fetal trisomies 21 and 18 with the use of standard screening and cfDNA testing. Birth outcomes or karyotypes were the reference standard.

Results.—The primary series included 1914 women (mean age, 29.6 years) with an eligible sample, a singleton fetus without aneuploidy, results from cfDNA testing, and a risk classification based on standard screening. For trisomies 21 and 18, the false positive rates with cfDNA testing were significantly lower than those with standard screening (0.3% vs. 3.6% for trisomy 21, $P < 0.001$; and 0.2% vs. 0.6% for trisomy 18, $P = 0.03$). The use of cfDNA testing detected all cases of aneuploidy (5 for trisomy 21, 2 for trisomy 18, and 1 for trisomy 13; negative predictive value, 100% [95% confidence interval, 99.8 to 100]). The positive predictive values for cfDNA testing versus standard screening were 45.5% versus 4.2% for trisomy 21 and 40.0% versus 8.3% for trisomy 18.

Conclusions.—In a general obstetrical population, prenatal testing with the use of cfDNA had significantly lower false positive rates and higher positive predictive values for detection of trisomies 21 and 18 than standard screening. (Funded by Illumina; ClinicalTrials.gov number, NCT01663350.)

► It is exciting to observe the emergence of new noninvasive technology that performs in a superior manner to the previous gold standard that involved invasive testing with the risk of fetal loss. It is also necessary to learn new abbreviations so when the residents/fellows are presenting, you are aware that "NIPT" stands for noninvasive prenatal testing. Also, the CARE study refers to the Comparison of Aneuploidy Risk Evaluations, a prospective, blinded, multicenter observational study comparing the results of noninvasive prenatal cfDNA (cell-free DNA) testing for fetal autosomal aneuploidy with the results of conventional screening for trisomy 21 (Down syndrome) and trisomy 18 (Edwards syndrome) in a general obstetrical population.

All previous clinical validation had revealed high-sensitivity, high-specificity, and negative predicative values for detection of the most common autosomal aneuploidies sufficiently robust for societies to render committee opinions stating that cfDNA testing could be offered to pregnant women at high risk for fetal aneuploidy as a screening option after counseling.[1-3] Bianchi's study has many strengths, not the least of which is that it is prospective, masked, monitored by an independent statistician, and represents racial and ethnic diversity from 21 US sites.

The main weakness is the small number of true positive results and reliance on clinical follow-up alone. Also 28.5% of the results of cfDNA testing were obtained in the third trimester. The fetal fraction increases with gestational age, and this might bias the results in favor of cfDNA testing. However, exclusion of the samples drawn in the third trimester did not have a significant effect on the false-positive rates. Because 0.9% of cfDNA tests did not provide results, the possibility of test failure should be presented to the family during pretest counseling. Such test failure can be repeated and is far better than the loss of a fetus following amniocentesis.

It was reassuring that the noninvasive prenatal cfDNA testing performed better than standard screening methods. A 10-fold improvement in the positive predictive value for trisomy 21 in a predominantly low-risk patient population is nothing short of spectacular. Bianchi noted that "The major advantage of using cfDNA testing was the reduction in rates of false-positive results (see Tables 2 and 3 in the original article). She suggested that on the basis of the current evidence, supported by this study, "cfDNA testing merits serious consideration as a primary screening method for fetal autosomal aneuploidy."

A. A. Fanaroff, MD, FRCPE

References

1. Benn P, Borell A, Chiu R, et al. Position statement from the aneuploidy screening committee on behalf of the board of the international society for prenatal diagnosis. *Prenat Diagn.* 2013;33:622-629.
2. Devers PL, Cronister A, Ormond KE, Facio F, Brasington CK, Flodman P. Noninvasive prenatal testing/noninvasive prenatal diagnosis: the position of the National Society of Genetic Counselors. *J Genet Couns.* 2013;22:291-295.
3. American College of Obstetricians and Gynecologists Committee on Genetics. Committee Opinion No. 545: noninvasive prenatal testing for fetal aneuploidy. *Obstet Gynecol.* 2012;120:1532-1534.

Minor Anomalies: Can They Predict Specific Major Defects? A Study Based on 23 Major and 14 Minor Anomalies in Over 25,000 Newborns with Birth Defects

Campaña H, Rittler M, Poletta FA, et al (Multidisciplinary Inst of Cellular Biology (IMBICE), La Plata, Argentina; Hosp Univ of Buenos Aires, Argentina; Ctr for Med Education and Clinical Res (CEMIC), Buenos Aires, Argentina)

Am J Perinatol 31:447-454, 2014

Background.—Minor anomalies (mAs) are morphological features with little clinical relevance that have been mentioned as possible predictors of major defects (MDs).

Objectives.—To identify the preferential associations between selected MDs and mAs and to establish if mAs can serve as predictors for specific MDs.

Study Design.—Information of newborns with birth defects was obtained from the ECLAMC (Latin American Collaborative Study of Congenital Malformations) database. The sample consisted of 27,247 live- and stillborn newborns with multiple malformations that included at least one of the selected MDs or mAs. The odds ratio and predictive values were calculated for significant associations, and concurrence rates in first degree relatives.

Results.—A total of 33 significant minor-major associations were identified. Single umbilical artery (SUA) and preauricular tags were the most frequent mAs; the former was associated with 10 MDs, the latter only with microtia. The highest positive predictive value was shown by SUA for anal atresia. Newborns with preauricular tags had significantly more relatives with microtia than expected.

Conclusions.—No new relevant associations between MDs and mAs were identified and few mAs seem to serve as predictors for specific MDs in the same newborn. However, preauricular tags can predict the occurrence of microtia in other family members.

► The initial examination of a newly born infant provides an opportunity to identify any minor or major malformations. Most of the so-called minor malformations are readily identified in approximately 15% of the population, whereas major birth defects are present in 2% of the population. However, minor malformations may be a clue that there are major, more serious disorders present. It has been estimated that 50% of infants with major anomalies will have accompanying minor anomalies. Not surprisingly, major malformations are more common in low birth weight and preterm infants. Today, malformations are the leading cause of neonatal mortality. In the report from Campaña, after probing a huge database, no earth-shattering revelations emerged. Their data reinforce the importance of looking for major malformations in pregnancies complicated by single umbilical arteries. The association between anorectal malformations and single umbilical artery (SUA) was relatively new. It has long been known that major cloacal and mermaid lesions have been accompanied by 2-vessel cord with only a single artery. Kim[1] found a high prevalence of ocular lesions in infants with a single umbilical artery including errors of refraction, so careful follow-up is necessary. Of some reassurance, our Spanish colleagues[2] have reported that the prognosis of the fetus with a SUA is determined by the presence or absence of associated major malformations. If the fetus has an isolated SUA with no signs of other malformations observed by an experienced sonographer, only a routine physical examination should be performed in newborns. Khalil et al[3] noted that pregnancy with isolated SUA was more likely to be complicated with polyhydramnios, preterm delivery < 34 weeks, birth weight < 10th percentile, cesarean delivery for fetal distress perinatal death, admission to the neonatal intensive care unit, and placental abnormalities, necessitating close monitoring of fetal growth and well-being.

Among the minor malformations, deep sacral dimples are common, and easily overlooked. They may signify underlying cord lesions and should be carefully monitored. The other take away message on minor malformations was that preauricular tags were associated with microtia and to look for microtia in other members of the family, but don't forget to check hearing as well.

A. A. Fanaroff, MD, FRCPE

References

1. Kim J, Park KH, Hwang JM. Ocular findings in children with single umbilical artery: a case series of 14 children. *Korean J Ophthalmol.* 2014;28:155-158.
2. Arcos-Machancoses JV, Marín-Reina P, Romaguera-Salort E, García-Camuñas Y, Pérez-Aytés A, Vento M. Postnatal development of fetuses with a single umbilical artery: differences between malformed and non-malformed infantsv. *World J Pediatr.* 2014 [Epub ahead of print].
3. Khalil MI, Sagr ER, Elrifaei RM, Abdelbasit OB, Halouly TA. Outcomes of an isolated single umbilical artery in singleton pregnancy: a large study from the Middle East and Gulf region. *Eur J Obstet Gynecol Reprod Biol.* 2013;171:277-280.

Fetal DNA Methylation Associates with Early Spontaneous Preterm Birth and Gestational Age

Parets SE, Conneely KN, Kilaru V, et al (Emory Univ, Atlanta, GA; Emory Univ School of Medicine, Atlanta, GA; et al)
PLoS One 8:e67489, 2013

Spontaneous preterm birth (PTB, <37 weeks gestation) is a major public health concern, and children born preterm have a higher risk of morbidity and mortality throughout their lives. Recent studies suggest that fetal DNA methylation of several genes varies across a range of gestational ages (GA), but it is not yet clear if fetal epigenetic changes associate with PTB. The objective of this study is to interrogate methylation patterns across the genome in fetal leukocyte DNA from African Americans with early PTB ($24^{1/7}$–$34^{0/7}$ weeks; N = 22) or term births ($39^{0/7}$–$40^{6/7}$ weeks; N = 28) and to evaluate the association of each CpG site with PTB and GA. DNA methylation was assessed across the genome with the HumanMethylation450 BeadChip. For each individual sample and CpG site, the proportion of DNA methylation was estimated. The associations between methylation and PTB or GA were evaluated by fitting a separate linear model for each CpG site, adjusting for relevant covariates. Overall, 29 CpG sites associated with PTB (FDR<.05; $5.7\times10^{-10}<p<2.9\times10^{-6}$) independent of GA. Also, 9637 sites associated with GA (FDR<.05; $9.5\times10^{-16}<p<1.0\times10^{-3}$), with 61.8% decreasing in methylation with shorter GA. GA-associated CpG sites were depleted in the CpG islands of their respective genes ($p<2.2\times10^{-16}$). Gene set enrichment analysis (GSEA) supported enrichment of GA-associated CpG sites in genes that play a role in embryonic development as well as the extracellular matrix. Additionally, this study replicated the association of several CpG sites associated with gestational age in other studies (*CRHBP, PIK3CD* and *AVP*). Dramatic differences in fetal DNA methylation are evident in fetuses born preterm versus at term, and the patterns established at birth may provide insight into the long-term consequences associated with PTB.

▶ Little is known about the epigenome and prematurity. *Epigenetics* refers to differences in gene expression in the absence of genetic variation. One of the most common epigenetic marks analyzed in epidemiologic studies is DNA methylation. Often, DNA methylation located in the promoters of genes is associated with silencing of expression. Parets et al studied cord blood DNA methylation from 22 preterm infants born spontaneously before $34^{1/7}$ weeks and 28 term infants 39 to less than 41 weeks. All infants were African-American. They used epigenome-wide technology to interrogate over 450 000 methylation sites across all (Illumina 450 K BeadChip). The authors found 29 CpG sites in which methylation differed in preterm compared with term infants. Intriguing findings included that preterm infants had lower DNA methylation of GSK3B (glycogen synthase kinase 3 β), which is involved in neuronal migration and negatively regulates MAML1 (mastermind-like 1). MAML1 is involved in the Notch pathway, which is responsible for maturation of several organ systems, including neurogenesis and intestinal development. Although this study was cross-sectional and cannot contribute to understanding causes of preterm birth, perhaps differential methylation by gestational age, even if a normal aspect of fetal development, may help explain preterm infants' susceptibility to long-term morbidities.

H. H. Burris, MD

Analysis of epigenetic changes in survivors of preterm birth reveals the effect of gestational age and evidence for a long term legacy

Cruickshank MN, Oshlack A, Theda C, et al (Royal Children's Hosp, Parkville, Victoria, Australia; et al)

Genome Med 5:96, 2013

Background.—Preterm birth confers a high risk of adverse long term health outcomes for survivors, yet the underlying molecular mechanisms are unclear. We hypothesized that effects of preterm birth can be mediated through measurable epigenomic changes throughout development. We therefore used a longitudinal birth cohort to measure the epigenetic mark of DNA methylation at birth and 18 years comparing survivors of extremely preterm birth with infants born at term.

Methods.—Using 12 extreme preterm birth cases and 12 matched, term controls, we extracted DNA from archived neonatal blood spots and blood collected in a similar way at 18 years of age. DNA methylation was measured at 347,789 autosomal locations throughout the genome using Infinium HM450 arrays. Representative methylation differences were confirmed by Sequenom MassArray EpiTYPER.

Results.—At birth we found 1,555 sites with significant differences in methylation between term and preterm babies. At 18 years of age, these differences had largely resolved, suggesting that DNA methylation differences at birth are mainly driven by factors relating to gestational age, such as cell composition and/or maturity. Using matched longitudinal samples, we found evidence for an epigenetic legacy associated with preterm birth, identifying persistent methylation differences at ten genomic loci. Longitudinal comparisons of DNA methylation at birth and 18 years uncovered a significant overlap between sites that were differentially-methylated at birth and those that changed with age. However, we note that overlapping sites may either differ in the same (300/1,555) or opposite (431/1,555) direction during gestation and aging respectively.

Conclusions.—We present evidence for widespread methylation differences between extreme preterm and term infants at birth that are largely resolved by 18 years of age. These results are consistent with methylation changes associated with blood cell development, cellular composition, immune induction and age at these time points. Finally, we identified ten probes significantly associated with preterm individuals and with greater than 5% methylation discordance at birth and 18 years that may reflect a long term epigenetic legacy of preterm birth.

▶ This is a study of blood DNA methylation of 12 individuals born preterm and 12 full-term controls at birth and then at 18 years. DNA methylation is one epigenetic mechanism that affects gene expression in the absence of genetic sequence variation. The investigators used an epigenomewide approach using the Infinium HM450 array, which analyzes more than 450 000 methylation sites simultaneously. There were many (>1500) sites that differed at birth between preterm infants and full-term controls and none that significantly differed by 18 years of age. This finding mirrors what we observe clinically, with differences between preterm infants and term infants eroding with the passage of decades. Differences at birth between preterm and full-term neonates are not surprising, as early development is associated with rapid changes in DNA methylation, and the health states of both a mother delivering preterm and an infant exposed to the extrauterine environment prematurely would be expected to affect DNA methylation. As an additional exploratory analysis, the investigators pooled the birth and 18-year samples into preterm and term strata and found

109 sites that differentiated the 2 groups. In this analysis, there were 8 probes not identified in the original birth sample comparisons. The authors postulate that larger studies might uncover an epigenetic legacy of prematurity. If so, epigenetics could shed light on the pathophysiology of the long-term health sequelae observed among ex-preterm infants.

H. H. Burris, MD

Neonatal Genome-Wide Methylation Patterns in Relation to Birth Weight in the Norwegian Mother and Child Cohort

Engel SM, Joubert BR, Wu MC, et al (Univ of North Carolina at Chapel Hill; Nat Inst of Environmental Health Sciences, Research Triangle Park, NC; et al)
Am J Epidemiol 179:834-842, 2014

Although epigenetic regulation plays a critical role in embryonic development, few studies have examined the relationship of epigenome-wide methylation with fetal growth. Using the Infinium HumanMethylation450 BeadChip (Illumina, Inc., San Diego, California) in a substudy of 1,046 infants from the Norwegian Mother and Child Cohort Study (MoBa) enrolled between 1999 and 2008, we examined epigenome-wide cord blood DNA methylation in relation to birth weight. In multivariable-adjusted robust linear regression models, we identified differential methylation at 19 cytosine-guanine dinucleotides (CpGs) associated with either decreased (AT-rich interactive domain 5B (*MRF1*-like) (*ARID5B*), 2 CpGs) or increased (x-ray repair complementing defective repair in Chinese hamster cells 3 (*XRCC3*), 4 CpGs) birth weight. *ARID5B* knockout mice have less adipose tissue and significantly lower weight in the postnatal period. *XRCC3* plays a key role in the maintenance of chromosome stability and the repair of DNA damage. Although there are fewer data on the other implicated genes, many of these genes have been shown to have roles in developmental processes. This constitutes the largest and most robust study of birth weight using an epigenome-wide methylation platform and offers potential insights into epigenetic mechanisms of fetal growth.

► Investigators analyzed associations of birth weight and genome-wide DNA methylation obtained from umbilical cord blood of 1046 infants participating in the Norwegian Mother and Child Cohort Study (MoBa) enrolled between 1999 and 2008. Study participants were a subset of the overall cohort (> 100 000 participants). Infants included in this subset were part of a nested case-cohort study designed to study asthma at 3 years of age. The authors then adjusted for asthma (a later-presenting variable) to adjust for the study design. Differential DNA methylation of 19 cytosine-guanine dinucleotide (CpG) sites was found to be associated with birth weight. Of the CpG identified, 13 were within genes and 6 were within intergenic regions. The authors concluded that "using cord blood DNA, we identified a small number of CpGs in 9 genes, including multiple significant CpGs in *ARID5B* and *XRCC3*, which are associated with birth weight in a large population-based cohort. Some biological plausibility for a role for *ARID5B* in particular in fetal growth is provided by associations with postnatal growth and lipid accumulation in mice." This article heralds numerous epigenome-wide association studies (EWAS) to come. We are entering an era, similar to the earlier genome-wide association studies era a decade ago, in which investigators will analyze DNA methylation patterns associated with the development of complex diseases. For neonatology, this likely means EWAS for all of the 3-letter acronyms: RDS, NEC, BPD, ROP (ie, respiratory distress syndrome, necrotizing enterocolitis, bronchopulmonary dysplasia, retinopathy of prematurity), and more. Translating findings to improve clinical care and outcomes will be the next challenge.

H. H. Burris, MD

Additional value of prenatal genomic array testing in fetuses with isolated structural ultrasound abnormalities and a normal karyotype: a systematic review of the literature

de Wit MC, Srebniak MI, Govaerts LCP, et al (Erasmus Med Centre, Rotterdam, The Netherlands)

Ultrasound Obstet Gynecol 43:139-146, 2014

Objective.—To establish the prevalence of submicroscopic genetic copy number variants (CNVs) in fetuses with a structural ultrasound anomaly (restricted to one anatomical system) and a normal karyotype. The aim was to determine the diagnostic and prognostic value of genomic array testing in these pregnancies.

Methods.—Embase and PubMed databases were systematically searched for all relevant articles on prevalence of pathogenic submicroscopic CNVs in fetuses with ultrasound anomalies. Reported cases were sorted into groups according to anatomical site of the detected ultrasound anomaly. The prevalence of causative submicroscopic CNVs was calculated for each group.

Results.—Combined data of the reviewed studies ($n = 18$) indicated that fetuses with an ultrasound anomaly restricted to one anatomical system ($n = 2220$) had a 3.1–7.9% chance of carrying a causative submicroscopic CNV, depending on the anatomical system affected. This chance increased to 9.1% for fetuses with multiple ultrasound anomalies ($n = 1139$).

Conclusion.—This review indicates that 3.1–7.9% of fetuses with a structural ultrasound anomaly restricted to one anatomical system and a normal karyotype will show a submicroscopic CNV, which explains its phenotype and provides information for fetal prognosis. Therefore, we conclude that microarray has considerable diagnostic and prognostic value in these pregnancies.

▶ Until recently, karyotyping has been the gold standard in prenatal diagnosis. Advances are occurring at blinding speed so that it is now commonplace to recognize genetic abnormalities using microarray techniques. These chromosomal changes were not identifiable with the cruder methodologies then in use. Genomic microarray achieves a much higher resolution than does karyotyping, revealing submicroscopic copy number variants (CNVs). These small CNVs are common in the human genome and may be relevant in congenital malformations and syndromes.

As a result, the authors of this report note that "some prenatal centers implemented genomic microarray as a diagnostic tool in the prenatal setting, instead of, or in addition to, karyotyping."

Furthermore, with more experienced technicians and better ultrasound equipment, more structural fetal malformations are being recognized. The authors wished to determine whether microarray techniques were worth doing on fetuses with single-organ abnormalities. Their aim was to establish the prevalence of submicroscopic genetic CNVs in fetuses with a structural ultrasound anomaly (restricted to one anatomic system) and a normal karyotype. Ultrasound anomalies (ie, single umbilical artery, echogenic bowel, echogenic cardiac focus, pyelectasis, short long bones, choroid plexus cysts, clinodactyly and nuchal translucency ≥3.5 mm) as well as undefined fetal hydrops, growth abnormalities, amniotic fluid alterations, and fetal akinesia, were considered as nonstructural abnormalities.

After a thorough literature review and detailed analysis, the authors reported that 5.6% (95% confidence interval [CI], 4.7%–6.6%) of 2220 fetuses with an ultrasound anomaly restricted to one anatomic system and 9.1% (95% CI, 7.5%–10.8%) of fetuses (n = 1139) with multiple anomalies carried a pathogenic submicroscopic CNV.

The authors, thus, confirm that there is additional benefit to performing a microarray in fetuses with single-organ ultrasound anomalies. With the cost of these measurements ever decreasing, one can anticipate that this will be used even more frequently with less rigid criteria to perform the test.

A. A. Fanaroff, MD, FRCPE

Anomalies associated with gastroschisis and omphalocele: Analysis of 2825 cases from the Texas Birth Defects Registry

Benjamin B, Wilson GN (Texas Tech Univ Health Science Ctr, Amarillo)
J Pediatr Surg 49:514-519, 2014

Background/Purpose.—The increasing prevalence of abdominal wall defects prompted analysis of anomalies associated with gastroschisis and omphalocele in the Texas Birth Defects Registry (TDBR).

Methods.—Cases of gastroschisis (ICD9 code 756.71), omphalocele (756.70), and/or unspecified anomalies of the abdominal wall (756.79) were obtained from the TDBR after IRB approval and analyzed using Microsoft Access© and Excel© databases.

Results.—Analysis began with 2825 cases including 1831 of gastroschisis, 814 of omphalocele, and 180 of unspecified abdominal wall defects plus 9680 associated anomalies that were classified according to system. The overall prevalence of abdominal wall defects among 3,806,299

Texas births from 1999 to 2008 was 7.4 per 10,000 with 4.8 per 10,000 for gastroschisis and 2.1 for omphalocele. After excluding ambiguous cases (8.5% possibly misclassified), anomaly spectra were similar for the two AWD with musculoskeletal (limb contractures or defects), cardiovascular, gastrointestinal, urogenital, and central nervous system defects being most common. Of 1831 cases with gastroschisis, 594 (32%) had associated anomalies compared to 654 (80%) of 814 omphalocele cases.

Conclusions.—Gastroschisis as well as omphalocele has significant associated anomalies that are important to appreciate during pre- and postnatal management.

▶ Increased availability and usage of ultrasound screening have led to improved identification of fetal structural abnormalities prenatally. The most common fetal abdominal wall defects are gastroschisis and omphalocele, with a respective prevalence of about 5 and 2 per 10 000 births. Prenatal ultrasound has a high sensitivity for these abnormalities, which may be recognized already at the time of the first trimester so-called nuchal scan. Before this report, the prevailing consensus was that major unrelated defects (mainly cardiac and gastrointestinal) were associated with gastroschisis in about 10% of cases, whereas omphalocele is associated with many more including chromosomal or genetic abnormalities. Using the Texas database, which included almost 4 million births between 1999 and 2008, Benjamin and Wilson have identified a huge cohort of cases of gastroschisis, omphalocele, and other abdominal wall defects. Although it has been well recognized that omphalocele is associated with other defects, and this was true in this series (80%), the finding that 32% of cases with gastroschisis had anomalies was surprising and new information. The prevailing teaching has been that, as noted above, gastroschisis was not associated with other anomalies. These data serve as a call for action to rule out other malformations in babies with gastroschisis.

A major challenge with gastroschisis is the prevention of late intrauterine death, whereas with omphalocele, it is vital to be aware of all the associated conditions, recognizing that not all can be diagnosed prenatally. Other abdominal wall defects such as inguinal hernia and umbilical hernia are common and encountered frequently in the neonatal intensive care unit and well-baby nursery.

Rarer forms of abdominal wall defects are pentalogy of Cantrell, omphalocele, bladder exstrophy, imperforate anus, spina bifida complex, Eagle-Barrett syndrome, body stalk anomaly, and bladder and cloacal exstrophy. These require multidisciplinary management and extensive counseling. It is worth looking at the number of vessels in the cord because many of these defects may be associated with a 2-vessel cord.

A. A. Fanaroff, MD, FRCPE

Accuracy of Ultrasonography at 11–14 Weeks of Gestation for Detection of Fetal Structural Anomalies: A Systematic Review

Rossi AC, Prefumo F (Univ of Bari, Italy; Univ of Brescia, Italy)
Obstet Gynecol 122:1160-1167, 2013

Objective.—To review the literature concerning the efficacy of early ultrasonography (at 11–14 weeks of gestation) to identify fetal malformations.

Data Sources.—A search in PubMed, MEDLINE, Embase, Cochrane Library, and ClinicalTrials.gov was performed (January 2000 to December 2012). Keywords were: fetal anatomy, fetal echocardiography, nuchal translucency, fetal structural anomalies, fetal malformations, prenatal diagnosis, prenatal screening, and first-trimester ultrasonography.

Methods of Study Selection.—Inclusion criteria were: fetal anatomy examination at early ultrasonography and diagnosis of fetal malformations confirmed by postnatal or postmortem examination. Data abstracted were: sample size, location of structural defect, ultrasound modality, presence of multiple defects, and study population. Pooled detection rate was calculated for each malformation and compared with χ^2. Differences were considered statistically significant if $P < .05$.

Tabulation, Integration, and Results.—From 1,203 articles, 19 were included. Overall, we pooled 78,002 fetuses undergoing ultrasonography at 11–14 weeks, of which 996 were malformed, leading to prevalence of malformation of 12 per 1,000. The overall detection rate was 472 of 957 (51%). The highest detection rate was achieved for neck anomalies (92%), whereas limbs (34%), face (34%), and genitourinary anomalies (34%) were associated with the lowest detection rate. At 14 weeks of gestation or less, fetal echocardiography detected 53% of congenital heart disease compared with 43% by complete scan ($P = .040$). The use of Doppler did not improve the detection rate for congenital heart defects (52% compared with 44%, respectively; $P = .11$). Multiple defects were identified more frequently than isolated malformations (60% compared with 44%; $P = .005$). The detection rate was higher combining transabdominal and transvaginal techniques (62%) than either abdominal (51%) or transvaginal (34%; $P < .001$). Detection rate was higher in women at high risk (65%) than unselected population (50% $P = .001$).

Conclusion.—Because of the natural history of fetal defects and the late development of some organ systems, a number of fetal malformations remain undetected by early ultrasonography (Box 1).

▶ This is an interesting article from a number of perspectives. Most importantly, overall, only 50% of malformations are identified at the 11- to 14-week screening, hence, the importance of the full anatomic scan at around 20 weeks and careful physical examination of all newborns within 24 hours of delivery. Secondly, this careful review screened more than 1200 articles and found only 19 worthy of inclusion in the review. Message: there are many publications but few of the highest quality when it comes to comprehensive reviews, metaanalyses

Box 1: Detection Rate of Fetal Malformations in the First Trimester

100% detection rate
- Acrania, anencephaly, ectopia cordis, encephalocele

50–99% detection rate
- Cystic hygroma, double-outlet right ventricular flow, Fallot, gastroschisis, omphalocele, holoprosencephaly, hypoplastic left heart syndrome, limb reduction, megacystis, polydactyly, septal defects, transposition of great vessels, valvular disease

1–49% detection rate
- Spina bifida, hydrocephalus, skeletal dysplasia, facial cleft, Dandy-Walker, aortic coarctation, arthrogryposis

0% detection rate
- Corpus callosum agenesia, bladder exstrophy, congenital cyst adenomatoid malformation, cerebellar hypoplasia, duodenal atresia, hydronephrosis, renal agenesia, duplex kidneys, bowel obstruction, extralobar sequestration

and the Cochrane reviews. Also there is marked inconsistency in the manner in which the results are presented, making it a major task for the authors to sift through the reports and find the relevant data. Recall that all the malformations needed to be validated either at autopsy or examination after delivery. Thirdly, there is great variability in the detection rate—depending on the site. Hence, most neck lesions are identified (92%), but only a third of face, genitourinary, and limb anomalies are identified. The manner of screening is important, and combining abdominal and vaginal probes increases the detection rate for malformations from 51% to 63%. Cardiac anomalies elude detection before 14 weeks of gestation in 47% of the fetuses. Box 1 is helpful in recognizing the chances of detecting anomalies before 14 weeks, which range from 100% for an encephalocele to 0% for duodenal atresia or exstrophy of the bladder. Major advances in magnification imaging and signal processing have enhanced visualization of fetal anatomy, yet only half the malformations are recognized before 14 weeks. Nevertheless, it is worthwhile to search for a wide range of fetal anomalies at the time of nuchal translucency scan by transabdominal, transvaginal or transvaginal and transabdominal ultrasonography.

A. A. Fanaroff, MD, FRCPE

4 Labor and Delivery

Triggers of Spontaneous Preterm Delivery – Why Today?

Hernández-Díaz S, Boeke CE, Romans AT, et al (Harvard School of Public Health, Boston, MA; Massachusetts General Hosp, Boston; et al)

Paediatr Perinat Epidemiol 28:79-87, 2014

Background.—Our goal is to study the triggers of spontaneous preterm delivery using a case-crossover design.

Methods.—In a pilot study, we enrolled 50 women with spontaneous preterm labour (PTL) and 50 with preterm premature rupture of membranes (PPROM) between 2011 and 2012. To assess non-transient risk factors, we also enrolled a control group of 158 pregnant women at their regular prenatal care visits matched to cases by gestational age and calendar time. The index time was defined as the onset of PTL/PPROM (for cases) or interview (for controls). Detailed data were collected through structured interviews regarding factors of interest during the 72 h that preceded the index time. Within case subjects, we compared the frequency of transient factors from 0 to 24 h before index time with that from 48 to 72 h before index time, and estimated matched odds ratios (OR) and 95% confidence intervals (CI).

Results.—Previously hypothesised chronic risk factors for spontaneous preterm delivery, including mood disorders and stressful events, were more common among cases than among controls. Within cases, skipped meals [OR 4.3, 95% CI 1.2, 15.2], disturbed sleep [OR 4.5, 95% CI 1.5, 13.3], sexual activity [OR 6.0, 95% CI 0.7, 69.8], and intake of spicy foods [OR 7.0, 95% CI 1.6, 30.8] were associated with an increased risk for PTL/PPROM within the subsequent 24 h. For physical exertion and other potential risk factors evaluated, the OR was close to the null.

Conclusion.—Skipping meals and disturbed sleep may be associated with imminent PTL/PPROM; sexual activity and spicy food may trigger PTL/PPROM in susceptible women. Larger case-crossover studies will be able to evaluate the impact of modifiable risk factors and acute predictors of PTL/PPROM, and might help guide obstetrical management.

▶ During the course of a neonatology antepartum consultation for a woman in preterm labor, the questions often arise, "Why me?" or "Why now?" This thoughtful study attempts to address the latter. The investigators enrolled 50 women with preterm labor; 50 women with preterm, premature rupture of membranes; and 158 control women during the course of prenatal care, matched by gestational age. The risk factors within the 72 hours before the case events that were significantly associated with spontaneous preterm delivery included skipping meals and poor sleep. Physical activity was not associated with case status. This study, like most case-control studies, may have suffered from recall bias, specifically for the positive associations. However, the null finding with respect to physical activity might help reassure mothers, who often feel guilty about exercise or physical labor the day or two before their preterm delivery, that the preterm birth was not their fault.

H. H. Burris, MD

Behavioural, educational and respiratory outcomes of antenatal betamethasone for term caesarean section (ASTECS trial)

Stutchfield PR, Whitaker R, Gliddon AE, et al (Betsi Cadwaladr Univ Health Board, Rhyl, UK; Bangor Univ, UK; NISCHR CRC, Rhyl, UK; et al)

Arch Dis Child Fetal Neonatal Ed 98:F195-F200, 2013

Objectives.—To determine whether antenatal betamethasone prior to elective term caesarean section (CS) affects long term behavioural, cognitive or developmental outcome, and whether the risk of asthma or atopic disease is reduced.

Design.—A questionnaire based follow-up of a multicentre randomised controlled trial (Antenatal Steroids for Term Elective Caesarean Section, BMJ 2005).

Setting.—Four UK study centres from the original trial.

Participants.—862 participants from the four largest recruiting centres, 92% of the original study. 824 (96%) were traced and 799 (93%) were successfully contacted. Fifty-one percent (407/799) completed and returned the questionnaire. The children were aged 8–15 years (median 12.2 years, 52% girls). 386 gave consent to contact schools with 352 (91%) reports received.

Main Outcome Measures.—Questionnaires including a strengths and difficulties questionnaire, International Study of Asthma and Allergies in Childhood, general health and school performance.

Results.—There were no significant differences between children whose mothers received betamethasone and controls for the mean total strengths and difficulties questionnaire scores and subscores for hyperactivity, emotional symptoms, prosocial behaviour, conduct or peer problems. 25 (12%) children whose mothers received betamethasone had reported learning difficulties compared with 27 (14%) control children. The proportion of children who achieved standard assessment tests KS2 exams level 4 or above for mathematics, English or science was similar as were the rates of ever reported wheeze (30% vs 30%), asthma (24% vs 21%), eczema (34% vs 37%) and hay fever (25% vs 27%).

Conclusions.—Antenatal betamethasone did not result in any adverse outcomes or reduction in asthma or atopy. It should be considered for elective CS at 37–38 weeks of gestation.

Trial Registration.—Original trial was preregistration, the trial publication is BMJ. 2005 Sep 24;331(7518):662.

▶ The ASTECS trial, conducted in the United Kingdom, was a randomized controlled clinical trial of 2 doses of betamethasone given 24 hours apart to mothers who were within 48 hours of delivery by elective cesarean section at 37 or greater weeks of gestation. The original study[1] enrolled 998 subjects in 10 units and found, among the treated group, a benefit in reduction in the primary outcome: risk of neonatal admission for respiratory distress. The current study collected data by questionnaire that focused on strengths and difficulties, asthma and allergies, general health, and school performance. Fifty-one percent of 862 potentially eligible participants completed and returned the questionnaires. Results showed no benefit of antenatal betamethasone in reducing asthma or allergy and no adverse effects on health, development, or academic achievement, as reflected by the questionnaire responses. Nevertheless, the rate of reported "health problems" was relatively high at 36% in each group, and the response rate leaves unanswered the possibility that selection bias might have contributed to the results. As a result, I don't find these data fully reassuring and would favor the current approach recommended by the American College of Obstetrics and Gynecology of postponing elective cesarean section until at least 39 weeks of gestation over administration of antenatal steroids. On the other hand, these data might well set the stage for further study among mothers who experience selected complications of pregnancy that are indications for late preterm delivery yet offer the possibility of a 48-hour latency before delivery must proceed.

L. J. Van Marter, MD, MPH

Reference

1. Stutchfield P, Whitaker R, Russell I. Antenatal betamethasone and incidence of neonatal respiratory distress after elective caesarean section: pragmatic randomised trial. *BMJ*. 2005;331:662.

The effect of obstetric practice change to reduce early term delivery on perinatal outcome

Little SE, Robinson JN, Puopolo KM, et al (Brigham and Women's Hosp, Boston, MA)

J Perinatol 34:176-180, 2014

Objective.—To investigate whether the national emphasis on attaining ≥39 weeks gestation has altered obstetric practice, and if so whether this has affected perinatal morbidity.

Study Design.—We examined trends in gestational age, neonatal morbidity, maternal complications and stillbirth for a retrospective cohort of singleton, live births between 37+0 and 39+6 weeks of gestation over a 5-year period at a single tertiary care center.

Result.—There were 21 343 eligible deliveries. The proportion of deliveries in the early term (<39 weeks) decreased from 47.8 to 40.2% ($P < 0.01$). The reduction was most pronounced for elective inductions (27.5 to 8.0%; $P < 0.01$) and scheduled cesareans (56.9 to 24.9%; $P < 0.01$), although a similar trend was seen for nonelective inductions (51.2 to 47.9%; $P = 0.03$). In multivariable analysis, there was a 10% decreased odds of early term delivery per year ($P < 0.01$). There were no changes in the rates of neonatal intensive care unit (NICU) evaluation (29.8 to 28.1%; $P = 0.11$), pre-eclampsia (7.6 to 8.5%; $P = 0.06$) or stillbirth (11.5 to 14.4 per 10 000; $P = 0.55$).

Conclusion.—A 10% annual decline in the odds of early term delivery was not accompanied by significant changes in perinatal morbidity.

▶ Little and colleagues examined trends in gestational age, neonatal morbidity and maternal complications/stillbirths among singleton pregnancies between 37 0/7 weeks of gestation and 39 6/7 weeks of gestation at a single tertiary care center in Boston from 2006 to 2011 after changes to obstetric guidelines to avoid elective deliveries before 39 weeks of gestation. The authors analyzed 21 343 births and found that early-term deliveries (<39 weeks) declined from 47.8% to 40.2%, and this reduction was mostly caused by the reduction of elective inductions and cesarean sections. There was no change in the proportion of children evaluated in the neonatal intensive care unit (29.8%—28.1%, $P = .11$) or the incidence of preeclampsia or stillbirth. The study concluded with a statement that the reduction of elective early delivery was not accompanied by differences in perinatal morbidity. The authors speculate that this was because of a lack of meaningful delays in delivery from just less than 39 weeks of gestation to just more than 39 weeks of gestation. However, the authors were rightly reassured that the policy shift to avoid early elective inductions/cesarean deliveries did not lead to worsening maternal morbidity or higher rates of still birth. This study nicely illustrates the value of an electronic medical record for mining perinatal outcomes, as massive quality improvement efforts may have unanticipated consequences that could be monitored using similar methods.

H. H. Burris, MD, MPH

Immersion in Water During Labor and Delivery

American Academy of Pediatrics Committee on Fetus and Newborn; American College of Obstetricians and Gynecologists Committee on Obstetric Practice ()
Pediatrics 133:758-761, 2014

Immersion in water has been suggested as a beneficial alternative for labor, delivery, or both and over the past decades has gained popularity in many parts of the world. Immersion in water during the first stage of labor may be associated with decreased pain or use of anesthesia and decreased duration of labor. However, there is no evidence that immersion in water during the first stage of labor otherwise improves perinatal outcomes, and it should not prevent or inhibit other elements of care. The safety and efficacy of immersion in water during the second stage of labor have not been established, and immersion in water during the second stage of labor has not been associated with maternal or fetal benefit. Given these facts and case reports of rare but serious adverse effects in the newborn, the practice of immersion in the second stage of labor (underwater delivery) should be considered an experimental procedure that only should be performed within the context of an appropriately designed clinical trial with informed consent. Facilities that plan to offer immersion in the first stage of labor need to establish rigorous protocols for candidate selection, maintenance and cleaning of tubs and immersion pools, infection control procedures, monitoring of mothers and fetuses at appropriate intervals while immersed, and immediately and safely moving women out of the tubs if maternal or fetal concerns develop.

▶ With the movement to demedicalize childbirth, water births have become more common. In referral centers, neonatologists witness the results of water births that have resulted in perinatal depression or respiratory failure. In April 2014, the American Academy of Pediatrics (AAP) Committee on Fetus and Newborn and the American College of Obstetricians and Gynecologists (ACOG) Committee on Obstetric Practice joined forces to publish a clinical report on water births. After a thorough review of the literature regarding immersion in water during labor and delivery, the AAP and ACOG conclude that "immersion in the second stage of labor (underwater delivery) should be considered an experimental procedure that only should be performed within the context of an appropriately designed clinical trial with informed consent." The report highlights concerns about the lack of power within the published studies to detect differences in rare adverse effects and, thus, asserts that safety of immersion in water during labor and delivery has not yet been demonstrated. The authors recognize that some studies found that during the first stage of labor, pain may be minimized by immersion, thus, lowering the need for anesthesia. However, the authors go on to assert that "facilities that plan to offer immersion in the first stage of labor need to establish rigorous protocols for candidate selection, maintenance and cleaning of tubs ... and protocols for moving women from tubs if urgent maternal or fetal concerns develop." This joint AAP/ACOG report on water births serves as a warning to patients and providers to immerse at their own risk.

H. H. Burris, MD, MPH

Effect of Delayed vs Early Umbilical Cord Clamping on Iron Status and Neurodevelopment at Age 12 Months: A Randomized Clinical Trial

Andersson O, Domellöf M, Andersson D, et al (Hosp of Halland, Sweden; Umeå Univ, Sweden; et al)

JAMA Pediatr 168:547-554, 2014

Importance.—Prevention of iron deficiency in infancy may promote neurodevelopment. Delayed cord clamping (DCC) can prevent iron deficiency during the first 6 months of life. However, no data are available on long-term effects on infant outcomes in relation to time for umbilical cord clamping.

Objective.—To investigate effects of DCC, as compared with early cord clamping (ECC), on infant iron status and neurodevelopment at age 12 months in a European setting.

Design, Setting, and Participants.—Randomized clinical trial of 382 full-term infants born after a low-risk pregnancy at a Swedish county hospital. Follow-up at 12 months included evaluation of iron status (ferritin level, transferrin saturation, transferrin receptor level, reticulocyte hemoglobin level, and mean cell volume) and parental assessment of neurodevelopment by the Ages and Stages Questionnaire, second edition (ASQ).

Interventions.—Infants were randomized to DCC (≥180 seconds after delivery) or ECC (≤10 seconds after delivery).

Main Outcomes and Measures.—The main outcome was iron status at age 12 months; the secondary outcome was ASQ score.

Results.—In total, 347 of 382 infants (90.8%) were assessed. The DCC and ECC groups did not differ in iron status (mean ferritin level, 35.4 vs 33.6 ng/mL, respectively; $P = .40$) or neurodevelopment (mean ASQ total score, 229.6 vs 233.1, respectively; $P = .42$) at age 12 months. Predictors of ferritin levels were infant sex and ferritin in umbilical cord blood. Predictors of ASQ score were infant sex and breast feeding within 1 hour after birth. For both outcomes, being a boy was associated with lower results. Interaction analysis showed that DCC was associated with an ASQ score 5 points higher among boys (mean [SD] score, 229 [43] for DCC vs 224 [39] for ECC) but 12 points lower among girls (mean [SD] score, 230 [39] for DCC vs 242 [36] for ECC), out of a maximum of 300 points ($P = .04$ for the interaction term).

Conclusions and Relevance.—Delayed cord clamping did not affect iron status or neurodevelopment at age 12 months in a selected population of healthy term-born infants. However, it may not be possible to demonstrate minor effects on neurodevelopment with the size of the study population and the chosen method for assessment. The current data indicate that sex may influence the effects on infant development after DCC in different directions. Themagnitude and biological reason for this finding remain to be investigated.

Trial Registration.—clinicaltrials.gov Identifier: NCT01245296.

▶ Delaying the clamping of the cord for 2 to 3 minutes after birth (delayed cord clamping [DCC]) results in a 30% increase in neonatal blood volume when compared with early cord clamping (ECC). Over the last decade, several studies found that DCC resulted in higher ferritin levels and less iron deficiency (ID) at 4 to 6 months of age. However, no previous studies evaluated the effects of DCC on iron status or neurodevelopmental outcomes at or after 12 months of age. In this study, Andersson et al assessed iron status and parent-reported infant development (using the Ages and Stages Questionnaire) in 347 infants 12 months after they were randomly assigned to DCC or ECC. Against their hypothesis, the authors did not find any differences in iron status or neurodevelopment between the 2 groups. Importantly, only one infant in the study fulfilled the criteria for ID anemia, a prevalence much lower than that found in a previous Swedish study in 12-month old children. This finding was likely due to a recently implemented national movement toward avoiding cow's milk and promoting iron-fortified cereals during the second half of the first year of life. It is, therefore, possible that DCC could have a more significant effect on iron status at 12 months of age in parts of the world in which iron intake is less promoted. A surprising finding of this study was that DCC was associated with a 12-point lower ASQ score in girls, and a 5-point higher score in boys. In a previous study, liberal red cell transfusion practices in preterm neonates were associated with more substantial decreases in intracranial volume in 12-year-old girls compared with boys.[1] Taken together, these findings raise the possibility of gender-related differences in the effects of iron on brain development, a hypothesis that requires further testing.

M. Sola-Visner, MD

Reference

1. Nopoulos PC, Conrad AL, Bell EF, et al. Long-term outcome of brain structure in premature infants: effects of liberal vs restricted red blood cell transfusions. *Arch Pediatr Adolesc Med.* 2011;165:443-450.

The effects of umbilical cord milking in extremely preterm infants: a randomized controlled trial

March MI, Hacker MR, Parson AW, et al (Beth Israel Deaconess Med Ctr, Boston, MA; Hampton Roads Ob/Gyn Ctr, Norfolk, VA; et al)

J Perinatol 33:763-767, 2013

Objective.—Delayed cord clamping has been shown to decrease the need for transfusion in preterm neonates, but may delay resuscitation. The aim of this study was to determine whether umbilical cord milking compared with immediate cord clamping in extremely preterm deliveries reduces the need for neonatal red blood cell transfusion.

Study Design.—Women admitted to a tertiary care center and expected to deliver between 24 to 28 completed weeks of gestation were randomized to cord milking before clamping or immediate cord clamping. The primary outcome was the risk of neonatal transfusion, reported as risk ratio (RR) and 95% confidence interval (CI).

Result.—Of 113 women who were enrolled and randomized, 56 were assigned to cord milking with 36 remaining eligible and completing the study and 57 were assigned to the control group with 39 remaining eligible and completing the study. Albeit not statistically significant, neonates in the cord milking group were less likely to require transfusion compared with those in the control group (RR: 0.86; 95% CI: 0.73 to 1.0). Neonates whose cords were milked had higher hematocrits at birth ($P = 0.004$) and were less likely to develop an intraventricular hemorrhage ($P = 0.0195$).

Conclusion.—Milking the umbilical cord of a preterm neonate is an easy intervention with the potential to improve perinatal outcomes. Our results suggest that milking of the cord increases the neonate's initial hematocrit and may lessen the need for transfusion in the neonatal period. The observed reduction in the incidence of intraventricular hemorrhage may have important long-term implications that warrant further study.

▶ This report of a pilot trial of umbilical cord milking upon delivery of infants at 24 to 28 weeks of gestation adds to the growing body of evidence that enhancement of placentofetal transfusion at birth is associated with a lower rate of intraventricular hemorrhage (IVH). In this trial, the rate of intraventricular hemorrhage of all grades was significantly lower after cord milking (odds ratio [OR], 0.32; 95% confidence interval [CI], 0.12–0.84), but the sample size was not adequate to show a significant effect on grade 3 to 4 IVH (OR, 0.50; 95% CI, 0.13–2.00). The effects of cord milking for preterm infants, compared with immediate cord clamping, has previously been reported only in another small trial (20 subjects in each arm) from Japan, which described a similar, but also statistically nonsignificant, reduction in the incidence of grade 3 to 4 IVH (OR, 0.44; 95% CI, 0.08–2.42).[1] These observations are tantalizing, as few other interventions that promise to reduce rates of severe IVH have been identified. Although we anticipate accrual of data confirming these effects, the optimal methodologies for cord milking (length of cord and number of times to milk) or passive placentofetal transfusion with delayed cord clamping (level of the baby, interval from delivery to clamping) also need further exploration, and these approaches should be directly compared with one another. These questions are ripe for randomized trials adequately powered to show differences in long-term neurodevelopmental outcomes as well as the more immediate outcome of survival without sonographic evidence of brain injury (grade 3–4 intraventricular hemorrhage or periventricular leukomalacia). It will be important to enroll subjects in such trials before incremental accrual of weaker evidence leads to loss of equipoise about the potential benefits of these strategies.

W. E. Benitz, MD

Reference

1. Hosono S, Mugishima H, Fujita H, et al. Umbilical cord milking reduces the need for red cell transfusions and improves neonatal adaptation in infants born at less than 29 weeks' gestation: a randomised controlled trial. *Arch Dis Child Fetal Neonatal Ed.* 2008;93:F14-F19.

Rapid target allopurinol concentrations in the hypoxic fetus after maternal administration during labour

Kaandorp JJ, for the ALLO-trial Study Group (Univ Med Centre, Utrecht, The Netherlands; et al)

Arch Dis Child Fetal Neonatal Ed 99:F144-F148, 2014

Objective.—Perinatal hypoxia-induced free radical formation is an important cause of hypoxic-ischaemic encephalopathy and subsequent neurodevelopmental disabilities. Allopurinol reduces the formation of free radicals, which potentially limits hypoxia-induced brain damage. We investigated placental transfer and safety of allopurinol after maternal allopurinol treatment during labour to evaluate its potential role as a neuroprotective agent in suspected fetal hypoxia.

Design.—We used data from a randomised, double-blind multicentre trial comparing maternal allopurinol versus placebo in case of imminent fetal hypoxia (NCT00189007).

Patients.—We studied 58 women in labour at term, with suspected fetal hypoxia prompting immediate delivery, in the intervention arm of the study.

Setting.—Delivery rooms of 11 Dutch hospitals.

Intervention.—500 mg allopurinol, intravenously to the mother, immediately prior to delivery.

Main Outcome Measures.—Drug disposition (maternal plasma concentrations, cord blood concentrations) and drug safety (maternal and fetal adverse events).

Results.—Within 5 min after the end of maternal allopurinol infusion, target plasma concentrations of allopurinol of ≥2 mg/L were present in cord blood. Of all analysed cord blood samples, 95% (52/55) had a target allopurinol plasma concentration at the moment of delivery. No adverse events were observed in the neonates. Two mothers had a red and/or painful arm during infusion.

Conclusions.—A dose of 500 mg intravenous allopurinol rapidly crosses the placenta and provides target concentrations in 95% of the fetuses at the moment of delivery, which makes it potentially useful as a neuroprotective agent in perinatology with very little side effects.

Trial Registration.—The study is registered in the Dutch Trial Register (NTR1383) and the Clinical Trials protocol registration system (NCT00189007).

▶ Therapeutic hypothermia is an effective therapy for hypoxic-ischemic encephalopathy (HIE). However, the rate of death or disability after treatment with cooling remains high (approximately 40%), and there is an urgent need for additional therapies to further improve outcomes of infants who have acute encephalopathy. Because most fetuses at risk for HIE are not identified until a mother is in active labor, a neuroprotective therapy that could be administered before delivery, readily crosses the placenta, and is not harmful to mother or fetus would be ideal. In the above study the investigators assessed the feasibility and safety of maternal allopurinol, an agent which, in animal models of asphyxia, limits hypoxia-induced brain injury. The study population is a subset of women who participated in a randomized, double-blind, placebo-controlled, multicenter trial assessing the effect of maternally administered allopurinol on free radical production and markers of neuronal damage in infants at risk for HIE (NCT00189007). The dose of allopurinol was based on a previous study in healthy pregnant women. Women were eligible for the study if fetal hypoxia was suspected (abnormal or nonreassuring fetal heart tracing, significant ST-wave abnormalities detected by

STAN monitor or a fetal blood scalp sample with pH < 7.20). A single intravenous dose of allopurinol was administered 10 minutes before delivery, and venous cord blood and maternal blood samples were obtained immediately after delivery. Approximately one-third of participating women did not receive the whole dose of allopurinol before birth. Although the authors found that it is feasible and safe to deliver a putative neuroprotective therapeutic agent to a fetus at risk of HIE by intravenously administering the agent to a woman in labor, it still needs to be shown that the agent (allopurinol) is, indeed, effective in preventing or mitigating neonatal brain injury.

L. A. Papile, MD

Vaginal delivery versus caesarean section in preterm breech delivery: a systematic review

Bergenhenegouwen LA, Meertens LJE, Schaaf J, et al (Ziekenhuis Groep Twente, The Netherlands; Maastricht Univ, The Netherlands; Amsterdam Med Centre, The Netherlands; et al)

Eur J Obstet Gynecol Reprod Biol 172:1-6, 2014

There is controversy on the preferred mode of delivery (vaginal delivery (VD) versus caesarean section (CS)) in preterm breech delivery in relation to neonatal outcome. While CS is supposed to be safer for the fetus, arguments against CS can be the increased risk of maternal morbidity, risks for future pregnancies, and costs. Moreover, neonatal respiratory distress syndrome occurs more frequently after CS compared to VD.

In the past, several RCTs have been started on this subject, but they were all preliminary and stopped due to recruitment difficulties. As the Cochrane review of these RCT's reported on 116 women only, knowledge on the effectiveness of CS and VD can at present only be obtained from non-randomized studies.

We performed a systematic review and meta-analysis of non-randomized studies that assessed the association between mode of delivery and neonatal mortality in women with preterm breech presentation. We searched Pubmed, Embase and the Cochrane library for articles comparing neonatal mortality after VD versus CS in preterm breech presentation (gestational age 25^{+0} till 36^{+6} weeks). Seven studies, involving a total of 3557 women, met the eligibility criteria and were included in this systematic review. The weighted risk of neonatal mortality was 3.8% in the CS group and 11.5% in the VD group (pooled RR 0.63 (95% CI 0.48–0.81)). We conclude that cohort studies indicate that CS reduces neonatal mortality as compared to VD.

▶ I was somewhat surprised to come across this publication from Holland. After all, the definitive publication from Hannah and colleagues[1] in 2000 presented overwhelming data indicating that cesarean sections were safer than vaginal births for breech delivery. To refresh you on the information: "Data were received for 2083 women. Of the 1041 women assigned planned caesarean section, 941

(90·4%) were delivered by caesarean section. Of the 1042 women assigned planned vaginal birth, 591 (56·7%) delivered vaginally. Perinatal mortality, neonatal mortality, or serious neonatal morbidity was significantly lower for the planned caesarean section group than for the planned vaginal birth group (17 of 1039 [1·6%] vs 52 of 1039 [5·0%]; relative risk 0·33 [95% CI 0·19—0·56]; $p < .0001$). There were no differences between groups in terms of maternal mortality or serious maternal morbidity (41 of 1041 [3·9%] vs 33 of 1042 [3·2%]; 1·24 [0·79—1·95]; $p = .35$)." Since then, breech deliveries in the United States have become rare, and trauma associated with these breech deliveries has been remarkably reduced. What about preterm infants? The authors raise concerns about the increased incidence of respiratory distress in babies delivered by cesarean section together with maternal morbidity and costs. Several randomized trials had been started but not completed because of lack of enrollment, so the authors had to include the data from nonrandomized trials resulting in some heterogeneity. For example, time to death varies from 7 days to a month. However, death is a very concrete endpoint, and the weighted mortality risk clearly factored the operative deliveries. We recognize that the timing of the cesarean section is difficult and that sometimes with extreme prematurity, labor progresses so rapidly that it is not possible to set up and do a section even in the best-equipped medical center. However, there is a clear message that mortality was 37% lower, 1- and 5-minute Apgar scores were higher, and there was less respiratory morbidity in those delivered by cesarean section.

Although a randomized trial would yield firmer evidence, I don't believe that it is justifiable given the available data.

A. A. Fanaroff, MD, FRCPE

Reference

1. Hannah ME, Hannah WJ, Hewson SA, Hodnett ED, Saigal S, Willan AR. Planned caesarean section versus planned vaginal birth for breech presentation at term: a randomised multicentre trial. Term Breech Trial Collaborative Group. *Lancet.* 2000;356:1375-1383.

Resuscitation intensity at birth is associated with changes in brain metabolic development in preterm neonates

Duerden EG, Brown-Lum M, Chau V, et al (Univ of Toronto, Ontario, Canada; Univ of British Columbia, Vancouver, Canada)

Neuroradiology 55:S47-S54, 2013

Introduction.—Intensive resuscitation at birth has been linked to intraventricular haemorrhage (IVH) in the preterm neonate. However, the impact of less intensive resuscitation on more subtle alterations in brain metabolic development is largely unknown. Our objective was to determine the relationship between the intensity of neonatal resuscitation following preterm birth on brain metabolic development.

Methods.—One hundred thirty-three very preterm-born neonates (median gestational age [GA] 27 ± 2 weeks) underwent MR spectroscopic imaging early in life (median postmenstrual age 32 weeks) and again at term-equivalent age (median 40 weeks). Severity of white matter injury, IVH and cerebellar haemorrhage on magnetic resonance imaging were scored. Ratios of N-acetylaspartate (NAA) and lactate to choline (Cho) were calculated in eight regions of interest and were assessed in relation to intensiveness of resuscitation strategy (bag and mask, continuous positive airway pressure [CPAP], intubation, cardiopulmonary resuscitation [CPR]).

Results.—Within the first hour of life, 14 newborns had no intervention, 3 received bag and mask, 30 had CPAP, 79 were intubated and 7 had CPR. Resuscitated infants were more likely to have IVH ($p = 0.02$). More intensive resuscitation was associated with decreased NAA/Cho maturation ($p < 0.001$, adjusting for birth GA). Metabolic development was similar in neonates requiring CPAP in comparison to those receiving no intervention. The change in lactate/Cho did not differ across resuscitation categories ($p = 0.8$).

Conclusions.—Intensity of resuscitation at birth is related to changes in metabolic brain development from early in life to term-equivalent age. Results suggest that preventing the need for intensive neonatal resuscitation may provide an opportunity to improve brain development in preterm neonates.

▶ As survival improves, there are continued challenges to reduce the morbidity in the tiniest of the preemies. The focus has shifted from treatments in the neonatal intensive care unit, to the first hour of life—the golden hour. The management in the delivery room can have lifelong implications, and there has been a gradual but a definite shift from aggressive respiratory management (intubation and surfactant) to a minimalistic approach (stabilizing with continuous positive airway pressure [CPAP])—"less is more!" Convincing data show that preterm babies receiving aggressive cardiopulmonary resuscitation in the delivery room have a higher incidence of intraventricular hemorrhage; however, the brain metabolite derangement has not been adequately studied. Animal primate models show lesser brain injury in animals receiving CPAP when compared with mechanical ventilation and positive pressure ventilation. In another animal model, CPAP is also shown to have a neuroprotective effect. This immediate period soon after birth is a critical time not just for respiratory outcomes (first few large assisted breaths and bronchopulmonary dysplasia) but also for neurodevelopmental outcome as is hypothesized in this study.

Miller et al showed earlier abnormal brain outcomes with postnatal infection and procedural pain, and the ELGAN (extremely low gestational age neonates) study[1] showed critically ill preterm infants with poor physiologic scores (SNAP II and SNAPPE II) to have disrupted corticospinal tract development and poor motor outcomes. However, this is the first study looking at magnetic resonance spectroscopic imaging (MRSI) outcomes after intensive resuscitation at birth in preterm infants. MRSI studies showing increases in lactate and decrease in *N*-acetylaspartate (NAA) have been used as outcome predictors in full-term infants with neonatal encephalopathy. Their MRSI studies found metabolic disturbances leading to altered neuronal maturation in preterm infants receiving aggressive resuscitation at birth.

The changes in the *N*-acetylaspartate, possibly a marker of neuronal maturation, and lactate, may help predict the neurodevelopmental outcome in the future and move us one step closer to changing the golden hour into a crystal ball for the future. This study is pivotal in providing a glimpse into the brain metabolism during resuscitation; however, it may be a little preemptive to implicate the degree of resuscitation alone as a major factor. The authors have focused on postnatal infections and other morbidities; whereas, we are aware that inflammatory cytokines play a key role in the development of cerebral palsy in preterm infants.[2] This study did not include the prenatal factors and uterine milieu as an independent factor contributing to the need for extensive resuscitation (sicker babies) and unfavorable outcomes. For future studies, it would be very helpful to include the prenatal risk factors, including placental insufficiency, infections and possibly the placental pathology too. As the authors have acknowledged, this is just a preliminary study, and other factors, including oxygen saturation and partial pressure of carbon dioxide together with other parameters, such as blood pressure and cardiac output, need to be considered as variables when looking at resuscitation outcomes.

M. Bhola, MD

References

1. Dammann O, Naples M, Bednarek F, et al. SNAP-II and SNAPPE-II and the risk of structural and functional brain disorders in extremely low gestational age newborns: the ELGAN study. *Neonatology.* 2010;97:71-82.
2. Carlo WA, McDonald SA, Tyson JE, et al; for the Eunice Kennedy Shriver National Institute of Child Health and Human Development Neonatal Research Network. Cytokines and neurodevelopmental outcomes in extremely low birth weight. *J Pediatr.* 2011;159:919-925.e3.

Terminal Fetal Heart Decelerations and Neonatal Outcomes

Cahill AG, Caughey AB, Roehl KA, et al (Washington Univ School of Medicine, St Louis, MO; Oregon Health and Science Univ, Portland)
Obstet Gynecol 122:1070-1076, 2013

Objective.—To describe the incidence and characteristics of terminal fetal heart rate decelerations and to estimate their association with acidemia.

Methods.—A 5-year retrospective cohort study of all women with singleton, nonanomalous gestations who labored and reached complete dilation at or after 37 weeks of gestation. The 30 minutes of electronic fetal monitoring before delivery were interpreted by two formally trained research nurses, blind to clinical data, using American College of Obstetricians and Gynecologists guidelines. Terminal decelerations (decelerations without recovery of 120 seconds or more) defined the exposure. Terminal bradycardia (10 minutes or more) was secondarily explored. Univariable and multivariable analyses were performed to estimate risk of acidemia (umbilical cord gas arterial pH level 7.10 or less).

Results.—Of 5,388 women meeting inclusion criteria, 951 (17.7%) experienced a terminal deceleration whereas 4,437 (82.3%) did not. The incidence of acidemia among the 951 women with a terminal deceleration was low (1.3%; n = 12). However, acidemia (adjusted odds ratio [OR] 18.6; 95% confidence [CI] 5.0–68.9) and higher-level nursery admission (adjusted OR 5.4; 95% CI 1.9–15.3) were more likely if the terminal deceleration was 10 minutes or more. Terminal decelerations were longer among neonates with acidemia (6.7 minutes compared with 3.2 minutes; $P < .01$). For every additional 120 seconds of duration beyond the first 120 seconds, there was a corresponding decrease in umbilical cord gas pH level by 0.042 (95% CI 0.040–0.048; $P < .01$).

Conclusions.—More than 98% of term fetuses with terminal decelerations deliver with normal umbilical cord gas pH levels. However, bradycardia is associated with increased risk of acidemia and higher-level nursery admission. This information can be incorporated into clinical decision-making regarding urgency of delivery.

Level of Evidence.—II.

▶ Development of a prolonged fetal bradycardia late in the course of labor is a common and anxiety-provoking event. Although it is well known that fetal heart rate monitoring has poor predictive value for cerebral palsy, these situations often lead to delivery by urgent cesarean section. In fact, surprisingly little empirical data are available to guide decision making in these difficult circumstances or to inform counseling of new parents in their aftermath. Historically, these considerations have relied on data gathered from infants born after uterine rupture and more recently from babies delivered by cesarean after a trial of labor. Extrapolation of such experiences to the general population of women in labor is difficult; however, as risks may follow from the underlying process (eg, uterine rupture), the characteristics of fetal heart rate changes may not be completely described, and small sample sizes preclude assessment of specific details of the fetal heart rate (FHR) findings, such as severity or duration of the bradycardia. This work attempts to fill some of that void in our knowledge. These authors found that terminal decelerations (heart rate deceleration of 15 beats per minute (bpm) or more below baseline for 120 seconds to 10 minutes) were common but were not associated with fetal acidemia (arterial cord blood pH <7.10 or <7.05), low Apgar score at 5 minutes, or neonatal intensive care unit admissions. Terminal bradycardia (FHR less than 110 bpm for 10 minutes or more) did increase the probability of those complications and did not reliably predict acidemia (sensitivity, 33.3%; positive predictive value, 12.9%). Decelerations longer than 120 seconds were modestly predictive of fetal acidemia, with reduction of cord blood pH by 0.042 for every 120 seconds of bradycardia beyond that threshold. Infants born after bradycardia episodes in the highest quartile (longer than 4.7 minutes) were significantly more likely ($P < .01$ by χ^2 test for trend) to be acidemic (pH ≤7.10), but the prevalence of acidemia in that group was still quite low (only 3.5%). Thus, although anxieties about terminal bradycardias may not be assuaged to the extent that urgent cesarean sections will disappear, these data do provide reassurance that obstetricians have some time to evaluate such findings as they play out, and that pediatricians and neonatologists can confidently assure parents that terminal bradycardia episodes rarely result in fetal acidemia and even more rarely in fetal injury.

W. E. Benitz, MD

Delay in intervention increases neonatal morbidity in births monitored with cardiotocography and ST-waveform analysis

Kessler J, Moster D, Albrechtsen S (Haukeland Univ Hosp, Bergen, Norway; Univ of Bergen, Norway)

Acta Obstet Gynecol Scand 93:175-181, 2014

Objective.—To assess the effect of the time interval from indication of hypoxia to delivery on neonatal outcome in high-risk pregnancies monitored with cardiotocography (CTG) and ST-waveform analysis.

Design.—Prospective observational study.

Setting.—University hospital, Norway, 2004–08.

Population.—Singleton high-risk births with a gestational age above 35^{+6} weeks, monitored with CTG and ST-waveform analysis.

Methods.—Logistic regression analysis and Kaplan–Meier survival plots.

Main Outcome Measure.—Neonatal morbidity in relation to the rapidity of intervention.

Results.—Of 6010 deliveries monitored with ST-waveform analysis, 1131 (19%) had an indication to intervene for fetal distress according to clinical guidelines. Those fetuses were at increased risk of an adverse neonatal outcome, and if delivered later than 20 min after the indication of hypoxia their risk increased further; i.e. transfer to the neonatal intensive care unit (NICU) from an odds ratio of 1.6 (95% confidence interval 1.2–2.2) to an odds ratio of 3.3 (95% confidence interval 2.5–4.3). The indication-to-delivery interval was longer for neonates with a 5-min Apgar score of <7, transfer to NICU and neonatal encephalopathy than for those without adverse outcome.

Conclusion.—In deliveries monitored with CTG and ST-waveform analysis, the risk of an adverse neonatal outcome was dependent on the time between indication of hypoxia and delivery. Nonadherence to the specific clinical guidelines increased the risk of neonatal morbidity.

▶ Despite its limitations, fetal heart rate monitoring persists as the dominant form of assessing fetal well-being for high-risk pregnancies. Cardiotocography (CTG) has been the gold standard for fetal surveillance of these pregnancies in labor in many countries for decades. There is agreement that the test has a high sensitivity but a low specificity, which probably has resulted in many unnecessary operative deliveries for "pseudo" fetal distress. By adding analysis of ST and T-wave changes of the fetal electrocardiogram, the predictive value of fetal heart rate assessments have improved. However, there have only been a handful of randomized trials of inconsistent quality. Although the data suggest that CTG combined with ST-interval analysis (STAN) is better than CTG alone, there is still much discussion of the topic. Olofsson et al performed a critical appraisal of all 5 published systematic reviews assessing the effect of CTG + STAN versus CTG only on neonatal and maternal outcomes.[1,2] "In the CTG + ST[AN] study arms, the larger Plymouth, Swedish and Dutch trials showed lower operative delivery and metabolic acidosis rates, while the smaller Finnish and French trials showed minor differences in operative delivery and higher metabolic acidosis rates."[1] The review of the 5 metaanalyses was problematic in that trials that should have been included were excluded from some of the metaanalyses; however, they did favor the combined CTG + STAN with fewer scalp blood sampling, fewer operative deliveries, and less metabolic acidosis.

A significant part of the problem is the interpretation of the monitoring strips. Using 9 observers, Rhöse et al found poor interobserver agreement on CTG classification and on clinical management.[3] The article by Kessler et al reinforces the value of combining CTG and STAN. When there was evidence of fetal distress, delay in delivering the baby resulted in adverse outcomes. Adverse neonatal outcome was defined by cord blood metabolic acidosis (arterial pH <7.05 and base deficit >12 mmol/L [severe]; arterial pH <7.15, <10th centile [moderate]; low 5-minute Apgar [<7]), transfer to the neonatal intensive care unit, and moderate or severe neonatal encephalopathy. When there was evidence of fetal distress, delivery had to occur within 20 minutes to minimize the risks. The bottom line is that we need continued vigilance of the fetus and better recognition of fetal stress and distress.

A. A. Fanaroff, MD, FRCPE

References

1. Olofsson P, Ayres-de-Campos D, Kessler J, Tendal B, Yli BM, Devoe L. A critical appraisal of the evidence for using cardiotocography plus ECG ST interval analysis for fetal surveillance in labor. Part I: the randomized controlled trials. *Acta Obstet Gynecol Scand.* 2014;93:556-568.
2. Olofsson P, Ayres-de-Campos D, Kessler J, Tendal B, Yli BM, Devoe L. A critical appraisal of the evidence for using cardiotocography plus ECG ST interval analysis for fetal surveillance in labor. Part II: the meta-analyses. *Acta Obstet Gynecol Scand.* 2014;93:571-586.
3. Rhöse S, Heinis AM, Vandenbussche F, van Drongelen J, van Dillen J. Inter- and intra-observer agreement of non-reassuring cardiotocography analysis and subsequent clinical management. *Acta Obstet Gynecol Scand.* 2014;93:596-602.

The impact of introducing universal umbilical cord blood gas analysis and lactate measurement at delivery

White CRH, Doherty DA, Newnham JP, et al (Univ of Western Australia, Australia)

Aust N Z J Obstet Gynaecol 54:71-78, 2014

Background.—There is growing support for umbilical cord blood gas analysis (UCBGA) to be conducted at delivery. A recent study in a tertiary level obstetric unit found that universal UCBGA was associated with improved perinatal outcomes, but there is less evidence of benefit in lower-risk environments. In such settings, lactate analysis may be a suitable alternative.

Aims.—This study evaluated the introduction of universal UCBGA into a secondary obstetric unit and universal umbilical cord lactate analysis program into primary and secondary units.

Methods.—After education, universal UCBGA or lactate analysis was introduced into one primary and two secondary level obstetric units. Univariate and adjusted analysis assessed changes in UCBGA values and Apgar scores over the study period.

Results.—There were no significant changes in mean blood gas and lactate values at any centre following introduction of universal UCBGA or lactate analysis. However, there was at the primary level obstetric unit a significant reduction in the proportion of neonates with moderate to severe elevations in umbilical artery lactate values. There was a non-significant reduction in arterial pH values less than 7.10 at the secondary metropolitan centre.

Conclusion.—The data presented in this study suggest that the benefits of introducing UCBGA into a tertiary obstetric centre may be reproduced in a primary obstetric centre within 12 months of implementation. Larger studies are required in secondary units to assess infrequent adverse obstetric and neonatal outcomes.

▶ Quality improvement is a key buzzword in medical circles today. It is reassuring to learn that the introduction of a simple, reliable, inexpensive measurement such as cord blood lactate can improve the quality of care in nonacademic medical centers. The condition of the babies at delivery as measured by a number of parameters improved after the routine introduction of cord blood measurements. The data presented demonstrate a 61% reduction in arterial lactate levels greater than the population-based 95th percentile and a 69% reduction in arterial lactate levels greater than the 99th percentile. There was also reduction in the rate of metabolic acidemia in the primary obstetric center of similar magnitude to the tertiary center.

The authors were concerned that it would be too expensive and require more sophisticated equipment to measure complete cord blood gas and had been reassured by White's[1] data that lactate alone was a good predictor of outcome. Indeed White, using a large cohort, demonstrated that combining data from umbilical artery lactate levels and neonatal resuscitation level produces the most effective predictor of moderate to severe hypoxic-ischemic encephalopathy, with a sensitivity of 85% and a specificity of 99%.

A single measure of lactate was extremely helpful. The authors speculate on why the obstetrical management improved and concluded that awareness and education were probably the primary factors. I would add that concern of being watched and monitored will result in a much less cavalier approach to deliveries, and this is reflected by the outcomes in this report.

Previous reports suggested that there were medicolegal, financial, neonatal, or educational benefits of universal cord blood gas analysis.[2,3] This is probably true for cord blood lactate as well. Potential barriers to the universal introduction of cord blood measurements include "insufficient time following delivery, increased workload and encroachment of technology into birth."[4]

A. A. Fanaroff, MD, FRCPE

References

1. White CR, Doherty DA, Henderson JJ, Kohan R, Newnham JP, Pennell CE. Accurate prediction of hypoxic-ischaemic encephalopathy at delivery: a cohort study. *J Matern Fetal Neonatal Med.* 2012;25:1653-1659.
2. White CR, Doherty DA, Henderson JJ, et al. Benefits of introducing universal umbilical cord blood gas and lactate analysis into an obstetric unit. *Aust N Z J Obstet Gynaecol.* 2010;50:318-328.
3. Garibaldi JM, Westgate JA, Ifeachor EC. The evaluation of an expert system for the analysis of umbilical cord blood. *Artif Intell Med.* 1999;17:109-130.
4. White CR, Kohan R, Doherty DA, Newnham JP, Pennell CE. Attitudes and barriers to the introduction of umbilical cord blood gas and lactate analysis at birth. *Aust N Z J Obstet Gynaecol.* 2013;53:271-276.

Training Neonatal Cardiopulmonary Resuscitation: Can It Be Improved by Playing a Musical Prompt? A Pilot Study

Dold SK, Schmölzer GM, Kelm M, et al (Charité Univ Med Centre, Berlin, Germany; The Royal Women's Hosp, Melbourne, Australia)
Am J Perinatol 31:245-248, 2014

Objective.—Effective neonatal cardiopulmonary resuscitation (CPR) requires 3:1 coordinated manual inflations (MI) and chest compressions (CC). We hypothesized that playing a musical prompt would help coordinate CC and MI during CPR.

Study Design.—In this pilot trial we studied the effect the "Radetzky-marsch" (110 beats per minute) on neonatal CPR. Thirty-six medical professionals performed CPR on a neonatal manikin. CC and MI were recorded with and without the music played, using a respiratory function monitor and a tally counter. Statistical analysis included Wilcoxon test.

Results.—Without music, the median (interquartile range) rate of CC was 115 (100 to 129) per minute and the rate of MI was 38 (32 to 42) per minute. When listening to the auditory prompt, the rate of CC decreased significantly to 96 (96 to 100) per minute ($p = 0.002$) and the rate of MI to 32 (30 to 34) per minute ($p = 0.001$). The interquartile range of interoperator variability decreased up to 86%.

Conclusion.—Listening to an auditory prompt improved compliance with the recommended delivery rates of CC and MI during neonatal CPR.

▶ "I gave it a 93. Great beat and I can resuscitate to it." This is an interesting article that demonstrated the (perhaps) subliminal effect of playing music during a simulated resuscitation. A pair of subjects, 1 performing manual inflations and 1 performing chest compressions, was observed with and without music (a portion of the "Radetzkymarsch") playing in the background. Resuscitative maneuvers were more consistent and with much less variability during the music-assisted resuscitation and adhered much more closely to recommended guidelines.

This simulation trial will of course need to be replicated in the actual delivery room setting. It could open up a whole new set of strategies. Those checking the resuscitation crash carts will need to be sure the MP4 players are fully charged, and maybe we'll need to bring a DJ with us.

S. M. Donn, MD

Improving Delivery Room Management for Very Preterm Infants

DeMauro SB, Douglas E, Karp K, et al (The Children's Hosp of Philadelphia, PA; The Hosp of the Univ of Pennsylvania, Philadelphia)

Pediatrics 132:e1018-e1025, 2013

Background and Objectives.—Events in the delivery room significantly impact the outcomes of preterm infants. We developed evidence-based guidelines to prevent heat loss, reduce exposure to supplemental oxygen, and increase use of noninvasive respiratory support to improve the care and outcomes of infants with birth weight ≤1250 g at our institution.

Methods.—The guidelines were implemented through multidisciplinary conferences, routine use of a checklist, appointment of a dedicated resuscitation nurse, and frequent feedback to clinicians. This cohort study compares a historical group ($n = 80$) to a prospective group ($n = 80$, after guidelines were implemented). Primary outcome was axillary temperature at admission to the intensive care nursery. Secondary outcomes measured adherence to the guidelines and changes in clinically relevant patient outcomes.

Results.—Baseline characteristics of the groups were similar. After introduction of the guidelines, average admission temperatures increased (36.4°C vs 36.7°C, $P < .001$) and the proportion of infants admitted with moderate/severe hypothermia fell (14% vs 1%, $P = .003$). Infants were exposed to less oxygen during the first 10 minutes ($P < .001$), with similar oxygen saturations. Although more patients were tried on continuous positive airway pressure (40% vs 61%, $P = .007$), the intubation rate was not significantly different (64% vs 54%, $P = .20$). Median durations of invasive ventilation and hospitalization decreased after the quality initiative (5 vs 1 days [$P = .008$] and 80 vs 60 days [$P = .02$], respectively).

Conclusions.—We have demonstrated significantly improved quality of delivery room care for very preterm infants after introduction of evidence-based delivery room guidelines. Multidisciplinary involvement and continuous education and reinforcement of the guidelines permitted sustained change.

▶ Few doubters would resist attesting to the benefits of introducing quality improvement programs into the nursery. Quality improvement (QI) consists of systematic and continuous actions that lead to measurable improvement in health care services and the health status of targeted patient groups. The Institute of Medicine (IOM) defines quality in health care as a direct correlation between the level of improved health services and the desired health outcomes of individuals and population. Monitoring quality of care, comparing outcomes across different centers, and conducting collaborative quality improvement projects can quickly and dramatically change outcomes, translating into lower mortality, less morbidity and even shortened hospital stays. The economic benefits and cost savings are enormous.

A prime example is the goal of reducing the number of infants admitted to the neonatal intensive care unit (NICU) with moderate hypothermia, defined as a temperature less than 36°F.

In addition to the work of DeMauro, abstracted above, there are other recent publications with similar outcomes.

DeMauro and colleagues developed evidence-based guidelines to prevent heat loss, reduce exposure to supplemental oxygen, and increase use of noninvasive respiratory support to improve the care and outcomes of infants with birth weight ≤1250 g. They developed a team structure with ongoing education and feedback to the staff that were committed to the process. The outcomes were spectacularly good. Not only were fewer babies admitted with moderate hypothermia (1% vs 14% prior to the QI initiative), but the duration of exposure to oxygen in the first 10 minutes was reduced, as were the duration of intubation and length of hospital stay. An integral part of the therapy was to warm the dedicated resuscitation area to 76° to 77° F. The authors emphasized the roles of multidisciplinary involvement and continuous education in sustaining the change. Hospital administrators may not be happy with a 20-days reduced hospital stay, but the parents and the insurance companies are thrilled.

Pinheiro and colleagues[1] developed a thermoregulation bundle that resulted in a sustained decrease in the number of hypothermic babies admitted to the NICU without increasing the number of hyperthermic babies (> 37.5°F = 2.5%).

Pinheiro et al[1] and Mathew et al[2] reported that vinyl bags and warming mattress are equally effective in improving admission temperature in extremely low gestational age neonates. Overall, QI projects related to neonatal hypothermia are inexpensive yet supremely cost effective.

A. A. Fanaroff, MD, FRCPE

References

1. Pinheiro JM, Furdon SA, Boynton S, Dugan R, Reu-Donlon C, Jensen S. Decreasing hypothermia during delivery room stabilization of preterm neonates. *Pediatrics*. 2014;133:e218-e226.
2. Mathew B, Lakshminrusimha S, Sengupta S, Carrion V. Randomized controlled trial of vinyl bags versus thermal mattress to prevent hypothermia in extremely low-gestational-age infants. *Am J Perinatol*. 2013;30:317-322.

Perinatal outcomes for extremely preterm babies in relation to place of birth in England: the EPICure 2 study

Marlow N, Bennett C, Draper ES, et al (UCL Inst for Women's Health, UK; Univ of Leicester, UK; et al)

Arch Dis Child Fetal Neonatal Ed 99:F181-F188, 2014

Background.—Expertise and resources may be important determinants of outcome for extremely preterm babies. We evaluated the effect of place of birth and perinatal transfer on survival and neonatal morbidity within a prospective cohort of births between 22 and 26 weeks of gestation in England during 2006.

Methods.—We studied the whole population of 2460 births where the fetus was alive at the admission of the mother to hospital for delivery. Outcomes to discharge were compared between level 3 (most intensive) and level 2 maternity services, with and without transfers, and by activity level of level 3 neonatal unit; ORs were adjusted for gestation at birth and birthweight for gestation (adjusted ORs (aOR)).

Findings.—Of this national birth cohort, 56% were born in maternity services with level 3 and 34% with level 2 neonatal units; 10% were born in a setting without ongoing intensive care facilities (level 1). When compared with level 2 settings, risk of death in level 3 services was reduced (aOR 0.73 (95% CI 0.59 to 0.90)), but the proportion surviving without neonatal morbidity was similar (aOR 1.27 (0.93 to 1.74)). Analysis by intended hospital of birth confirmed reduced mortality in level 3 services. Following antenatal transfer into a level 3 setting, there were fewer intrapartum or labour ward deaths, and overall mortality was higher for those remaining in level 2 services (aOR 1.44 (1.09 to 1.90)). Among level 3 services, those with higher activity had fewer deaths overall (aOR 0.68 (0.52 to 0.89)).

Interpretation.—Despite national policy, only 56% of births between 22 and 26 weeks of gestation occurred in maternity services with a level 3 neonatal facility. Survival was significantly enhanced following birth in level 3 services, particularly those with high activity; this was not at the cost of increased neonatal morbidity.

▶ It is well accepted that hospital expertise is an important factor in improved outcomes for high-risk pregnancies with threatened very preterm birth. Center experience as measured by neonatal intensive care volume may also be an effective indicator of quality of neonatal care; however, data related to volume are sparse. In this population-based report the authors provide additional evidence that survival is greater in specialist hospitals with the highest activity services.

The EPICure 2 study involved the prospective collection of the details of all births reported between 22 and 26 weeks of gestation in all maternity hospitals in England during 2006. Because the study was based on the complete population of mothers with a live fetus at the point of hospital admission that led to delivery, data regarding antenatal death and delivery-room deaths were included in the data set. Neonatal morbidity was defined as 1 or more of retinopathy of prematurity requiring retinal surgery, moderate or severe bronchopulmonary dysplasia (oxygen or respiratory support at 36 weeks' gestational age), severe brain injury (hemorrhagic parenchymal infarct, cystic changes, or hydrocephalus on cerebral ultrasound), or necrotizing enterocolitis managed by laparotomy.

Time-specific mortality risk indicated that in higher level of care facilities, there was a reduced mortality occurring around delivery and during the first 7 days after birth; however mortality after 7 days of age or before delivery did not differ. In contrast to mortality, neonatal morbidity did not vary with place of birth. High-activity, high-level units had a lower overall mortality compared with medium-activity, high-level facilities, but there was no difference in time-specific mortality, nor was there any difference in survival without morbidity. These data support the concept that care in the perinatal period and during the first week after birth in a high-activity, high-level facility is particularly important in reducing mortality of babies born extremely early.

L. A. Papile, MD

Selected perinatal outcomes associated with planned home births in the United States

Cheng YW, Snowden JM, King TL, et al (Univ of California, San Francisco, School of Medicine; Oregon Health and Science Univ School of Medicine, Portland)

Am J Obstet Gynecol 209:325.e1-325.e8, 2013

Objective.—More women are planning home birth in the United States, although safety remains unclear. We examined outcomes that were associated with planned home compared with hospital births.

Study Design.—We conducted a retrospective cohort study of term singleton live births in 2008 in the United States. Deliveries were categorized by location: hospitals or intended home births. Neonatal outcomes were compared with the use of the χ^2 test and multivariable logistic regression.

Results.—There were 2,081,753 births that met the study criteria. Of these, 12,039 births (0.58%) were planned home births. More planned home births had 5-minute Apgar score <4 (0.37%) compared with hospital births (0.24%; adjusted odds ratio, 1.87; 95% confidence interval, 1.36–2.58) and neonatal seizure (0.06% vs 0.02%, respectively; adjusted odds ratio, 3.08; 95% confidence interval, 1.44–6.58). Women with planned home birth had fewer interventions, including operative vaginal delivery and labor induction/augmentation.

Conclusion.—Planned home births were associated with increased neonatal complications but fewer obstetric interventions. The trade-off between maternal preferences and neonatal outcomes should be weighed thoughtfully.

▶ After a period of decline through the 1990s, planned home births have been increasing since 2004. Recognition of this fact prompted the American Academy of Pediatrics to weigh in with recommendations for postnatal care of infants born at home.[1] Although not endorsing home births as intrinsically safe, the statement advocates care for the neonate born at home that adheres to the same standards that apply to in-hospital births and supports the American Congress of Obstetricians and Gynecologists recommendation that home births should be supervised only by midwives certified by the American Midwifery Certification Board. This analysis of national data on low-risk births in 2008 provides valuable information to inform this ongoing controversy. The available data did not include the most important endpoint, that of neonatal mortality rates. Prior analyses have found a 3-fold increase in the adjusted odds of mortality for nonanomalous neonates in association with planned birth at home[2]; the absolute increase in mortality rate was about 1 additional death per 1000 births. This study presents data that also may be taken as either worrisome or reassuring, depending on the disposition of the viewer. Although the odds ratios for both adverse outcomes were significantly greater than 1, the incremental risk of a 5-minute Apgar score less than 4 was 1 per 1000 births and that for neonatal seizures was about 1 in 2500 births. Women may look at those odds and feel that the risks of home birth for the baby are reassuringly small. Moreover, home births are associated with about one-quarter the risk of neonatal intensive care unit admission for the baby and many fewer obstetric interventions for the mother. The importance of midwife training and certification is highlighted by data not presented in the abstract of this article but included in the full text: neonatal complication rates were not higher for planned home births attended by certified nurse-midwives, but infants delivered by other midwives were more likely to have 5-minute Apgar scores less than 4 (adjusted odds ratio [OR], 1.62; 95% confidence interval [CI], 1.01–1.83) or neonatal seizure (adjusted OR, 3.29; 95% CI, 1.22–8.87) compared with neonates born in a hospital. It is not clear whether this difference results from differences in skill level, a lower threshold for abandonment of the plan for birth at home, or more stringent criteria for attempting home birth by those practitioners. Does this mean that home births are safe in general? In brief, no. The message here is that selective home births for women at low risk, with appropriate provisions for timely and rapid transfer to a hospital if complications arise, under the supervision of an appropriately trained midwife, can be achieved with modest neonatal risks, which may be deemed reasonable by well-informed parents. It is likely that the relative safety of planned home births results from selective use of this option by women who have been carefully screened to ensure that they are at low risk. Our job as advocates for the neonate is to ensure that those standards are understood, respected, and continuously refined.

W. E. Benitz, MD

References

1. Committee on Fetus and Newborn. Planned home birth. *Pediatrics.* 2013;131:1016-1020.
2. Wax JR, Lucas FL, Lamont M, Pinette MG, Cartin A, Blackstone J. Maternal and newborn outcomes in planned home birth vs planned hospital births: a metaanalysis. *Am J Obstet Gynecol.* 2010;203:243.e241-243.e248.

5 Infectious Disease and Immunology

Stratification of Risk of Early-Onset Sepsis in Newborns ≥34 Weeks' Gestation

Escobar GJ, Puopolo KM, Wi S, et al (Kaiser Permanente Division of Res, Oakland, CA; Brigham and Women's Hosp, Boston, MA; et al)

Pediatrics 133:30-36, 2014

Objective.—To define a quantitative stratification algorithm for the risk of early-onset sepsis (EOS) in newborns ≤34 weeks' gestation.

Methods.—We conducted a retrospective nested case-control study that used split validation. Data collected on each infant included sepsis risk at birth based on objective maternal factors, demographics, specific clinical milestones, and vital signs during the first 24 hours after birth. Using a combination of recursive partitioning and logistic regression, we developed a risk classification scheme for EOS on the derivation dataset. This scheme was then applied to the validation dataset.

Results.—Using a base population of 608 014 live births ≤34 weeks' gestation at 14 hospitals between 1993 and 2007, we identified all 350 EOS cases <72 hours of age and frequency matched them by hospital and year of birth to 1063 controls. Using maternal and neonatal data, we defined a risk stratification scheme that divided the neonatal population into 3 groups: treat empirically (4.1% of all live births, 60.8% of all EOS cases, sepsis incidence of 8.4/1000 live births), observe and evaluate (11.1% of births, 23.4% of cases, 1.2/1000), and continued observation (84.8% of births, 15.7% of cases, incidence 0.11/1000).

Conclusions.—It is possible to combine objective maternal data with evolving objective neonatal clinical findings to define more efficient strategies for the evaluation and treatment of EOS in term and late preterm infants. Judicious application of our scheme could result in decreased antibiotic treatment in 80 000 to 240 000 US newborns each year (Table 1).

► This elegant and powerful analysis of data from more than 600 000 newborn infants provides a model for use of clinical databases to guide improvements in clinical practice. It is likely to be one of the most influential articles in neonatal medicine in 2014, and deservedly so. In previous work, these authors developed a regression model for prediction of the risk of early-onset sepsis based on the obstetric factors that have traditionally provided the basis for

TABLE 1.—Hierarchical Classification of Clinical Signs[a]

Clinical Presentation[b]	Description
Clinical illness	In the first 12 h of age, the infant had a 5-min Apgar <5; received nasal continuous positive airway pressure or mechanical ventilation; received continuous infusion of vasoactive drugs; had a clinical seizure; or had significant respiratory distress (nasal flaring, grunting, or retractions were present and the infant received supplemental oxygen within the first 6 h)
Equivocal presentation	In the first 12 h of age, the infant experienced at least 2 instances of 1 of the following, with "instance"[c] meaning that there were ≥2 measurements ≥2 h apart:
	Heart rate ≥160
	Respiratory rate ≥60
	Temperature ≥100.4°F or <97.5°F
	Respiratory distress (grunting, flaring, or retracting)
Well appearing	The infant did not fall into one of the above 2 groups in the first 12 h of age

[a]Clinical presentations shown in the table are mutually exclusive and the scheme is applied sequentially, with infants removed from the group before applying the next category.

[b]To quantify the duration of clinical instability and avoid classifying infants based on transient abnormalities, we used the concept of "instance" for vital signs and respiratory distress (grunting, flaring, or retractions). An instance was the occurrence of a second abnormal value at least 2 hours after the first occurrence of an abnormal index value. Abnormal values after the index measurement counted as a new instance if they were followed by another abnormal measurement at least 2 hours later. Instances were sign-specific (ie, an abnormal temperature followed by an abnormal respiratory rate 2.1 hours later would not count as an instance for either temperature or respiratory rate).

[c]See text, Supplemental Information, and reference 2 for a description of data collection protocol.

neonatal treatment choices: gestational age, highest maternal intrapartum temperature, duration of rupture of membranes, group B *Streptococcus* colonization status, and nature and duration of intrapartum antibiotic exposure. Even optimal use of those risk indicators fails to provide sufficient predictive power to guide management, as the number needed to treat to ascertain only half of the cases of early onset sepsis exceeds 300. To improve performance of the algorithm, that work has now been extended to incorporate information about the neonate's condition at birth and over the subsequent 12 hours. Using a rigorous process of recursive partitioning and logistic regression, they stratified risk according to the model based on maternal factors alone (sepsis risk < 0.65, 0.65–1.54, and ≥1.54 per 1000 births) and according to the presence and severity of clinical signs of illness in the neonate (Table 1). They propose a strategy for consolidating the resulting 3-by-3 matrix into 3 risk groups, for which treatment (4% of infants, 61% of cases, number needed to treat [NNT] 118), evaluation (11% of infants, 23% of cases, NNT 823), or observation alone (85% of infants, 16% of cases, NNT 9370) are recommended. This risk stratification represents a significant advance but remains unsatisfactory because of the large number of infants who require treatment (> 100) or evaluation (> 800) for each case of early onset sepsis. An alternative strategy might select infants who are ill appearing and have an a priori risk estimate of ≥0.65 per 1000 for treatment (0.4% of infants, 18% of cases, NNT 38), those who are well appearing with an a priori risk less than 1.54 per 1000 and those with equivocal signs and an a priori risk less than 0.65 per 1000 for observation (96% of the population, 39% of cases, NNT 4250), and the remainder for evaluation (4% of infants, 43% of cases, NNT 152).

These options frame the conundrum: even with such carefully crafted paradigms for risk stratification, too many babies need treatment or diagnostic testing for each baby who actually is septic. This does not mean that our traditional approaches were wrong but rather reflects an enormous change in this landscape over the last 2 decades. The determined efforts of our obstetric colleagues have reduced the rate of early-onset sepsis from 3 to 5 to 0.5 to 0.6 cases per 1000 births (as in this large cohort). In this era, it is inescapable that one-third of the cases occur in infants who appear well and more than half occur in infants who have few or no maternal risk factors, compelling adoption of a fundamentally different approach. The shape of that is not yet apparent, but it likely will incorporate close monitoring for clinical signs of infection, sensitive diagnostic tests based on early components of the innate immune system, and a more restrained use of empiric antibiotic therapy.

W. E. Benitz, MD

Effect of Fluconazole Prophylaxis on Candidiasis and Mortality in Premature Infants: A Randomized Clinical Trial

Benjamin DK Jr, for the Fluconazole Prophylaxis Study Team (Duke Clinical Res Inst, Durham, NC; et al)

JAMA 311:1742-1749, 2014

Importance.—Invasive candidiasis in premature infants causes death and neurodevelopmental impairment. Fluconazole prophylaxis reduces candidiasis, but its effect on mortality and the safety of fluconazole are unknown.

Objective.—To evaluate the efficacy and safety of fluconazole in preventing death or invasive candidiasis in extremely low-birth-weight infants.

Design, Setting, and Patients.—This study was a randomized, blinded, placebo-controlled trial of fluconazole in premature infants. Infants weighing less than 750 g at birth (N = 361) from 32 neonatal intensive care units (NICUs) in the United States were randomly assigned to receive either fluconazole or placebo twice weekly for 42 days. Surviving infants were evaluated at 18 to 22 months corrected age for neurodevelopmental outcomes. The study was conducted between November 2008 and February 2013.

Interventions.—Fluconazole (6 mg/kg of body weight) or placebo.

Main Outcomes and Measures.—The primary end point was a composite of death or definite or probable invasive candidiasis prior to study day 49 (1 week after completion of study drug). Secondary and safety outcomes included invasive candidiasis, liver function, bacterial infection, length of stay, intracranial hemorrhage, periventricular leukomalacia, chronic lung disease, patent ductus arteriosus requiring surgery, retinopathy of prematurity requiring surgery, necrotizing enterocolitis, spontaneous intestinal perforation, and neurodevelopmental outcomes—defined as a Bayley-III cognition composite score of less than 70, blindness, deafness, or cerebral palsy at 18 to 22 months corrected age.

Results.—Among infants receiving fluconazole, the composite primary end point of death or invasive candidiasis was 16% (95% CI, 11%-22%) vs 21% in the placebo group (95% CI, 15%-28%; odds ratio, 0.73 [95% CI, 0.43-1.23]; $P=.24$; treatment difference, −5% [95% CI, −13% to 3%]). Invasive candidiasis occurred less frequently in the fluconazole group (3% [95% CI, 1%-6%]) vs the placebo group (9% [95% CI, 5%-14%]; $P=.02$; treatment difference, −6% [95% CI, −11% to −1%]). The cumulative incidences of other secondary outcomes were not statistically different between groups. Neurodevelopmental impairment did not differ between the groups (fluconazole, 31% [95% CI, 21%-41%] vs placebo, 27% [95% CI, 18%-37%]; $P=.60$; treatment difference, 4% [95% CI, −10% to 17%]).

Conclusions and Relevance.—Among infants with a birth weight of less than 750 g, 42 days of fluconazole prophylaxis compared with placebo did not result in a lower incidence of the composite of death or invasive candidiasis. These findings do not support the universal use of prophylactic fluconazole in extremely low-birth-weight infants.

Trial Registration.—clinicaltrials.gov Identifier: NCT00734539.

▶ Invasive candidiasis frequently causes death or neurodevelopmental impairment in preterm infants. Although fluconazole prophylaxis has been widely demonstrated to reduce the incidence of invasive candidiasis, its effects on morbidity and mortality are unknown. This trial was a randomized, blinded, placebo-controlled trial of fluconazole prophylaxis in 361 premature infants weighing <750 grams at birth. Infants were randomized to 42 days of fluconazole 6 mg/kg twice weekly or placebo. The primary end point was a composite of death or invasive candidiasis before study day 49. Secondary endpoints included evaluations of morbidity, drug safety, and neurodevelopmental outcomes at 18 to 22 months corrected age. Fluconazole prophylaxis had no impact on the primary endpoint (16% vs 21%, $P=.24$), although invasive candidiasis occurred less frequently in the fluconazole group (3% vs 9%, $P=.02$). Fluconazole prophylaxis did not impact secondary end points, including the incidence of neurodevelopmental impairment at 18 to 22 months corrected age (31% vs 27%, $P=.60$). This trial further supports the efficacy of fluconazole prophylaxis but does not support universal implementation in premature infants weighing <750 g at birth. The low incidence of culture-proven candidiasis in the placebo group of this high-risk population contrasts with previous trials and may signal the importance of environmental control measures emerging as standards of neonatal intensive care (decreased use of broad-spectrum antibiotics, increased use of line bundles, improved hand washing). Identification and implementation of noninvasive methods to reduce the incidence of candidiasis in the neonatal intensive care may further limit the utility of routine fluconazole prophylaxis. However, early identification of moderate-to-high risk infants who may benefit from fluconazole prophylaxis remains a research priority.

C. C. McPherson, PharmD

Using vaginal Group B *Streptococcus* colonisation in women with preterm premature rupture of membranes to guide the decision for immediate delivery: a secondary analysis of the PPROMEXIL trials

Tajik P, van der Ham DP, Zafarmand MH, et al (Academic Med Centre, Amsterdam, the Netherlands; Maastricht Univ Med Centre, the Netherlands; et al)

BJOG 2014 [Epub ahead of print]

Objective.—To investigate whether vaginal Group B *Streptococcus* (GBS) colonisation or other baseline characteristics of women with preterm premature rupture of membranes (PPROM) can help in identifying subgroups of women who would benefit from immediate delivery.

Design.—Secondary analysis of the PPROMEXIL trials.

Setting.—Sixty hospitals in the Netherlands.

Population.—Women with PPROM between 34 and 37 weeks of gestation.

Methods.—Random assignment of 723 women to immediate delivery or expectant management.

Main Outcome Measures.—Early onset neonatal sepsis.

Results.—Vaginal GBS colonisation status was the only marker which was significantly associated with the benefit of immediate delivery (*P* for interaction: 0.04). GBS colonisation was observed in 14% of women. The risk of early onset neonatal sepsis in GBS-positive women was high (15.2%) when they were managed expectantly but this risk was reduced to 1.8% with immediate delivery. The early onset neonatal sepsis risk was much lower in neonates of GBS-negative women: 2.6% after expectant management and 2.9% with immediate delivery. We estimated that by inducing labour only in GBS-positive women, there would be a 10.4% increase in term delivery rate, while keeping neonatal sepsis and caesarean delivery rates comparable to a strategy of labour induction for all.

Conclusions.—Our *post hoc* findings suggest that women with PROM between 34 and 37 weeks might benefit from immediate delivery if they have GBS vaginal colonisation, while in GBS-negative women labour induction could be delayed until 37 weeks.

▶ The management of pregnancies complicated by preterm prolonged rupture of membranes (PPROM) remains controversial. Delivery at specific gestational age cutoffs has been advocated to decrease the risk of neonatal early-onset sepsis. The 2 previously published PPROMEXIL trials randomized 723 women with singleton or twin pregnancies and PPROM that occurred after 26 weeks' gestation to delivery at 34 0/7 weeks (or within 48 hours of PROM if this occurred after 34 0/7 weeks) or to expectant management until 37 0/7 weeks' gestation, with induction of labor or indicated cesarean delivery at that point. The PPROMEXIL trials revealed no difference in the incidence of neonatal death, sepsis, or any other major neonatal morbidity between the 2 strategies, despite a significant difference in gestational age and weight at birth. In the current study, the authors used logistic regression to model the interaction among maternal group B

Streptococcus (GBS) status, neonatal sepsis, and maternal treatment group in a secondary analysis of the original PPROMEXIL data set. Among infants born to the 103 GBS-colonized study women, the risk of neonatal sepsis was 15.2% among those born to women managed expectantly but only 1.8% among those born to women in the immediate delivery group (odds ratio 0.10; 95% confidence interval: 0.01–0.84). The trials did not specify the whether antibiotic prophylaxis before or during labor should be administered to GBS-colonized women. Variable types of oral or IV antibiotics were observed to be administered within the trial, but no statistically valid conclusions could be made regarding the effect of maternal antibiotic administration. The authors suggest that expectant management of PPROM to 37 0/7 weeks may be safe only for women who are not GBS colonized and advocate an immediate-delivery strategy at ≥34 0/7 weeks' gestation for GBS-colonized women pending confirmation of their findings.

K. M. Puopolo, MD, PhD

Maternal Antibody at Delivery Protects Neonates From Early Onset Group B Streptococcal Disease

Baker CJ, Carey VJ, Rench MA, et al (Baylor College of Medicine, Houston, TX; Harvard Med School and Harvard Pilgrim Health Care Inst, Boston, MA)
J Infect Dis 209:781-788, 2014

Background.—Further reduction in the group B streptococcal (GBS) disease burden in neonates in the United States awaits an additional prevention strategy, such as maternal immunization.

Methods.—We performed a prospective, multicenter, case-control study of 33 mothers delivering neonates with early onset GBS infection (cases), and 99 age- and ethnicity-matched mothers colonized with the same capsular polysaccharide (CPS) types delivering healthy neonates (controls). Relative risk and absolute risk were calculated for early onset disease associated with concentrations of type Ia, III, or V CPS-specific antibody in maternal serum.

Results.—For GBS types Ia and III, maternal CPS–specific antibody concentrations of ≥0.5 g/mL were associated with a relative risk of approximately 0.1 (95% confidence intervals [CIs], .01–.74 and 0–.72, respectively; *P* = .02 for each), corresponding to a 90% risk reduction (by logistic regression). For type V, the relative risk was 0.3 (95% CI, .01–3.1), corresponding to a 70% risk reduction. By Bayesian modeling, the risk of early onset disease would decrease by 70% if maternal CPS-specific antibody concentrations for these 3 GBS types were ≥1 μg/mL.

Conclusions.—Maternal CPS-specific antibody serum concentrations of ≥1 μg/mL at the time of delivery appear to protect most neonates from early onset GBS type Ia and III disease.

▶ One of the enduring enigmas of early-onset neonatal group B streptococcal (GBS) infection is the very large disparity between the proportion of babies who are exposed to GBS (25%–30%) and the rate of actual infection with this organism (1–3 per 1000 births). Passively acquired immunity has long been known to be a significant factor in this, as low titers of type-specific antibody correlate with susceptibility to GBS infections. This report affirms those decades-old observations and extends them to serotype V, which was not common in that earlier era. Noting that the strategy of intrapartum prophylaxis has reduced the attack rate by more than 80%, but not to zero, these authors suggest that immunization to achieve protective antibody levels in pregnant women may provide an opportunity for further reduction in the incidence of this disease. Given the current low attack rate for early-onset GBS sepsis, the efficacy of a vaccination strategy is likely to be very difficult to demonstrate, however. This challenge may be compounded by another enigma: the babies who are at greatest risk appear to be those born to mothers who have heavy vaginal GBS colonization, suggesting that their low antibody titers may not result simply from lack of antigen exposure. The case for an immunization strategy would be greatly strengthened by demonstration that vaccines can elicit protective antibody production in heavily colonized women with low levels of GBS-specific IgG, particularly in those who have given birth to an affected infant. That is not the only potential application of these important results, however. We should not be sanguine about the effects of exposing a quarter to a third of our newborn babies to antibiotic prophylaxis, which has as yet unknown but potentially adverse effects on acquisition of a healthy microbiome. Development of rapid bedside tests that could determine whether a women beginning labor is colonized with GBS and if she has serum levels of specific immunoglobulin adequate to protect her baby against infection with her colonizing organism might allow much more selective use of intrapartum prophylaxis, for example. The authors of this work should be commended for not resting on the considerable success of current prevention strategies and in their efforts to find ways to do even better.

W. E. Benitz, MD

Impact of Perinatal Practices for Early-onset Group B Streptococcal Disease Prevention

Berardi A, on behalf of the GBS Prevention Working Group, Emilia-Romagna (Azienda Ospedaliero-Universitaria Policlinico, Modena, Italy; et al)
Pediatr Infect Dis J 32:e265-e271, 2013

Background.—Prevention of residual cases of neonatal group B streptococcus (GBS) early-onset disease (EOGBS) has become a goal in the past decade. This study is aimed at evaluating changes in the incidence of EOGBS over a 9-year period after the implementation of a screening-based approach and comparing 2 different protocols for managing healthy-appearing at-risk newborns (ARNs).

Methods.—A screening-based strategy was introduced in Emilia-Romagna (Italy) in 2003. A prospective, cohort study was conducted from 2003 to 2011; culture-proven EOGBS cases were analyzed in 2 periods: period 1 (2003 to 2008) and period 2 (2009 to 2011). ARNs (≥35 weeks' gestation) were managed according to 2 different protocols: laboratory testing plus observation (period 1) was replaced with expectant observation alone (period 2).

Results.—Ninety-one EOGBS cases were observed (incidence rate: 0.26/1000 live births). The incidence in full-term babies declined from 0.30 (period 1) to 0.14/1000 live births (period 2, $P = 0.04$). Recto-vaginal screening cultures in full-term mothers increased significantly from 10/45 (period 1) to 10/14 (period 2, $P = 0.002$). EOGBS was diagnosed earlier in ARNs than in not-at-risk newborns (mean age 5.5 versus 14.5 hours, $P = 0.007$). There were no differences in age at diagnosis irrespective of whether ARNs were managed with laboratory testing plus observation (mean 3.5 hours, period 1) or with expectant observation alone (mean 2.4 hours, period 2).

Conclusions.—When screening cultures were handled according to standard protocols, cases of EOGBS in full-term newborns simultaneously decreased. ARNs were diagnosed in a timely manner through both strategies. The clinical yield of laboratory testing was negligible.

▶ Efforts to prevent early-onset group B streptococcal (EOGBS) sepsis beginning in the mid-1900s reduced the attack rate in the United States from about 1.8 to fewer than 0.3 per 1000 live births. This success, based on provision of intrapartum antibiotic prophylaxis (IPAP) for women at increased risk for neonatal infection, has fundamentally changed the landscape of early-onset neonatal bacterial infections, especially among late-preterm and term infants. Because of the efficacy of this prevention strategy, most infants with EOGBS disease now are born to women without identified risk factors. Consequently, assessment of obstetric risk factors is no longer reliable for ascertainment of infants who will develop EOGBS sepsis. The lower attack rate (prior probability of disease), further compromises the already poor predictive value of common diagnostic tests. Although recent modifications of consensus guidelines from the Centers for Disease Control (CDC) and American Academy of Pediatrics have moved away from reliance on laboratory testing, screening using laboratory tests remains an important, but increasingly anachronistic, component of those protocols.

This important report of a regional experience from Northern Italy, covering 9 years and more than 350 000 births, provides a view into the future. Two substantial changes in practice were implemented during that interval. First, progressive implementation of the CDC-recommended regimen for antepartum screening cultures and IPAP reduced the rate of EOGBS sepsis in term infants (52 of 209 949 [0.24/1000] from 2003–2008 vs 16 of 117 494 [0.14/1000] from 2009–2011; $P = .046$) but not in preterm infants (15 of 16 788 [0.89/1000] vs 8 of 9567 [0.83/1000]; P value not significant). Second, the evaluation protocol for at-risk infants changed from a limited evaluation (complete blood count, blood culture, and C-reactive protein level at 6–12 hours of age) to expectant observation (focused assessments of general well-being, skin color and perfusion, and respiratory signs, 6 times over the first 36 hours and at discharge). At-risk neonates were defined as those born to women who met CDC criteria for IPAP but were not treated, received treatment less than 4 hours before delivery, or received an antibiotic other than ampicillin or cefazolin (penicillin was not used). Babies with signs of illness or a history of chorioamnionitis were treated with antibiotics in both periods. The extent to which transition to expectant observation reduced diagnostic testing is not reported, but it likely was substantial.

In this cohort, 91 infants had blood cultures positive for group B streptococcus: 14 had asymptomatic bacteremia, 16 were less than 35 weeks of gestation, and 33 were term infants with no identified risk factors. Of the 28 cases of EOGBS sepsis diagnosed in at-risk newborns born at ≥35 weeks of gestation, 14 had signs of illness at birth and 8 had signs at less than 12 hours of age (before screening tests were or would have been performed under the limited evaluation protocol). Of the remaining 6 at-risk infants, 4 had diagnostic testing (abnormal in only 2) before onset of clinical signs and 2 had clinical signs at 36 and 39 hours of age after missed screening testing (during the limited evaluation period). Identification of infants with sepsis based on serial clinical examinations, each taking less than 60 seconds to perform, had a sensitivity of at least 93% (95% CI, 76%–99%), outperforming any currently available laboratory test, without delaying diagnosis. Seven newborns with EOGBS died, including 6 born before 35 weeks of gestation and 1 term infant not identified as at risk; none would have been identified by laboratory testing based on identification of risk factors. The benefits of laboratory testing in this large cohort were, therefore, negligible. The time for abandonment of those outdated practices appears to be upon us.

W. E. Benitz, MD

The microbiota regulates neutrophil homeostasis and host resistance to *Escherichia coli* K1 sepsis in neonatal mice

Deshmukh HS, Liu Y, Menkiti OR, et al (Children's Hosp of Philadelphia, PA; et al)

Nat Med 20:524-530, 2014

Neonatal colonization by microbes, which begins immediately after birth, is influenced by gestational age and the mother's microbiota and is modified by exposure to antibiotics. In neonates, prolonged duration of antibiotic therapy is associated with increased risk of late-onset sepsis (LOS), a disorder controlled by neutrophils. A role for the microbiota in regulating neutrophil development and susceptibility to sepsis in the neonate remains unclear. We exposed pregnant mouse dams to antibiotics in drinking water to limit transfer of maternal microbes to the neonates. Antibiotic exposure of dams decreased the total number and composition of microbes in the intestine of the neonates. This was associated with decreased numbers of circulating and bone marrow neutrophils and granulocyte/macrophage–restricted progenitor cells in the bone marrow of antibiotic-treated and germ-free neonates. Antibiotic exposure of dams reduced the number of interleukin-17 (IL-17)-producing cells in the intestine and production of granulocyte colony–stimulating factor (G-CSF). Granulocytopenia was associated with impaired host defense and increased susceptibility to *Escherichia coli* K1 and *Klebsiella pneumoniae* sepsis in

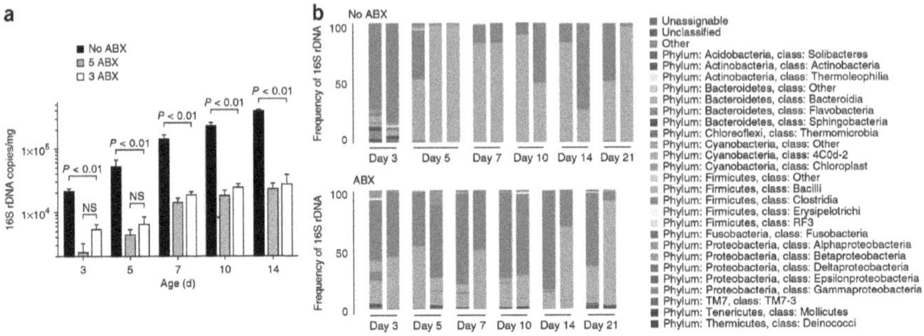

FIGURE 1.—Perinatal antibiotic exposure alters the pattern of microbial colonization in the intestine and attenuates postnatal granulocytosis. (**a**) 16S ribosomal DNA (rDNA) copy numbers from the intestinal contents of neonatal mice exposed to a combination of three (3 ABX) or five (5 ABX) antibiotics or no antibiotics (No ABX), as determined using real-time PCR. $n = 10$ for all groups. NS, not significant. (**b**) Relative abundance of phylum- and class-level commensal bacteria obtained from 16S rDNA pyrosequencing of the intestinal contents of age- and sex-matched neonatal mice exposed to five antibiotics (ABX) or no antibiotics. Each bar represents the pooled intestinal contents from 9 age-defined neonatal mice from 4 different litters. (Reprinted from Deshmukh HS, Liu Y, Menkiti OR, et al. The microbiota regulates neutrophil homeostasis and host resistance to Escherichia coli K1 sepsis in neonatal mice. *Nat Med.* 2014;20:524-530.)

antibiotic-treated neonates, which could be partially reversed by administration of G-CSF. Transfer of a normal microbiota into antibiotic-treated neonates induced IL-17 production by group 3 innate lymphoid cells (ILCs) in the intestine, increasing plasma G-CSF levels and neutrophil numbers in a Toll-like receptor 4 (TLR4)— and myeloid differentiation factor 88 (MyD88)—dependent manner and restored IL-17—dependent resistance to sepsis. Specific depletion of ILCs prevented IL-17— and G-CSF—dependent granulocytosis and resistance to sepsis. These data support a role for the intestinal microbiota in regulation of granulocytosis, neutrophil homeostasis and host resistance to sepsis in neonates (Fig 1a, b).

▶ The use of perinatal as well as neonatal antibiotics especially in premature infants is widespread. The concern that this may actually be causing harm has been increasing over the past few years because of the concern for late-onset sepsis with more resistant micro-organisms as well as a more recent finding that duration of postnatal antibiotics in preterm infants may actually result in increased odds of necrotizing enterocolitis. The mechanisms for such findings have not been rigorously evaluated. This study in mice shows a mechanistic relationship between antibiotic therapy in the perinatal period, the resulting alterations in the microbiota of the intestine, and the role of these alterations in regulating neutrophil development and subsequent susceptibility to sepsis. In this study, antibiotic exposure to pregnant mothers decreased the total number and the composition of microbes in the neonatal intestine. When evaluating the differences in phylum and class of bacteria over the first 3 weeks in the antibiotic-treated versus on non-antibiotic-treated groups, marked differences were found (Fig 1a, b). Concurrent with these differences, the antibiotic exposed mice had a lower number of interleukin 17—producing cells in the intestine and granulocytopenia. Two pathogens, *Escherichia coli* K1 and *Klebsiella pneumoniae*, were found associated with increased sepsis in the antibiotic-treated groups. This study is important because it shows a mechanistic relationship between perinatal antibiotic use and lower resistance to sepsis in neonates via a pathway that is dependent on the types of microbes present in the intestine. Further evaluation of this pathway could lead to specific microbial manipulation strategies that could decrease antibiotic-induced intestinal microbiota dysbiosis and decrease both morbidity and mortality in these infants.

J. Neu, MD

Probiotic Effects on Late-onset Sepsis in Very Preterm Infants: A Randomized Controlled Trial

Jacobs SE, for the ProPrems Study Group (The Royal Women's Hosp, Melbourne, Australia; et al)

Pediatrics 132:1055-1062, 2013

Background and Objective.—Late-onset sepsis frequently complicates prematurity, contributing to morbidity and mortality. Probiotics may reduce mortality and necrotizing enterocolitis (NEC) in preterm infants, with unclear effect on late-onset sepsis. This study aimed to determine the effect of administering a specific combination of probiotics to very preterm infants on culture-proven late-onset sepsis.

Methods.—A prospective multicenter, double-blinded, placebocontrolled, randomized trial compared daily administration of a probiotic combination (*Bifidobacterium infantis, Streptococcus thermophilus*, and *Bifidobacterium lactis*, containing 1×10^9 total organisms) with placebo (maltodextrin) in infants born before 32 completed weeks' gestation weighing <1500 g. The primary outcome was at least 1 episode of definite late-onset sepsis.

Results.—Between October 2007 and November 2011, 1099 very preterm infants from Australia and New Zealand were randomized. Rates of definite late-onset sepsis (16.2%), NEC of Bell stage 2 or more (4.4%), and mortality (5.1%) were low in controls, with high breast milk feeding rates (96.9%). No significant difference in definite late-onset sepsis or all-cause mortality was found, but this probiotic combination reduced NEC of Bell stage 2 or more (2.0% versus 4.4%; relative risk 0.46, 95% confidence interval 0.23 to 0.93, $P = .03$; number needed to treat 43, 95% confidence interval 23 to 333).

Conclusions.—The probiotics *B infantis, S thermophilus,* and *B lactis* significantly reduced NEC of Bell stage 2 or more in very preterm infants, but not definite late-onset sepsis or mortality. Treatment with this combination of probiotics appears to be safe.

► More than 5000 infants have been enrolled in more than 22 randomized, controlled trials (RCTs) of probiotic preparations for preterm infants. Systematic reviews of these trials have documented a major reduction in necrotizing enterocolitis (NEC) and a reduction in death with the routine use of probiotics in high-risk preterm infants.[1] However, these reviews, including several probiotic strains and combinations administered at varying gestational ages, do not report a significant reduction in late-onset sepsis.

The study from Jacobs et al focuses on the fact that because preterm infants acquire their colonizing gastrointestinal bacteria from the neonatal intensive care unit (NICU) environment rather than from their mothers' flora or breast milk, they colonize with potentially pathogenic bacteria (*Escherichia coli, Enterococcus* spp and *Klebsiella pneumonia*). This is made even worse with the widespread and potentially prolonged courses of antibiotics these infants receive and the possibility that this increases the risk of both NEC and late-onset sepsis.

The Jacobs study, an RCT from 10 centers in Australia and New Zealand, included 1100 very low-birth-weight infants, less than 1500 g, receiving probiotics within 72 hours of birth. This ProPrems trial used the ABC Dophilus Probiotic Powder from Solgar, Leonia, New Jersey. This contained *Bifidobacterium infantis, Streptococcus thermophiles*, and *Bifidobacterium lactis*. The primary outcome was at least one episode of definite late-onset sepsis using very stringent criteria for "definite sepsis" as a positive isolation of organisms from blood, urine, or spinal fluid. "Clinical sepsis" is defined as a negative blood culture but elevated C-reactive protein plus elevated immature-to-total neutrophil ratio and receipt of antibiotics. There was no reduction in late-onset sepsis with the probiotics. However, these 1100 patients with approximate gestational age of 28 weeks add to the experience with probiotics and NEC, showing a reduction in NEC from 4.4% in control to 2.0% for those receiving the probiotics. More than 95% of the infants were receiving human milk in the study.

Our only problem with probiotics is that no one has determined which probiotic is the most effective, what combinations work best, when they should be used, or the duration of administration. The combination of probiotics in the Jacobs study appears to be safe, cheap, and readily implemented. Probiotics may be of greatest value globally in neonatal settings with high rates of NEC, mortality, and late-onset sepsis. In fact, a recent cohort study of probiotics in the first North American NICU using a mixture of 4 probiotics showed a reduction in NEC from almost 10% to 5% among almost 300 infants compared with 317 not receiving probiotics for the previous 17 months.[1] These authors conclude that a reliable preparation is available in Canada and available for the United States and that probiotics should be considered standard of care and used routinely in all preterm infants less than 32 weeks of gestation. As noted below, this will not happen in the United States until a randomized trial confirming these other studies has been completed. We are, in fact, rediscovering the wheel.

A trial has finally commenced in the United States. In the meantime, the US Food and Drug Administration has renamed probiotics for these infants *live biotherapeutic products*. This designation underscores that the scrutiny for these agents will continue to be much more intense and demanding than probiotics, which are promoted on more general nutritional claims and less pathogen testing.

Here is our conundrum. It doesn't appear that the live biotherapeutics are going to become available without further intense study in the United States, that is, we can't rely on the 5000 patients already studied to choose an agent, and it will take many years to choose a dose and combination of these microbes. Multiple therapies show promise, such as lactoferrin, which has an IND for research use as the recombinant form, but the product is no longer being manufactured. The bovine lactoferrin also has potential, but it too has not been approved for experimentation in the United States. All of these alternative methods need to be studied and evaluated further if we are to make progress in the field.

D. H. Adamkin, MD

Reference

1. Janvier A, Malo J, Barrington KJ. Cohort study of probiotics in a North American neonatal intensive care unit. *J Pediatr.* 2014;164:980-985.

Toll-like receptor genetic variants are associated with gram-negative infections in VLBW infants

Sampath V, Mulrooney NP, Garland JS, et al (Med College of Wisconsin, Milwaukee; Children's Hosps and Clinics of Minnesota, Minneapolis; Wheaton Franciscan Health Care, Milwaukee, WI; et al)
J Perinatol 33:772-777, 2013

Objective.—To test the hypothesis that single-nucleotide polymorphisms (SNPs) in Toll-like receptor (TLR) genes alter susceptibility to bacterial infections and modulate white blood cell (WBC) counts during infections in very low birth weight (VLBW) infants (birth weight <1500 g).

Study Design.—VLBW infants recruited in a multicenter study were genotyped for nine functional *TLR* SNPs and associations between SNPs and infection rates examined. WBC counts obtained during infections were compared among infants with and without SNPs.

Result.—In our cohort ($n = 408$), 90 infants developed bacterial infections. Presence of *TLR4* (rs4986790 and rs4986791) variants were associated with Gram-negative (G−ve) infections. Female infants heterozygous for the X-linked *IRAK1* (rs1059703) SNP had less G−ve infections. In regression models controlling for confounders, the *TLR4* (rs4986790) SNP was associated with increased G−ve infections. The *TLR5* (rs5744105) variant was associated with elevated WBC counts during infections.

Conclusion.—*TLR* genetic variants can contribute to increased risk of bacterial infections and altered immune responses in VLBW infants.

► Toll-like receptors (TLRs) are a family of cell surface receptors that recognize a variety of pathogen-associated molecular patterns (PAMPs), leading to activation of the innate immune system in a protective response to the presence of potentially invasive pathogenic organisms. Each TLR is specific for particular classes of PAMPs. For example, TLR2 (in concert with TLR1 or TLR6) recognizes molecules associated with gram-positive bacteria, and TLR4 recognizes products of gram-negative bacteria. In this work, the authors have identified an association between invasive gram-negative infections in very low-birth-weight infants and particular single-nucleotide polymorphisms in the TLR4 gene. These observations suggest that the traditional approach to understanding the biological basis of neonatal infection may have been framed using the wrong question. The tendency has been to ask what it is about babies or preterm babies that makes them, as a group, more vulnerable to bacterial infection? It may be more fruitful to ask what it is about babies who develop serious bacterial infections that distinguishes them from their peers who do not become infected, despite exposure to the same potential pathogens? After all, for every baby who has early-onset group B streptococcal sepsis, 50 or more are exposed to that organism but do not become infected. Adult TLR2 knockout mice have compromised host resistance to infection with GBS, resulting in earlier and greater mortality,[1] suggesting a potential role for TLR2 polymorphisms in neonatal vulnerability to that infection. We may also be asking the wrong question when we ponder the slower, more blunted time course of the C-reactive protein response to coagulase-negative Staphylococcal infection in preterm infants. Perhaps the subset of infants who become infected with those organisms do so because their innate immune response to *Staphylococci* is specifically compromised, rather than because the properties of that organism lead to a generally more moderate immune response in all babies. Development of more tightly targeted approaches to risk assessment, diagnostic evaluation, and empiric treatment of sepsis in newborn infants will benefit greatly from detailed exploration these individual genetic proclivities.

W. E. Benitz, MD

Reference

1. Puliti M, Uematsu S, Akira S, Bistoni F, Tissi L. Toll-like receptor 2 deficiency is associated with enhanced severity of group B streptococcal disease. *Infect Immun*. 2009;77:1524-1531.

Neutrophil CD64 for Daily Surveillance of Systemic Infection and Necrotizing Enterocolitis in Preterm Infants

Lam HS, Cheung HM, Poon TCW, et al (The Chinese Univ of Hong Kong, China)

Clin Chem 59:1753-1760, 2013

Background.—Early detection and treatment of infected preterm infants could decrease morbidity and mortality. Neutrophil CD64 has been shown to be an excellent early diagnostic biomarker of late-onset sepsis (LOS) and necrotizing enterocolitis (NEC). We aimed to study whether using CD64 as a daily surveillance biomarker could predict LOS/NEC before clinical manifestation.

Methods.—We collected 0.1 mL whole blood from very low birth weight (VLBW) infants from day 7 postnatal age until routine daily blood tests were no longer required. Four categories of responses were defined: proven sepsis, clinical sepsis, nonsepsis/non-NEC, and asymptomatic CD64 activation.

Results.—A total of 146 infants were consecutively recruited and 155 episodes of sepsis evaluation were performed. The biomarker screening utility, sensitivity, specificity, positive predictive value, and negative predictive value for surveillance of LOS/NEC using a cutoff of 5655 antibody-PE (phycoerythrin) molecules bound/cell were 89%, 98%, 41%, and 99.8%, respectively. LOS/NEC was detected a mean of 1.5 days before clinical presentation. However, 63 episodes of CD64 activation occurred in asymptomatic infants who would not otherwise have required sepsis evaluations.

Conclusions.—As a surveillance biomarker, neutrophil CD64 detected LOS/NEC 1.5 days before clinical presentation, but at the expense of performing 41% additional sepsis evaluations. This was mainly attributed to an unexpected group of asymptomatic infants with CD64 activation, who recovered spontaneously and did not require antimicrobial treatment. The latter group has not been previously recognized in VLBW infants and could represent subclinical infection secondary to transient bacterial translocation or mild viral infection (Fig 2).

▶ This important report provides essential new information about a rapidly maturing new technology for diagnosis of serious bacterial infection in newborns: quantitation of markers of cellular differentiation on the surface of neutrophils. In this instance, the marker in question is CD64, a high affinity receptor for the Fc portion of immunoglobulin G, which is rapidly upregulated on the surface of granulocytes in response to exposure to bacterial products. In this report, measurement of CD64 expression in more than 4500 daily samples obtained from 146 very low birth weight (VLBW) infants during their neonatal intensive care unit hospitalization, including 55 instances of late-onset sepsis and 155 diagnostic evaluations for sepsis, allowed delineation of 4 temporal patterns of CD64 expression (Fig 2). Infants with proven or probable sepsis showed elevations in CD64 expression beginning 1 to 2 days before recognition of clinical signs of illness, with levels returning to normal about 7 days later. A smaller and more transient elevation of CD64 was observed in some infants who had no other clinical signs of sepsis, and an absence of CD64 elevation correlated with absence of infection. There was no difference between the expression profiles for infants with proven or clinical sepsis, suggesting a sensitivity of blood cultures of only 60%, consistent with prior experience.

Although these data were gathered in VLBW infants at risk for late-onset infections, these profiles are probably representative of the expected response patterns in early-onset disease and in more mature infants and, therefore, provide a framework for integration of these measurements into clinical practice. Although the focus of this report is on use of CD64 for surveillance for infection, the performance of CD64 as a diagnostic test in infants with clinical signs of infection may be even more valuable; these authors report sensitivity and specificity of 89% and 95%, respectively, corresponding to positive and negative predictive values of 91% and 94%, respectively, in this cohort of infants

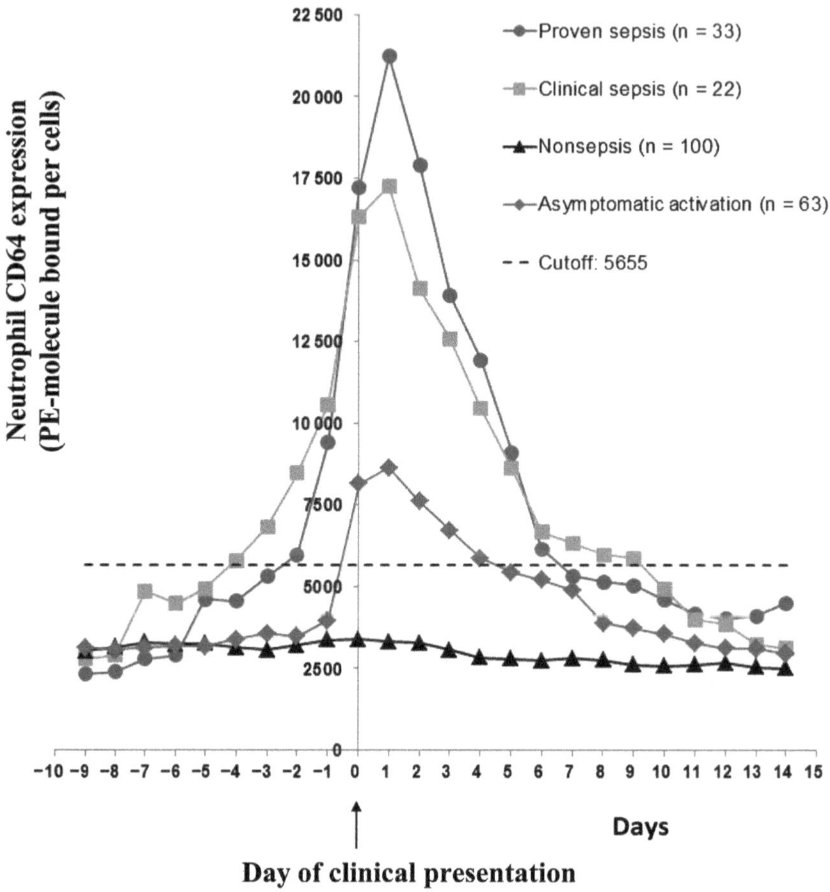

FIGURE 2.—Neutrophil CD64 expression before and after the onset of clinical presentation of LOS/NEC. The optimized cutoff (5655 PE units) is included for reference. For the asymptomatic activation (category 4) episodes, there was no definitive day of clinical presentation, and hence the peak of CD64 elevation was aligned to the CD64 peak of categories 1 and 2. (Reprinted from Lam HS, Cheung HM, Poon TCW, et al. Neutrophil CD64 for daily surveillance of systemic infection and necrotizing enterocolitis in preterm infants. *Clin Chem.* 2013;59:1753-1760, with permission from American Association for Clinical Chemistry.)

in whom the prevalence of proven or clinical sepsis was 36% (55 of 155). Among asymptomatic infants, the negative predictive value of a normal CD64 level was 99.8%. These data suggest 2 applications for this test. First, it may prove useful for screening for early-onset infection in asymptomatic infants with perinatal risk factors for infection. In this population of infants, who are at modest risk for sepsis, a normal CD64 level would provide sufficient reassurance to permit forgoing empirical antibiotic therapy. Second, normal CD64 measurements in infants with clinical findings consistent with either early- or late-onset sepsis may allow deferral of or early discontinuation of empiric treatment. Adoption of those strategies should result in substantial reduction in unnecessary treatment of infants for suspected neonatal sepsis.

It is essential to recognize that these results require the same meticulous attention to technique described by these authors, however. In particular, blood samples were placed in ice and transported to the laboratory for immediate processing. The analytical method incorporated QuantiBRITE beads to enable quantitation of the number of anti-CD64 antibodies bound per cell, rather than semiquantitative relative measurements reported in some other case series. Incorporation of this technology into routine neonatal care will require demonstration that these technical standards can be achieved by our regular bedside and laboratory staff on an everyday basis.

W. E. Benitz, MD

Concurrent Bloodstream Infections in Infants with Necrotizing Enterocolitis

Bizzarro MJ, Ehrenkranz RA, Gallagher PG (Yale Univ School of Medicine, New Haven, CT)

J Pediatr 164:61-66, 2014

Objective.—To determine the incidence, microbiology, risk factors, and outcomes related to bloodstream infections (BSIs) concurrent with the onset of necrotizing enterocolitis (NEC).

Study Design.—We performed a retrospective review of all cases of NEC in a single center over 20 years. BSI was categorized as "NEC-associated" if it occurred within 72 hours of the diagnosis of NEC and "post-NEC" if it occurred >72 hours afterwards. Demographics, hospital course data, microbiologic data, and outcomes were compared via univariate and multivariate analyses.

Results.—NEC occurred in 410 infants with mean gestational age and birth weight of 29 weeks and 1290 g, respectively; 158 infants were diagnosed with at least one BSI; 69 (43.7%) with NEC-associated BSI, and 89 (56.3%) with post-NEC BSI. Two-thirds of NEC-associated BSI were due to gram-negative bacilli compared with 31.9% of post-NEC BSI (OR: 4.27; 95% CI: 2.02, 9.03) and 28.5% of all BSI in infants without NEC (OR: 5.02; 95% CI: 2.82, 8.96). Infants with NEC-associated BSI had higher odds of requiring surgical intervention (aOR: 3.51; 95% CI: 1.98, 6.24) and death (aOR: 2.88; 95% CI: 1.39, 5.97) compared with those without BSI.

Conclusions.—BSI is a common, underappreciated complication of NEC occurring concurrent with the onset of disease and afterwards. The microbiologic etiology of NEC-associated BSI is different from post-NEC and late-onset BSI in infants without NEC with a predominance of gram-negative bacilli. Infants with NEC-associated BSI are significantly more likely to die than those with post-NEC BSI and NEC without BSI.

▶ This is a study of infants admitted to the neonatal intensive care unit at the Yale-New Haven hospital over an approximately 20-year period. Blood culture results were evaluated in infants who had necrotizing enterocolitis (NEC) within 72 hours of the positive blood culture results, infants who had positive blood culture results more than 72 hours after NEC, and infants who had late-onset positive blood stream infections without previous episode of NEC. The purpose of this study was to determine the risk factors and outcomes related to bloodstream infections if they are concurrent with the onset of NEC in these infants. Of little surprise, the authors observed a high rate of bloodstream infections in infants with NEC. Of interest, most cases of NEC-associated bloodstream infections were attributed to gram-negative bacilli with *Escherichia Coli*, and *Klebsiella pneumonia* was responsible for most microbial cases. Those infants who had positive bloodstream infections that were not associated with NEC had most of their cultures positive for gram positives such as coagulase-negative *Staphylococcus*.

The question arises as to where these organisms come from. Their most likely site of origin is the intestinal lumen with a breakdown of the intestinal barrier. However, the fact that sepsis without NEC is comprised primarily of the gram-positive microorganisms suggests that these microbes actually are also present in the gastrointestinal tract and may also translocate. The difference between NEC and non-NEC cases of positive blood stream infections may provide us with some information on the pathophysiology of NEC. A recent study using 16S sequencing of feces in preterm infants found a high association of *K pneumonia* before the onset of NEC.[1] It is possible that high levels of gram-negative microorganisms such as *K pneumonia* may actually predispose the gastrointestinal tract to greater inflammatory mediator injury, but studies to support this mechanism are still lacking. However, if support can be found for such a mechanism, this could provide clues to microbial therapeutic interventions leading to prevention.

J. Neu, MD

Reference

1. Torrazza RM, Ukhanova M, Wang X, et al. Intestinal microbial ecology and environmental factors affecting necrotizing enterocolitis. *PLoS One*. 2013;8:e83304.

6 Cardiovascular System

A randomised placebo-controlled trial of early treatment of the patent ductus arteriosus

Kluckow M, Jeffery M, Gill A, et al (Royal North Shore Hosp, Sydney, Australia; Univ of Western Australia, Perth, Australia; et al)

Arch Dis Child Fetal Neonatal Ed 99:F99-F104, 2014

Objective.—Failure of closure of the patent ductus arteriosus (PDA) may be associated with harm. Early cardiac ultrasound-targeted treatment of a large PDA may result in a reduction in adverse outcomes and need for later PDA closure with no increase in adverse effects.

Study Design.—Multicentre, double-blind, placebo-controlled randomised trial.

Setting.—Three neonatal intensive care units in Australia.

Patients and Interventions.—Eligible infants born <29 weeks were screened for a large PDA and received indomethacin or placebo before age 12 h.

Main Outcome.—Death or abnormal cranial ultrasound.

Results.—The trial ceased enrolment early due to lack of availability of indomethacin. 164 eligible infants were screened before 12 h; of the 92 infants with a large PDA, 44 were randomised to indomethacin and 48 to placebo. There was no difference in the main outcome between groups. Infants receiving early indomethacin had significantly less early pulmonary haemorrhage (PH) (2% vs 21%), a trend towards less periventricular/intraventricular haemorrhage (PIVH) (4.5% vs 12.5%) and were less likely to receive later open-label treatment for a PDA (20% vs 40%). The 72 non-randomised infants with a small PDA were at low risk of pulmonary haemorrhage and had an 80% spontaneous PDA closure rate.

Conclusions.—Early cardiac ultrasound-targeted treatment of a large PDA is feasible and safe, resulted in a reduction in early pulmonary haemorrhage and later medical treatment but had no effect on the primary outcome of death or abnormal cranial ultrasound.

Registered Trial.—Australian New Zealand Clinical Trials Registry (ACTRN12608000295347).

▶ Determination of the appropriate timing and extent of evaluation and treatment of patent ductus arteriosus (PDA) remains an active controversy in neonatal medicine. Choosing the optimal path in the diagnosis and treatment of PDA is especially challenging in managing extremely preterm infants among whom PDA is prevalent. For such infants, echocardiography can be a stressful intervention; furthermore, existing data suggest that neither treatment nor observation of a PDA is entirely risk free. This report by Kluckow and colleagues provides new insights that might assist clinicians caring for this population in their efforts to balance selected risks and benefits of PDA evaluation and treatment. This multicenter double-masked randomized clinical trial studied 164 infants born before 29 weeks' gestation in 1 of 3 Australian tertiary centers, screening them for PDA by ultrasound performed before 12 hours of age. Of these, 92 infants were found to have a large PDA and were randomized to receive either standard indomethacin treatment or placebo. The primary study outcome, death and/or abnormal cranial ultrasound, was not significantly different between the 2 study groups. On the other hand, infants who received early indomethacin treatment were at substantially lower risk of pulmonary hemorrhage and were less likely to require later open-label treatment for a PDA. Furthermore, early indomethacin treatment was associated with a trend toward reduction in risk of severe intracranial hemorrhage as well as reduced likelihood of the need for later treatment of the PDA. There was a high rate of spontaneous closure (80%) among infants found at the early echocardiogram to have a small PDA. As the authors note, low study power might have contributed to the failure to demonstrate a difference in the primary study outcome between groups. Another potential study limitation is the relatively high rate of pulmonary hemorrhage that might have set the stage for a positive effect of intervention. Still, I find novel and informative Kluckow and colleagues' data suggesting that, among extremely preterm infants, an early systematic approach to PDA evaluation fosters a selective therapeutic approach that maximizes benefit and minimizes risk of a least 1 known complication of PDA and additionally might obviate the need for later treatment.

L. J. Van Marter, MD, MPH

Comparison of Oral Paracetamol versus Ibuprofen in Premature Infants with Patent Ductus Arteriosus: A Randomized Controlled Trial

Dang D, Wang D, Zhang C, et al (The First Hosp of Jilin Univ, Changchun, China)

PLoS ONE 8:e77888, 2013

Trial Design.—Oral ibuprofen has demonstrated good effects on symptomatic patent ductus arteriosus (PDA) but with many contraindications and potential side-effects. In the past two years, oral paracetamol administration to several preterm infants with PDA has been reported. Here, a randomized, non-blinded, parallel-controlled and non-inferiority trial was designed to evaluate the efficacy and safety profiles of oral paracetamol to those of standard ibuprofen for PDA closure in premature infants.

Methods.—One hundred and sixty infants (gestational age ≤ 34 weeks) with echocardiographically confirmed PDA were randomly assigned to receive either oral paracetamol (n = 80) or ibuprofen (n = 80). After the initial treatment course in both groups, the need for a second course was determined by echocardiographic evaluation. The main outcome was rate of ductal closure, and secondary outcomes were adverse effects and complications.

Result.—The ductus was closed in 65 (81.2%) infants of the paracetamol group compared with 63 (78.8%) of the ibuprofen group. The 95% confidence interval of the difference between these groups was [−0.080, 0.128], demonstrating that the effectiveness of paracetamol treatment was not inferior to that of ibuprofen. In fact, the incidence of hyperbilirubinemia or gastrointestinal bleeding in the paracetamol group was significantly lower than that of the ibuprofen group. No significant differences in other clinical side effects or complications were noted.

Conclusion.—This comparison of drug efficacy and safety profiles in premature infants with PDA revealed that oral paracetamol was comparable to ibuprofen in terms of the rate of ductal closure and even showed a decreased risk of hyperbilirubinemia or gastrointestinal bleeding. Therefore, paracetamol may be accepted as a first-line drug treatment for PDA in preterm infants.

Trial Registration.—ChiCTR.org ChiCTR-TRC-12002177.

▶ Hemodynamically significant patent ductus arteriosus (PDA) may contribute to morbidity in preterm infants. Cyclooxygenase inhibitors (indomethacin and ibuprofen) are widely used to close a PDA but have well-described adverse effects. Case series have emerged suggesting paracetamol (also known as acetaminophen) as an alternative therapy to induce ductal closure with few adverse effects in symptomatic preterm infants. This randomized, controlled trial enrolled 90 preterm infants (≤30 weeks' gestational age, ≤1250 g, postnatal age 48–96 hours) with a clinically significant PDA confirmed by echocardiography. Infants were randomized to oral paracetamol (15 mg/kg every 6 hours for 3 days) or oral ibuprofen (10 mg/kg once, followed by 5 mg/kg at 24 and 48 hours). A second course of therapy was used for patients who failed to respond to the initial course or whose duct reopened after initial closure. PDA closure rates after a single course of therapy were similar between treatment groups (paracetamol 73% vs ibuprofen 78%, $P = .6$). There was a trend toward a higher rate of ductal reopening in the paracetamol group (24% vs 16%, $P = .43$) but no difference in the rate of surgical ligation (3% vs 5%, $P = .55$). The incidence of adverse effects, including measures of renal function and gastrointestinal irritation, did not differ between groups. This study provides important preliminary data regarding a novel approach to medical treatment of PDA. Concerns over the adverse effects of common therapies to treat PDA in preterm infants have led to a heated debate over the true clinical significance of the ductus arteriosus. Introduction of a relatively safe medical therapy may substantially alter the context of these debates of risk versus benefit. Future research is warranted to define the efficacy of oral or intravenous paracetamol compared with widely accepted standards of care (intravenous indomethacin and ibuprofen).

C. C. McPherson, PharmD

Oral Paracetamol versus Oral Ibuprofen in the Management of Patent Ductus Arteriosus in Preterm Infants: A Randomized Controlled Trial

Oncel MY, Yurttutan S, Erdeve O, et al (Zekai Tahir Burak Maternity Teaching Hosp, Ankara, Turkey; Ankara Univ School of Medicine, Turkey)
J Pediatr 164:510-514.e1, 2014

Objective.—To compare the efficacy and safety of oral paracetamol and oral ibuprofen for the pharmacological closure of patent ductus arteriosus (PDA) in preterm infants.

Study Design.—This prospective, randomized, controlled study enrolled 90 preterm infants with gestational age ≤30 weeks, birthweight ≤1250 g, and postnatal age 48 to 96 hours who had echocardiographically confirmed significant PDA. Each enrolled patient received either oral paracetamol (15 mg/kg every 6 hours for 3 days) or oral ibuprofen (initial dose of 10 mg/kg, followed by 5 mg/kg at 24 and 48 hours).

Results.—Spontaneous closure rate for the entire study group was 54%. After the first course of treatment, the PDA closed in 31 (77.5%) of the patients assigned to the oral ibuprofen group vs 29 (72.5%) of those enrolled in the oral paracetamol group (P =.6). The reopening rate was higher in the paracetamol group than in the ibuprofen group, but the reopening rates were not statistically different (24.1% [7 of 29] vs 16.1% [5 of 31]; P =.43). The cumulative closure rates after the second course of drugs were high in both groups. Only 2 patient (2.5%) in the paracetamol group and 3 patients (5%) in the ibuprofen group required surgical ligation.

Conclusion.—This randomized, controlled clinical study compared oral paracetamol with ibuprofen in preterm infants and demonstrated that paracetamol may be a medical alternative in the management of PDA.

▶ One of my coeditors has eloquently made a strong case that "Practitioners should tolerate ductal patency and learn to manage its causes and consequences rather than focusing on achievement of ductal closure."[1] He has extensively reviewed the literature, and although he acknowledges numerous morbidities, including bronchopulmonary dysplasia (BPD), associated with a patent ductus, he has been unable to find evidence that closing the ductus either pharmacologically or surgically reduces these complications. Furthermore, these treatments carry the risk of significant morbidity. He comments: "Persistence of ductal patency should be considered a sign of rather than a direct cause of the several morbidities with which it is clearly associated" and "Despite the potential shortcomings of those trials, they provide substantial cumulative evidence that early, routine treatment to close a persistently patent ductus arteriosus [PDA] in preterm infants does not improve outcomes and should therefore be abandoned." His case is strengthened by a report from Chock et al,[2] who investigated whether PDA treatment and other clinical or echocardiographic (ECHO) factors were associated with the development of death or BPD. They retrospectively studied clinical and ECHO characteristics of preterm infants with birth weight <1500 g and ECHO diagnosis of a PDA. Only lower gestational age, and not PDA treatment or ECHO score, was associated with the adverse outcome of death or

BPD. Chock suggested that "Further investigation of PDA management strategies and effects on adverse outcomes of prematurity is needed."

Oncel, Yurttutan, et al[3-5] have added a new agent for pharmacologic closure, Paracetamol, into the mix. They have demonstrated that both oral and intravenous paracetamol effectively closes the ductus. Paracetamol has few side effects, is inexpensive, readily available both enterally and intravenously, hence it may be superior to indomethacin or ibuprofen. In the randomized trial abstracted above, paracetamol was not inferior to ibuprofen. I would like to see the investigators heed Benitz's[1] recommendations and include a control group that receives none of these agents and look at the rates of spontaneous closure and morbidity. I hope this is not just a pipe dream.

A. A. Fanaroff, MD, FRCPE

References

1. Benitz WE. Patent ductus arteriosus: to treat or not to treat? *Arch Dis Child Fetal Neonatal Ed.* 2012;97:F80-F82.
2. Chock VY, Punn R, Oza A, et al. Predictors of bronchopulmonary dysplasia or death in premature infants with a patent ductus arteriosus. *Pediatr Res.* 2014; 75:570-575.
3. Oncel MY, Yurttutan S, Uras N, et al. An alternative drug (paracetamol) in the management of patent ductus arteriosus in ibuprofen-resistant or contraindicated preterm infants. *Arch Dis Child Fetal Neonatal Ed.* 2013;98:F94.
4. Oncel MY, Yurttutan S, Degirmencioglu H, et al. Intravenous paracetamol treatment in the management of patent ductus arteriosus in extremely low birth weight infants. *Neonatology.* 2013;103:166-169.
5. Yurttutan S, Oncel MY, Arayıcı S, et al. A different first-choice drug in the medical management of patent ductus arteriosus: oral paracetamol. *J Matern Fetal Neonatal Med.* 2013;26:825-827.

Hypotension in Preterm Neonates: Low Blood Pressure Alone Does Not Affect Neurodevelopmental Outcome

Alderliesten T, Lemmers PMA, van Haastert IC, et al (Wilhelmina Children's Hosp/Univ Med Ctr Utrecht, The Netherlands)

J Pediatr 164:986-991, 2014

Objective.—To compare neurodevelopmental outcome, mean arterial blood pressure (MABP), and regional cerebral oxygenation ($rSco_2$) between preterm neonates treated for hypotension and controls.

Study Design.—Preterm neonates (N = 66) with a gestational age (GA) ≤32 weeks, without a patent ductus arteriosus, treated for hypotension (dopamine ≥5 μg/kg/min) were included. Neonates were matched to controls for GA, birth weight, sex, and year of birth. The $rSco_2$ was determined by using near-infrared spectroscopy. Monitoring of MABP, $rSco_2$, and arterial saturation was started at admission and continued for at least 72 hours. Neurodevelopmental outcome was assessed at 18 and 24 months' corrected age by using the Griffiths Mental Development Scales or the Bayley Scales of Infant and Toddler Development, Third Edition.

Results.—Infants treated for hypotension spent more time with an MABP less than GA (median 9% vs 0%, $P < .001$) and time with an MABP/rSco_2 correlation >0.5 (27% vs 17%, $P < .001$). Time spent with an rSco_2 <50% and neurodevelopmental outcome at 18 and 24 months' corrected age were not significantly different between infants treated for hypotension and controls. The 26 neonates with an rSco_2 <50% for >10% of time had a lower neurodevelopmental outcome at 18 months (median 99 vs 104, $P = .02$).

Conclusion.—An MABP less than GA (in weeks) was not associated with lower rSco_2 or with lower neurodevelopmental outcome scores. However, regardless of MABP, low rSco_2 was associated with lower neurodevelopmental outcome scores. Perfusion/oxygenation variables could be of additional value in neonatal intensive care.

▶ One of my pet peeves is hearing that a preterm infant was given a bolus of fluid or started on a pressor for "hypotension," usually defined as a mean blood pressure less than the gestational age in weeks. Like pulse oximetry, we have become enamored by a measurable number, but one that does not necessarily connote the parameter we really need to know: tissue oxygen delivery.

In this nested, case-control study, the investigators examined the effects of low blood pressure and regional cerebral oxygenation (using near infrared spectroscopy) in infants less than 32 weeks' gestation who received dopamine for hypotension during the first 72 hours of life. Infants with a hemodynamically significant patent ductus arteriosus were excluded. Infants were compared with age-matched controls who were normotensive. Neurodevelopmental outcomes at 18 and 24 months of corrected age were assessed. No differences were found between hypotensive and normotensive infants. Neither regional cerebral oxygenation nor lower neurodevelopmental outcome scores correlated with low blood pressure.

The management of blood pressure is yet another example of the "numerocentricity" of most neonatologists. Despite compelling data that blood pressure (like saturation) will increase on its own in the first few hours of life, the overwhelming majority of babies who refuse to ride the 50th percentile are subjected to treatment with fluid boluses or pressors, but there is ample evidence that these are potentially harmful practices. This was shown in the ELGANS study, where 83% and 77% of all infants less than 23–24 and 25 weeks, respectively, received treatment for hypotension in the first 24 hours of life.[1] Alderliesten and colleagues demonstrated that cerebral oxygenation is generally unaffected by mean blood pressure, suggesting intact autoregulation, and again, a lack of a relationship between early neonatal mean arterial blood pressure and neurodevelopmental outcomes at 18 and 24 months' corrected age.

Blood pressure is but one determinant of tissue oxygen delivery. Further evaluation of functional echocardiography, vena caval blood flow, and near infrared spectroscopy may help to improve our understanding of this. Until then, don't just do something, stand there.

S. M. Donn, MD

Reference

1. Laughon M, Bose C, Allred E, et al. Factors associated with treatment for hypotension in extremely low gestational age newborns during the first postnatal week. *Pediatrics*. 2007;119:273-280.

Use of Antihypotensive Therapies in Extremely Preterm Infants

Batton B, for the Eunice Kennedy Shriver National Institute of Child Health & Human Development Neonatal Research Network (Case Western Reserve Univ, Cleveland, OH; et al)

Pediatrics 131:e1865-e1873, 2013

Objective.—To investigate the relationships among blood pressure (BP) values, antihypotensive therapies, and in-hospital outcomes to identify a BP threshold below which antihypotensive therapies may be beneficial.

Methods.—Prospective observational study of infants $23^{0/7}$ to $26^{6/7}$ weeks' gestational age. Hourly BP values and antihypotensive therapy use in the first 24 hours were recorded. Low BP was investigated by using 15 definitions. Outcomes were examined by using regression analysis controlling for gestational age, the number of low BP values, and illness severity.

Results.—Of 367 infants enrolled, 203 (55%) received at least 1 antihypotensive therapy. Treated infants were more likely to have low BP by any definition ($P < .001$), but for the 15 definitions of low BP investigated, therapy was not prescribed to 3% to 49% of infants with low BP and, paradoxically, was administered to 28% to 41% of infants without low BP. Treated infants were more likely than untreated infants to develop severe retinopathy of prematurity (15% vs 8%, $P = .03$) or severe intraventricular hemorrhage (22% vs 11%, $P < .01$) and less likely to survive (67% vs 78%, $P = .02$). However, with regression analysis, there were no significant differences between groups in survival or in-hospital morbidity rates.

Conclusions.—Factors other than BP contributed to the decision to use antihypotensive therapies. Infant outcomes were not improved with antihypotensive therapy for any of the 15 definitions of low BP investigated.

▶ As technical advances led to increased survival rates among infants with birth weight less than 1000 g in 1980s, neonatologists entered previously unexplored territory. With little or no direct experience to guide practice, many management concepts had to be extrapolated from what was known about critical care of older patients. This report is a stark reminder that we are still lost in that wilderness, at least with respect to our understanding of and ability to rationally manage low blood pressure in very low birth weight (VLBW) preterm infants. Like blood glucose levels, we are learning that what is common may not be salutary and, conversely, that which appears to be anomalous may not be hazardous. These authors use data collected from a multicenter cohort of VLBW infants to show that we have no useful criteria for diagnosis of hypotension, no consistent or demonstrably effective strategies for management of blood pressure perceived to be too low, no evidence that such interventions—even if successful in addressing blood pressure values—have beneficial effects on long term outcomes, and few ideas about what the long-term outcomes of interest might be. These observations should give pause to the idea that blood pressure measurement is a useful intermediary measure of well-being, leading to consideration of other approaches to hemodynamic evaluation, such as assessment of tissue perfusion by NIRS. While taking a circumspect and skeptical approach to intervention, such measures need to be correlated with adverse outcomes, which most likely should be intraventricular hemorrhage and periventricular leukomalacia in the short term and survival without neurodevelopmental impairment in the long term. Until well-designed trials show that particular treatments applied in infants with specific measures of hemodynamic disturbance result in better outcomes, we may have to abandon strategies that are dependent on measurement of potential intermediary process variables (eg, blood pressure, cerebral blood flow, cerebral regional oxygen saturation). It may be better to rely on evidence that certain management approaches result in better outcomes, while incidentally also affecting hemodynamic status and stability (timing cord clamping to permit placentofetal transfusion, for example). Now that we know what we don't know, it is important to remember these authors' admonition that "antihypotensive therapy should be used cautiously for these infants because treatment of low BP is associated with similar or worse infant outcomes."

W. E. Benitz, MD

Targeted neonatal echocardiography (TnECHO) service in a Canadian neonatal intensive care unit: a 4-year experience

El-Khuffash A, Herbozo C, Jain A, et al (The Rotunda Hosp, Dublin, Ireland; The Hosp for Sick Children, Toronto, Ontario, Canada)

J Perinatol 33:687-690, 2013

Objective.—To characterize the effect of a targeted neonatal echocardiography (TnECHO) program on decision making in a tertiary level unit.

Study Design.—Retrospective cohort study of neonates, admitted between September 2007 and April 2011. Details of the TnECHO, and the clinical decisions within 6 h of the consultation were recorded.

Result.—A total of 199 infants underwent 512 echocardiograms with a median (interquartile range) of 2 (1 to 3) TnECHO studies per infant. The indications included assessment for patent ductus arteriosus (PDA; $n = 261$, 51%), post-PDA ligation assessment ($n = 101$, 19%), pulmonary hemodynamics ($n = 81$, 16%), myocardial performance and systemic blood flow ($n = 52$, 10%), and central venous catheter tip position ($n = 6$, 1%). TnECHO consultation was followed by a change in clinical management in 212 cases (41%) and avoidance of a planned intervention in 112 cases (22%).

Conclusion.—TnECHO may be a useful tool to guide clinical decisions in the neonatal intensive care unit setting. Well-planned prospective studies are needed to assess the impact of TnECHO on outcomes.

► This single-center observation reports on the use of targeted neonatal echocardiography at the Hospital for Sick Children between 2007 and 2011. During this time, 512 echocardiographic studies were performed on 199 neonates. Importantly, the results of the studies were used to direct therapy in 41% of cases and to avoid a planned intervention in another 21%. Thus, in nearly two-thirds of cases, management was altered by performance of the test.

Targeted or functional echocardiography is seldom available in the United States, whereas it is widespread in other areas of the world, especially Australia and in Eastern and Central Europe, where pediatric cardiologists are scarce. Neonatologists in these areas are trained to perform functional echocardiography and use it to make decisions regarding hemodynamic manipulations based on metrics such as myocardial contractility, cardiac output, or superior vena cava flow. Decisions as to whether to use volume expansion or drugs to improve contractility, reduce afterload, or increase peripheral vascular resistance are facilitated by a better examination of cardiac physiology.

I suspect that the reason this has not happened in the United States is a turf battle between neonatologists and pediatric cardiologists, centered on billing issues. Yet is it really any different from reading a chest x-ray at 2 AM to rule out a pneumothorax or performing an amplitude-integrated electroencephalogram in the early hours to determine suitability for cooling? We are trained to do these procedures, and it is time for us, as a group, to have access to functional echocardiography on a 24/7 basis. Neonatal intensive care units never close. If the service cannot be made available to us, we should do it ourselves.

S. M. Donn, MD

Pulse oximetry screening for critical congenital heart defects in newborn infants: Should it be routine?

Ewer AK (Birmingham Women's Hosp, Edgbaston, UK)

Arch Dis Child Fetal Neonatal Ed 99:F93-F95, 2014

Screening with pulse oximetry for critical congenital heart defects is the subject of much recent debate. This review will explore the recent evidence for screening and discuss how implementation of screening might be best achieved.

► Critical congenital heart disease (CCHD) is a life-threatening problem with an incidence of 1–3 of 1000 live births. It warrants early diagnosis and timely referral.[1] Delay in diagnosis can affect survival and long-term outcome and increase parental anxiety. Early diagnostic techniques include fetal ultrasonography and newborn examination. Reports from the developed world suggest that only

25% to 50% of CCHD cases are diagnosed antenatally. These figures are even lower in developing, resource-limited countries.

Neonatal examination allows detection of heart murmurs but is limited by the fact that approximately 50% of CCHD does not present with murmurs in the immediate neonatal period.[2] Clinicians have been trying to find novel ways to use technology to improve early detection. Pulse oximetry was suggested for screening babies for CCHD, and although in use for nearly 15 years, the practice had been patchy and limited to observational studies.[3] After the publication of Ewer et al[4] and the prospective study of deWahl et al,[5] there has been increasing interest.

This article provides an overview of evidence and highlights the usefulness of pulse oximetry as a newborn screening tool. The author has recommended universal adoption. The review projected an incremental cost-effectiveness ratio of £24 000 (about $41 000) per timely diagnosis compared with clinical examination alone.

Pulse oximetry is reported to have a specificity of 99.9% (95% confidence interval [CI] 99.7–99.9), suggesting that if the SpO_2 is >95%, it is highly unlikely for an infant to have CCHD. The exceptions are lesions involving obstruction of aorta. These lesions are difficult to detect even with fetal echocardiography and newborn examination. The sensitivity is 76.5% (95% CI, 67.7% to 83.5%).[6] The false-positive test allows early detection of noncardiac conditions such as Group B streptococcal disease and maladaptation.

The arguments suggesting increased echocardiography workload from false positives can be resolved using clinical decision making in which systematic examination is used to identify noncardiac cases. The routine newborn examination to detect heart murmurs is known to have limitations over and above pulse oximetry screening. Murmurs detect only 37% of cardiac malformations, and most obstructive left heart lesions do not present with heart murmurs. Evaluation of murmurs during neonatal examination and fetal echocardiography for antenatal detection of CCHD continue to remain standard practices.

There are unresolved issues including agreement on performance of just postductal versus pre- and postductal screening, disposable versus nondisposable sensors, and age at screening because infants may be discharged within 6 to 12 hours.

Pulse oximetry as a screening tool should be adopted only after assessing the infrastructure and providing appropriate funding. Failing to recognize these problems could result in increased pressure on critical care services and the risk of litigation related to delayed diagnosis. These decisions are country-specific and depend on the health service model and availability of critical care services.

Efforts to improve early detection have the potential to identify >90% of CCHD before clinical manifestations. This could reduce mortality and long-term cardiovascular and neurologic morbidity. Various models can be evaluated to limit unnecessary transfers while minimizing the risks. One model suggests using a lower saturation target (SpO_2 <90%) for immediate cardiac assessment or referral to a pediatric cardiology center and a higher level (SpO_2 91%–95%)

for close observation, monitoring, and assessment, deferring discharge. These models require practice auditing and revision as necessary.

S. Gupta, DM, MD, FRCPCH, FRCPI

References

1. Acharya G, Sitras V, Maltau JM, et al. Major congenital heart disease in northern Norway: shortcomings of pre- and postnatal diagnosis. *Acta Obstet Gynecol Scand.* 2004;83:1124-1129.
2. Prudhoe S, Abu-Harb M, Richmond S, Wren C. Neonatal screening for critical cardiovascular anomalies using pulse oximetry. *Arch Dis Child Fetal Neonatal Ed.* 2013;98:F346-F350.
3. Richmond S, Reay G, Abu Harb M. Routine pulse oximetry in the asymptomatic newborn. *Arch Dis Child Fetal Neonatal Ed.* 2002;87:F83-F88.
4. Ewer AK, Middleton LJ, Furmston AT, et al. Pulse oximetry screening for congenital heart defects in newborn infants (PulseOx): a test accuracy study. *Lancet.* 2011;378:785-794.
5. de-Wahl Granelli A, Wennergren M, Sandberg K, et al. Impact of pulse oximetry screening on the detection of duct dependent congenital heart disease: a Swedish prospective screening study in 39,821 newborns. *BMJ.* 2009;338:a3037.
6. Thangaratinam S, Brown K, Zamora J, Khan KS, Ewer AK. Pulse oximetry screening for critical congenital heart defects in asymptomatic newborn babies: a systematic review and meta-analysis. *Lancet.* 2012;379:2459-2464.

Late Detection of Critical Congenital Heart Disease Among US Infants: Estimation of the Potential Impact of Proposed Universal Screening Using Pulse Oximetry

Peterson C, Ailes E, Riehle-Colarusso T, et al (Ctrs for Disease Control and Prevention, Atlanta, GA)

JAMA Pediatr 168:361-370, 2014

Importance.—Critical congenital heart disease (CCHD) was added to the Recommended Uniform Screening Panel for Newborns in the United States in 2011. Many states have recently adopted or are considering requirements for universal CCHD screening through pulse oximetry in birth hospitals. Limited previous research is directly applicable to the question of how many US infants with CCHD might be identified through screening.

Objectives.—To estimate the proportion of US infants with late detection of CCHD (>3 days after birth) based on existing clinical practice and to investigate factors associated with late detection.

Design, Setting, and Participants.—Descriptive and multivariable analysis. Data were obtained from a multisite population-based study of birth defects in the United States, the National Birth Defects Prevention Study (NBDPS). We included all live-born infants with estimated dates of delivery from January 1, 1998, through December 31, 2007, and nonsyndromic, clinically verified CCHD conditions potentially detectable through screening via pulse oximetry.

Main Outcomes and Measures.—The main outcome measure was the proportion of infants with late detection of CCHD through echocardiography or at autopsy under the assumption that universal screening at birth hospitals might reduce the number of such late diagnoses. Secondary outcome measures included prevalence ratios for associations between selected demographic and clinical factors and late detection of CCHD.

Results.—Of 3746 live-born infants with nonsyndromic CCHD, late detection occurred in 1106 (29.5% [95% CI, 28.1%-31.0%]), including 6 (0.2%) (0.1%-0.4%) first receiving a diagnosis at autopsy more than 3 days after birth. Late detection varied by CCHD type from 9 of 120 infants (7.5% [95% CI, 3.5%-13.8%]) with pulmonary atresia to 497 of 801 (62.0% [58.7%-65.4%]) with coarctation of the aorta. In multivariable analysis, late detection varied significantly by CCHD type and study site, and infants with extracardiac defects were significantly less likely to have late detection of CCHD (adjusted prevalence ratio, 0.58 [95% CI, 0.49-0.69]).

Conclusions and Relevance.—We estimate that 29.5%of live-born infants with nonsyndromic CCHD in the NBDPS received a diagnosis more than 3 days after birth and therefore might have benefited from routine CCHD screening at birth hospitals. The number of infants in whom CCHD was detected through screening likely varies by several factors, including CCHD type. Additional population-based studies of screening in practice are needed.

▶ The US Surgeon General has mandated pulse oximetry screening. It has proven to be safe, sensitive, and specific. The false positive rate is <1%, so that unnecessary echocardiography and family anxiety are held to a minimum. Indeed, many of the so-called false positives have proven to result from other illnesses that require attention and could easily have been missed. Ewer,[1] one of the early proponents of screening for critical congenital heart disease (CCHD), has written a position paper titled, "Pulse Oximetry Screening for Critical Congenital Heart Defects in Newborn Infants: Should It Be Routine?" He acknowledged that pulse oximetry screening is not a perfect test, with a sensitivity of approximately 75% for CCHD,[2] but he is of the strong opinion that, in combination with other routine screening procedures, the vast majority will be identified. He concludes: "Given the simplicity of the test and underlying principles, it is hard to argue against routine pulse oximetry screening." I find no argument with his logic and am supportive of the concept. Implementation in the United States is occurring at a good pace. Ewer also described a good business model justifying screening, which is a useful document for those introducing screening programs.[3] Peterson et al, in the manuscript abstracted here, have carefully examined the potential benefits of screening. They estimated that almost 30% of cases with nonsyndromic CCHD in the National Birth Defects Prevention Study might have benefited from routine CCHD screening at birth hospitals because their diagnoses were delayed by at least 3 days. The underlying heart disease obviously affected the rate, and coarctation of the aorta is the easiest diagnosis to miss.

It may be easy to mandate screening, but implementation presents a number of challenges. In Minnesota, a state with sophisticated health care and providers,

91 of 99 eligible centers participated in a survey, and 90 reported the ability to screen newborns in accordance with recommendations.[4] However, only 22 centers, with 63% of births, had access to echocardiography and routinely stocked prostaglandins for neonatal use. In their pilot study of 7549 newborns who were screened, 6 failed screens, and there was 1 CCHD diagnosis. Two of the failed screens were due to misinterpretation of the algorithm, 1 failed screen was not reported, and 4 failed screens were not recognized. Repeated screens were required for 115 newborns, with 29% of retesting due to misinterpretation of the algorithm. The mean nursing time required was 5.5 minutes, and the cost was $5.10 per screen. Bottom line, there is much learning and teaching yet to be done before we have universal screening in the United States. The authors suggested a central reporting mechanism.

The comments in this article related to screening for CCHD at sea level. What about moderate and high altitude? Well, you would guess that the number of false positives would be higher, because normal saturations at altitude would be lower and more variable. You would be correct. Wright et al[5] reported a higher failure rate for CCHD screening at altitude when using sea-level guidelines and pleaded for studies at moderate and high altitudes to develop the appropriate, adjusted screening protocols. They were of the opinion that the increased false positives placed an unnecessary burden on families, communities, and health resources.

While on the topic of congenital heart disease, Botto et al[6] explored the relationship between maternal fever in the first trimester and congenital heart disease. They found that genitourinary infections were associated with selected heart defects, particularly right-sided obstructive defects (odds ratios > 3) and possibly others, whereas common respiratory illnesses were associated with low-to-negligible risks for most heart defects. Elevated risk estimates could be mitigated by periconceptual multivitamin supplements.

A. A. Fanaroff, MD, FRCPE

References

1. Ewer AK. Pulse oximetry screening for critical congenital heart defects in newborn infants: Should it be routine? *Arch Dis Child Fetal Neonatal Ed.* 2014;99: F93-F95.
2. Thangaratinam S, Brown K, Zamora J, Khan KS, Ewer AK. Pulse oximetry screening for critical congenital heart defects in asymptomatic newborn babies: a systematic review and meta-analysis. *Lancet.* 2012;379:2459-2464.
3. Ewer AK. How to develop a business case to establish a neonatal pulse oximetry programme for screening of congenital heart defects. *Early Hum Dev.* 2012;88: 915-919.
4. Kochilas L, Lohr JL, Bruhn E, et al. Implementation of critical congenital heart disease screening in Minnesota. *Pediatrics.* 2013;132:e587-e594.
5. Wright J, Kohn M, Niermeyer S, Rausch CM. Feasibility of critical congenital heart disease newborn screening at moderate altitude. *Pediatrics.* 2014;133: e561-e569.
6. Botto LD, Panichello JD, Browne ML, et al. Congenital heart defects after maternal fever. *Am J Obstet Gynecol.* 2014;210:359.e1-359.e11.

Cardiovascular function in children who had chronic lung disease of prematurity

Joshi S, Wilson DG, Kotecha S, et al (Cardiff Univ, UK; Univ Hosp of Wales, Cardiff, UK)

Arch Dis Child Fetal Neonatal Ed 2014 [Epub ahead of print]

Objectives.—Although increased pulmonary arterial pressure is common in infancy in preterm infants who develop chronic lung disease of prematurity (CLD), it is unknown if the increase persists into childhood. We, therefore, assessed if 8–12-year-old children with documented CLD in infancy had evidence of right ventricular dysfunction or pulmonary arterial hypertension at rest or in response to acute hypoxia when compared to preterm and term-born controls.

Methods.—We studied 90 children: 60 born at ≤32 weeks of gestation (28 with CLD and 32 preterm controls), and 30 term-born controls. All had echocardiography including myocardial velocity imaging, at rest and while breathing 15% oxygen and 12% oxygen for 20 min each.

Results.—Baseline oxygen saturation, heart rate, blood pressure and echocardiographic markers of left and right ventricular function were similar in all three groups. While breathing 12% oxygen, the oxygen saturation decreased to 81.9% in the CLD group compared to 85.1% ($p < 0.05$) and 84.7% ($p < 0.01$) in the preterm and term controls, respectively. In response to hypoxia, all three groups showed increases in velocity of tricuspid regurgitation, end-diastolic velocity of pulmonary regurgitation, and right ventricular relaxation time; and decreases in pulmonary arterial acceleration time and the ratio of right ventricular acceleration time to ejection time. However, there were no differences between groups.

Conclusions.—Childhood survivors of CLD have comparable left and right ventricular function at 8–12 years of age to preterm and term-born children, and no evidence of increased pulmonary arterial pressure even after hypoxic exposure.

▶ I read this article with great interest in light of the current controversy surrounding the management of pulmonary hypertension (PAH) complicating bronchopulmonary dysplasia (BPD). There is little doubt that our colleagues in pediatric cardiology and pulmonology have become enamored with the use of sildenafil, despite warnings from the US Food and Drug Administration[1] after the STARTS trials, in which treatment of children with PAH had a higher mortality in the higher dose group.[2] It appears that many clinicians have jumped on the treatment bandwagon without a good understanding of the natural history of the disorder.

In this study, Joshi and colleagues examined 8- to 12-year follow-up of cardiovascular function in 60 preterm infants 32 weeks' gestation or less, half with BPD and half without, and 30 term control infants. Echocardiography was performed, and it included a hypoxic challenge. All 3 groups had comparable left and right ventricular function and no evidence of PAH even with a hypoxic challenge. Although it may be argued that the study had a selection bias and information regarding pulmonary arterial pressure at 36 weeks was not provided, it suggests that many infants who are oxygen-dependent at 36 weeks will have normal ventricular function at 8 to 12 years.

The sildenafil issue is troublesome, in that both safety and efficacy are unsupported by appropriate clinical evidence. Despite several admonishments, warnings, and opinions,[1,3,4] it continues to be administered to infants with BPD who have even mild PAH. This study suggests that there may be a shift in the risk: benefit ratio with more harm than good. Use of the drug outside of a randomized clinical trial is troublesome, potentially dangerous, and ill advised.

S. M. Donn, MD

References

1. FDA Drug Safety Communication: FDA recommends against use of Revatio (sildenafil) in children with pulmonary hypertension. http://www.fda.gov/Drugs/DrugSafety/ucm317123.htm. Accessed June 23, 2014.
2. Mourani PM, Sontag MK, Ivy DD, Abman SH. Effects of long-tern sildenafil treatment for pulmonary hypertension in infants with chronic lung disease. *J Pediatr.* 2009;154:379-384.
3. Berkelhamer SK, Mestan KK, Steinhorn RH. Pulmonary hypertension in bronchopulmonary dysplasia. *Semin Perinatol.* 2013;37:124-131.
4. Bhatt-Mehta V, Donn SM. Sildenafil for pulmonary hypertension complicating bronchopulmonary dysplasia. *Expert Rev Clin Pharmacol.* 2014;7:393-395.

Unilateral Vocal Fold Paralysis After Congenital Cardiothoracic Surgery: A Meta-analysis

Strychowsky JE, Rukholm G, Gupta MK, et al (McMaster Univ, Hamilton, Ontario, Canada)

Pediatrics 133:e1708-e1723, 2014

Background and Objective.—There is variation in the literature in regard to the occurrence of unilateral vocal fold paralysis (UVFP) after congenital cardiothoracic surgery. The objective of this study was to identify and appraise the evidence for the occurrence of UVFP after congenital cardiothoracic surgery in a meta-analysis.

Method.—A comprehensive search strategy in Medline, Embase, and the Cochrane Library was conducted, limited to English publications. Two independent reviewers screened studies for eligibility criteria. Of the 162 identified studies, 32 (20%) met the inclusion criteria. Using the Oxford Centre for Evidence-Based Medicine guidelines, 2 reviewers appraised the level of evidence, extracted data, and resolved discrepancies by consensus. Weighted pooled proportion and 95% confidence intervals (CIs) are reported.

Results.—Thirty-two studies ($n = 5625$ patients) were included. Levels of evidence varied from level 3 to 4. Among all studies, the weighted pooled proportion of UVFP was 9.3% (95% CI, 6.6% to 12.5%), and among 11 studies ($n = 584$ patients) that postoperatively evaluated patients with flexible nasopharyngolaryngoscopy to document presence of UVFP, the weighted pooled proportion of UVFP was 29.8% (95% CI, 18.5% to 42.5%). Twenty-one studies (*n* = 2748 patients) evaluated patients undergoing patent ductus arteriosus ligation surgery, and the weighted pooled proportion of UVFP was 8.7% (95% CI, 5.4% to 12.6%). Six of these (*n* = 274 patients) assessed all patients postoperatively, and the weighted pooled proportion of UVFP was 39% (95% CI, 18% to 63%). Pooled analyses of risk factors and comorbidities are reported. Heterogeneity and publication bias were detected.

Conclusions.—UVFP is a demonstrated risk of congenital cardiothoracic surgery. Routine postoperative nasopharyngolaryngoscopy for vocal fold assessment by an otolaryngologist is suggested.

▶ Unilateral vocal fold paralysis (UVFP) is a known complication of cardiothoracic surgery; however, large-scale reporting of data regarding the prevalence and associated risk factors has been lacking. In this meta-analysis conducted by Strychowsky and colleagues, investigators reviewed 162 and incorporated into analyses 32 studies that met their rigorous inclusion criteria. They found, among all studies, the weighted pooled proportion of UVFP was 9.3%; for infants undergoing patent ductus arteriosus ligation, it was 8.7%. What is striking in the subgroup analyses is that, among studies that systematically evaluated infants postoperatively with nasopharyngolaryngoscopy, these numbers rose to 29.8% and 39%, respectively. Risk factors for UVFP included lower gestational age, lower birth weight, and lighter weight at the time of surgery. The authors also report what they could glean from a subset of studies regarding the natural history of UVFP, the likelihood of recovery of vocal fold function, and medical and surgical treatment options. This meta-analysis suggests that UVFP might be far more common following PDA ligation and other cardiothoracic surgery than is appreciated on standard clinical assessment and warrants a more systematic approach to postoperative laryngeal evaluation than currently is commonplace. The work further underscores the need for intervention and follow-up studies of infants affected by postoperative UVFP.

L. J. Van Marter, MD, MPH

7 Respiratory Disorders

Effects of Targeting Higher vs Lower Arterial Oxygen Saturations on Death or Disability in Extremely Preterm Infants: A Randomized Clinical Trial

Schmidt B, for the Canadian Oxygen Trial (COT) Group (Univ of Pennsylvania, Philadelphia; et al)

JAMA 309:2111-2120, 2013

Importance.—The goal of oxygen therapy is to deliver sufficient oxygen to the tissues while minimizing oxygen toxicity and oxidative stress. It remains uncertain what values of arterial oxygen saturations achieve this balance in preterm infants.

Objective.—To compare the effects of targeting lower or higher arterial oxygen saturations on the rate of death or disability in extremely preterm infants.

Design, Setting, and Participants.—Randomized, double-blind trial in 25 hospitals in Canada, the United States, Argentina, Finland, Germany, and Israel in which 1201 infants with gestational ages of 23 weeks 0 days through 27 weeks 6 days were enrolled within 24 hours after birth between December 2006 and August 2010. Follow-up assessments began in October 2008 and ended in August 2012.

Interventions.—Study participants were monitored until postmenstrual ages of 36 to 40 weeks with pulse oximeters that displayed saturations of either 3% above or below the true values. Caregivers adjusted the concentration of oxygen to achieve saturations between 88% and 92%, which produced 2 treatment groups with true target saturations of 85% to 89% (n = 602) or 91% to 95% (n = 599). Alarms were triggered when displayed saturations decreased to 86% or increased to 94%.

Main Outcomes and Measures.—The primary outcome was a composite of death, gross motor disability, cognitive or language delay, severe hearing loss, or bilateral blindness at a corrected age of 18 months. Secondary outcomes included retinopathy of prematurity and brain injury.

Results.—Of the 578 infants with adequate data for the primary outcome who were assigned to the lower target range, 298 (51.6%) died or survived with disability compared with 283 of the 569 infants (49.7%) assigned to the higher target range (odds ratio adjusted for center, 1.08; 95% CI, 0.85 to 1.37; $P = .52$). The rates of death were 16.6% for those in the 85% to 89% group and 15.3% for those in the 91% to 95% group (adjusted odds ratio, 1.11; 95% CI, 0.80 to 1.54; $P = .54$). Targeting lower saturations reduced the postmenstrual age at last use of oxygen therapy (adjusted mean difference, −0.8 weeks; 95% CI, −1.5 to −0.1; $P=.03$) but did not alter any other outcomes.

Conclusion and Relevance.—In extremely preterm infants, targeting oxygen saturations of 85% to 89% compared with 91% to 95% had no significant effect on the rate of death or disability at 18 months. These results may help determine the optimal target oxygen saturation.

Trial Registrations.—ISRCTN Identifier: 62491227; ClinicalTrials.gov Identifier: NCT00637169.

▶ Just more than decade ago, the STOP-ROP and BOOST trials showed higher rates of adverse respiratory outcomes if pulse oximetry readings were targeted in the high compared with the low 90s. Attention then turned to ascertainment of the lower end of the optimum range for saturation targets in preterm infants. The first completed trial, SUPPORT, found that an SpO_2 target range of 85% to 89%, compared with 91% to 95%, was associated with a lower risk of severe retinopathy of prematurity (ROP) (relative risk [RR] 0.52; 95% confidence interval [CI], 0.37–0.73) but a higher risk of death before discharge (RR, 1.27; 95% CI, 1.10–1.60) and at 18 months of age (RR, 1.25; 95% CI, 1.00–1.55). The Canadian Oxygen Trial (COT) described in this report used a similar study design and enrolled a comparable number of subjects. The offsets in the pulse oximeter readouts that were used to generate the high and low target range groups were the same, but the alarm limits were narrower in the COT study (triggering at 86% and 94% rather than 84% and 96% for low and high readings, as in SUPPORT). That difference may account for better separation of the true arterial saturation distributions in the 2 target groups in the COT trial. Despite greater distinctness between study groups, COT did not replicate either a lower rate of severe ROP (odds ratio [OR], 0.95; 95% CI, 0.65–1.39) or a higher risk of death before 18 months of age (OR, 1.12; 95% CI, 0.78–1.61) in the lower target group. The reasons for these different results are not apparent. The overall rates of severe ROP (13.4% in SUPPORT, 13.0% in COT) were not different, but the mortality rate at 18 months of age was higher in the SUPPORT cohort (20.1% vs 15.9%, $P < .01$), suggesting that either the study populations or the clinical contexts may have been dissimilar. The COT authors speculate that differences between studies in the proportions of subjects who had median saturations less than 85% or greater than 95% might account for these differences. Although those proportions may differ between trials, there appears to be little difference between groups within trials, so it is not readily evident how or whether that might account for the failure to detect differential outcomes in COT. A larger concern is the transition in the Masimo analytical algorithm introduced about halfway through trial enrollment to correct underrepresentation of saturation values between 87% and 90%.[1] Although analysis did not find a significant impact of that change in this trial, it was consequential in BOOST II (see commentary on that report). The implications of this trial, therefore, remain ambiguous, pending more detailed analyses combining data from the SUPPORT, BOOST II, and COT trials.

W. E. Benitz, MD

Reference

1. Johnston ED, Boyle B, Juszczak E, King A, Brocklehurst P, Stenson BJ. Oxygen targeting in preterm infants using the Masimo SET Radical pulse oximeter. *Arch Dis Child Fetal Neonatal Ed*. 2011;96:F429-F433.

Respiratory Outcomes of the Surfactant Positive Pressure and Oximetry Randomized Trial (SUPPORT)

Stevens TP, on behalf of the SUPPORT Study Group of the *Eunice Kennedy Shriver* National Institute of Child Health and Human Development Neonatal Research Network (Univ of Rochester Med Ctr and Golisano Children's Hosp, NY; et al)

J Pediatr 2014 [Epub ahead of print]

Objective.—To explore the early childhood pulmonary outcomes of infants who participated in the National Institute of Child Health and Human Development's Surfactant Positive Airway Pressure and Pulse Oximetry Randomized Trial (SUPPORT), using a factorial design that randomized extremely preterm infants to lower vs higher oxygen saturation targets and delivery room continuous positive airway pressure (CPAP) vs intubation/ surfactant.

Study Design.—The Breathing Outcomes Study, a prospective secondary study to the Surfactant Positive Airway Pressure and Pulse Oximetry Randomized Trial, assessed respiratory morbidity at 6-month intervals from hospital discharge to 18-22 months corrected age (CA). Two prespecified primary outcomes—wheezing more than twice per week during the worst 2-week period and cough longer than 3 days without a cold—were compared for each randomized intervention.

Results.—One or more interviews were completed for 918 of the 922 eligible infants. The incidences of wheezing and cough were 47.9% and 31.0%, respectively, and did not differ between the study arms of either randomized intervention. Infants randomized to lower vs higher oxygen saturation targets had a similar risk of death or respiratory morbidity (except for croup and treatment with oxygen or diuretics at home). Infants randomized to CPAP vs intubation/surfactant had fewer episodes of wheezing without a cold (28.9% vs 36.5%; $P < .05$), respiratory illnesses diagnosed by a doctor (47.7% vs 55.2%; $P < .05$), and physician or emergency room visits for breathing problems (68.0% vs 72.9%; $P < .05$) by 18-22 months CA.

Conclusion.—Treatment with early CPAP rather than intubation/ surfactant is associated with less respiratory morbidity by 18-22 months CA. Longitudinal assessment of pulmonary morbidity is necessary to fully evaluate the potential benefits of respiratory interventions for neonates.

▶ This article reports the 18- to 22-month respiratory outcomes of survivors of the SUPPORT Trial, conducted from 2005 to 2011 by the Eunice Kennedy

Shriver National Institutes of Child Health and Human Development Neonatal Research Network. In this study, the investigators used a factorial design to evaluate outcomes among extremely preterm infants associated with randomization to continuous positive airway pressure (CPAP) versus intubation in the delivery room and 1 of 2 commonly used target ranges of oxygen saturation (85% to 89% and 91% to 95%). Results of the previously reported primary analyses showed a higher mortality rate and lower rate of retinopathy of prematurity among the group randomly assigned to the lower target range for oxygen saturation and no difference in the primary outcome (death or need for supplemental oxygen at 36 weeks post-menstrual age [PMA]) by delivery room respiratory management. The current analyses of data concerning later respiratory outcomes obtained by parental questionnaire showed, at 18 to 22 months of age, similar rates of wheezing and cough among all 4 study arms but higher rates of respiratory illness diagnosed by a doctor and wheezing in the absence of a cold; however, emergency room visits for respiratory illness were less frequent among infants randomly assigned to delivery room CPAP for respiratory support. These findings would not have been predicted based on the primary outcome and suggest that strategies in delivery room respiratory management might have important implications for health and quality of life, subsequent health risks, and long-term economic implications of extremely preterm birth. The results also suggest that even rigorous assessment of 36-week PMA pulmonary status is an imperfect surrogate for long-term pulmonary outcomes among survivors of extreme prematurity. These results highlight the ongoing contributions of the SUPPORT trial and underscoring the importance of the conduct of other well-designed and rigorously conducted randomized clinical trials that also incorporate long-term follow-up of extremely preterm infants.

L. J. Van Marter, MD, MPH

Oxygen Saturation and Outcomes in Preterm Infants

The BOOST II United Kingdom, Australia, and New Zealand Collaborative Groups (Univ of Edinburgh, UK; Univ of Sydney, New South Wales, Australia; et al)

N Engl J Med 368:2094-2104, 2013

Background.—The clinically appropriate range for oxygen saturation in preterm infants is unknown. Previous studies have shown that infants had reduced rates of retinopathy of prematurity when lower targets of oxygen saturation were used.

Methods.—In three international randomized, controlled trials, we evaluated the effects of targeting an oxygen saturation of 85 to 89%, as compared with a range of 91 to 95%, on disability-free survival at 2 years in infants born before 28 weeks' gestation. Halfway through the trials, the oximeter-calibration algorithm was revised. Recruitment was stopped early when an interim analysis showed an increased rate of death at 36 weeks in the group with a lower oxygen saturation. We analyzed pooled data from patients and now report hospital-discharge outcomes.

Results.—A total of 2448 infants were recruited. Among the 1187 infants whose treatment used the revised oximeter-calibration algorithm, the rate of death was significantly higher in the lower-target group than in the higher-target group (23.1% vs. 15.9%; relative risk in the lower-target group, 1.45; 95% confidence interval [CI], 1.15 to 1.84; $P = 0.002$). There was heterogeneity for mortality between the original algorithm and the revised algorithm ($P = 0.006$) but not for other outcomes. In all 2448 infants, those in the lower-target group for oxygen saturation had a reduced rate of retinopathy of prematurity (10.6% vs. 13.5%; relative risk, 0.79; 95% CI, 0.63 to 1.00; $P = 0.045$) and an increased rate of necrotizing enterocolitis (10.4% vs. 8.0%; relative risk, 1.31; 95% CI, 1.02 to 1.68; $P = 0.04$). There were no significant between-group differences in rates of other outcomes or adverse events.

Conclusions.—Targeting an oxygen saturation below 90% with the use of current oximeters in extremely preterm infants was associated with an increased risk of death. (Funded by the Australian National Health and Medical Research Council and others; BOOST II Current Controlled Trials number, ISRCTN00842661, and Australian New Zealand Clinical Trials Registry numbers, ACTRN12605000055606 and ACTRN12605000253606.)

► The year I was born, there was an epidemic of retinopathy of prematurity (RoP) attributed to excessive use of supplemental oxygen in treating premature infants. Had I been born preterm, I might well have sustained significant visual impairment or even complete loss of sight. As a visually oriented person, I cannot imagine such a fate—one that, even today, affects far too many babies born extremely preterm. These factors led to my keen interest in RoP and, especially, in therapeutic approaches that offer the promise of eradicating this terrible complication of prematurity. Restriction of the use of supplemental oxygen, made more straightforward by advent of accurate oximetry monitors, is 1 such approach. Because restricting supplemental oxygen in preterm infants to lower ranges of oxygen saturation was shown in observational studies to be associated with lower risk of RoP in preemies, at least 2 large randomized clinical trials were launched to test this hypothesis: SUPPORT 1 and BOOST II. The BOOST II study enrolled 2448 infants born before 28 weeks' gestation, randomizing them to lower (85%–89%) versus higher (91%–95%) oxygen saturations. The primary outcome was disability-free survival at age 2. As had previously been found in the SUPPORT 1[1] trial using similar oxygen saturation ranges, BOOST II found lower rates of RoP but greater likelihood of mortality among infants randomized to the lower oxygen saturation group. BOOST, in addition, found a greater rate of necrotizing enterocolitis among infants randomized to the lower oxygen saturation group. These 2 large trials clearly demonstrate that lowering oxygen saturation to 85% to 89% is too hazardous to warrant this approach for RoP prevention. Scientists clearly need to continue to identify effective ways to prevent preterm birth and to develop treatments to prevent RoP among those born extremely preterm.

L. J. Van Marter, MD, MPH

Reference

1. SUPPORT Study Group of the Eunice Kennedy Shriver NICHD Neonatal Research Network, Carlo WA, Finer NN, Walsh MC, et al. Target ranges of oxygen saturation in extremely preterm infants. *N Engl J Med.* 2010;362:1959-1969.

Oxygen Saturation and Outcomes in Preterm Infants

The BOOST II United Kingdom, Australia, and New Zealand Collaborative Groups (Univ of Edinburgh, Scotland, UK; Univ of Sydney, Australia; Univ of Otago, Christchurch, New Zealand; et al)

N Engl J Med 368:2094-2104, 2013

Background.—The clinically appropriate range for oxygen saturation in preterm infants is unknown. Previous studies have shown that infants had reduced rates of retinopathy of prematurity when lower targets of oxygen saturation were used.

Methods.—In three international randomized, controlled trials, we evaluated the effects of targeting an oxygen saturation of 85 to 89%, as compared with a range of 91 to 95%, on disability-free survival at 2 years in infants born before 28 weeks' gestation. Halfway through the trials, the oximeter-calibration algorithm was revised. Recruitment was stopped early when an interim analysis showed an increased rate of death at 36 weeks in the group with a lower oxygen saturation. We analyzed pooled data from patients and now report hospital-discharge outcomes.

Results.—A total of 2448 infants were recruited. Among the 1187 infants whose treatment used the revised oximeter-calibration algorithm, the rate of death was significantly higher in the lower-target group than in the higher-target group (23.1% vs. 15.9%; relative risk in the lower-target group, 1.45; 95% confidence interval [CI], 1.15 to 1.84; $P = 0.002$). There was heterogeneity for mortality between the original algorithm and the revised algorithm ($P = 0.006$) but not for other outcomes. In all 2448 infants, those in the lower-target group for oxygen saturation had a reduced rate of retinopathy of prematurity (10.6% vs. 13.5%; relative risk, 0.79; 95% CI, 0.63 to 1.00; $P = 0.045$) and an increased rate of necrotizing enterocolitis (10.4% vs. 8.0%; relative risk, 1.31; 95% CI, 1.02 to 1.68; $P = 0.04$). There were no significant between-group differences in rates of other outcomes or adverse events.

Conclusions.—Targeting an oxygen saturation below 90% with the use of current oximeters in extremely preterm infants was associated with an increased risk of death.

▶ This simultaneous report of results from parallel trials of low and high pulse oximetry targets (85%–89% vs 91%–95%, respectively) provides the third pillar of available data on this important matter, alongside the Surfactant, Positive

Pressure, and Pulse Oximetry Randomized Trial (SUPPORT) and COT trials. The necessity for modification of the Masimo analytical algorithm for calculation of oxygen saturation estimates about halfway through subject enrollment confounds interpretation of the results and any attempts to directly compare results with those of other trials (especially SUPPORT), but that correction may make these observations most cogent to current practice. These BOOST II trials from Australia, New Zealand, and the United Kingdom showed higher mortality among infants assigned to the low target range group after revision of the oximeter algorithm (relative risk [RR], 1.45; 95% confidence interval [CI], 1.15–1.84). Among all enrolled infants, those in the lower target group experienced a lower rate of severe retinopathy (retinopathy of prematurity [ROP] requiring treatment in accordance with ETROP criteria; RR, 0.79; 95% CI, 0.63–1.00) and a higher rate of necrotizing enterocolitis (RR, 1.31; 95% CI, 1.02–1.68). Although these results are similar to those from SUPPORT, there are important differences between those trials. In the BOOST trials, the offsets used to create differential true SpO_2 targets were slightly different, and alarm limits (where specified) were narrower (86–87 and 93–94 rather than 85 and 95, respectively). In SUPPORT, alarm limits of 85% and 95% corresponded to true saturations of 85% and 95%, but the narrower limits and conversion algorithm for the BOOST trials result in different alarm limits between groups: approximately 84 and 90 in the low target group vs 89 and 95 in the high target group. While these targets and alarm limits resulted in similar distributions of true SpO_2 measurements between 85% and 95%, the proportions of infants with measures outside that range were similar in the SUPPORT groups but differed in BOOST II, with more infants in the low target group having saturations less than 85% and more in the high group having saturations greater than 95%. These differences in the tails of the distribution may be responsible for the differential effects on outcomes in the BOOST II trials but would not account for the SUPPORT findings. Taken collectively, these trials suggest that mortality can be reduced by targeting pulse oximetry readings greater than 90%, with low and high oximeter alarm limits set at 90% and 95%, respectively. This lower mortality comes at the cost of a higher rate of severe ROP—a favorable trade-off of an unmanageable problem for a treatable one.

W. E. Benitz, MD

Temporal quantification of oxygen saturation ranges: an effort to reduce hyperoxia in the neonatal intensive care unit

Bizzarro MJ, Li FY, Katz K, et al (Yale Univ School of Medicine, New Haven, CT; Yale Ctr for Analytical Sciences, New Haven, CT)

J Perinatol 34:33-38, 2014

Objective.—To reduce exposure to hyperoxia and its associated morbidities in preterm neonates.

Study Design.—A multidisciplinary group was established to evaluate oxygen exposure in our neonatal intensive care unit. Infants were assigned target saturation ranges and signal extraction technology implemented to temporally quantify achievement of these ranges. The outcomes bronchopulmonary dysplasia/death, retinopathy of prematurity (ROP)/death, severe ROP and ROP requiring surgery were compared in a pre- versus post-intervention evaluation using multivariate analyses.

Result.—A total of 304 very low birth weight pre-initiative infants were compared with 396 post-initiative infants. Multivariate analyses revealed decreased odds of severe ROP (adjusted odds ratio (OR): 0.41; 95% confidence interval (CI): 0.24–0.72) and ROP requiring surgery (adjusted OR 0.31; 95% CI: 0.17–0.59) post-initiative. No differences in death were observed.

Conclusion.—Significant reductions in severe ROP and ROP requiring surgery were observed after staff education and implementation of new technology to quantify success in achieving targeted saturations and reinforce principles and practices.

▶ This retrospective study by Bizzarro et al analyzed the effect of a quality improvement (QI) initiative aimed at reducing exposure to hyperoxia in premature infants. The interventions included revised oxygen management guidelines, education about harm from hyperoxia, changes to delivery-room resuscitation practices, and the introduction of signal extraction technology to quantify time spent within a specified target range.

A comparison between 2 epochs was provided, and a significant reduction in severe retinopathy of prematurity (ROP) and ROP requiring laser surgery was demonstrated. No difference in bronchopulmonary dysplasia was seen.

The authors appropriately highlight the limitations of their retrospective review—namely, the inability to control for all variables contributing to the outcomes of interest. Efforts to decrease late-onset sepsis and improve nutrition were also underway during the study periods. However, their report certainly lends itself to "real-life" application in which most NICUs doing improvement work have several QI initiatives underway.

This report is certainly timely, with recent randomized controlled trials leaving the neonatal community uncertain about the optimal strategy to manage oxygen therapy to minimize harm from both hypoxia and hyperoxia. The authors state that application of pulse oximeters able to quantify time spent above, below, and within the target oxygen saturation range played a major role in this effort. The direct effect of this strategy cannot be deduced from the QI effort as a whole, but it would be interesting to investigate on a larger scale. The multipronged approach described to reduce exposure to hyperoxia clearly improved the local incidence of severe ROP and serves as a reference for other institutions with a similar goal.

R. J. Vartanian, MD

Transcribed oxygen saturation vs oximeter recordings in very low birth weight infants

Ruiz TL, Trzaski JM, Sink DW, et al (Trinity College, Hartford, CT; Connecticut Children's Med Ctr, Hartford)

J Perinatol 34:130-135, 2014

Objective.—The objective of this study was to compare hand-transcribed oxygen saturation (SpO_2) with electronic oximeter data in very low birth weight infants (VLBWI, <1500 g).

Study Design.—Oximeter data were downloaded from birth through 36 weeks postmenstrual age (PMA) for VLBWI before and after interventions to improve neonatal intensive care unit oxygen management. Transcribed SpO_2 values were obtained by chart review. Proportions of transcribed and oximetry data in target (85 to 93%), hypoxemic (80 to 84%), and hyperoxemic (≥98%) ranges before and after intervention were compared.

Result.—There were 30 441 oximetry hours before intervention and 54 538 oximetry hours after intervention. Transcribed SpO_2 values correlated strongly with oximeter overall. However, during hours on supplemental oxygen, transcribed values significantly overdocumented target range and underdocumented values 80 to 84 and ≥98%. This finding varied by respiratory support and PMA, and increased after intervention.

Conclusion.—Transcribed SpO_2 values overdocumented target range and underdocumented hyperoxemic and hypoxemic ranges compared with electronic oximeter data. These results support incorporating electronic oximeter data into medical records.

► Maintaining adequate and stable oxygenation in preterm infants continues to be a major challenge in clinical care. This is exacerbated by the fact that the optimal oxygen saturation range to maintain normal retinal development, reduce neurological impairment, and minimize lung injury is currently unknown. Recent data suggest that morbidity is associated with both low baseline[1] and fluctuations[2] in oxygen saturation and therefore should be avoided. Even with heightened awareness shown by Ruiz et al, studies have shown a need for improvement in both accurate transcription of oxygen saturation and maintaining infants within a given target range.

Clinical practice guidelines are needed and should encompass standards for pulse oximeter settings and accurate documentation of oxygen saturation. Prolonged averaging times (16 seconds), commonly used in the intensive care unit to reduce nuisance alarms, have been shown to falsely increase desaturation events of > 20 seconds, whereas Ruiz et al and others have shown the inaccuracies of nursing documentation. Therefore, improvements in clinical practice should include short averaging times to minimize false reporting of desaturation events of long duration, and pulse oximeter summary data electronic recordings, such as histogram downloads, to provide unbiased documentation of overall time at various levels of oxygen saturation. Unfortunately, these summary reports do not currently provide information on the incidence of fluctuations in oxygenation, which have been associated with oxidative stress during the reoxygenation phase. These intermittent hypoxemic events may be further influenced by both monitor alarm delays and the response time of clinical staff. Automated closed loop systems, shown to reduce both the need for manual adjustment of supplemental oxygenation and exposure to hyper- and hypoxemia,[3] may be a promising future tool for stabilization of oxygenation in this vulnerable patient cohort.

R. J. Martin, MD
J. M. Di Fiore, BSEE

References

1. SUPPORT Study Group of the Eunice Kennedy Shriver NICHD Neonatal Research Network, Carlo WA, Finer NN, Walsh MC, et al. Target ranges of oxygen saturation in extremely preterm infants. *N Engl J Med.* 2010;362:1959-1969.
2. Di Fiore JM, Bloom JN, Orge F, et al. A higher incidence of intermittent hypoxemic episodes is associated with severe retinopathy of prematurity. *J Pediatr.* 2010; 157:69-73.
3. Claure N, Bancalari E. Automated closed loop control of inspired oxygen concentration. *Respir Care.* 2013;58:151-161.

Reducing Unplanned Extubations in the NICU

Merkel L, Beers K, Lewis MM, et al (Penn State Hershey Children's Hosp, PA)
Pediatrics 133:e1367-e1372, 2014

Background and Objectives.—Unplanned extubation can be a significant event that places the patient at risk for adverse events. Our goal was to reduce unplanned extubations to <1 unplanned extubation per 100 patient-intubated days.

Methods.—All unplanned extubations in the NICU beginning in October 2009 were audited. Data collected included time of day, patient weight, and patient care activity at the time of the event. Bundles of potentially better practices were implemented in sequential Plan-Do-Study-Act cycles. Rates of unplanned extubation (number per patient-intubated day) for each month were analyzed by using control charts, and causes of unplanned extubation were analyzed by using Pareto charts.

Results.—We found a significant decrease in the unplanned extubation rate after implementation of the first bundle of potentially better practices in May 2010 (2.38 to 0.41 per 100 patient-intubated days). Several more Plan-Do-Study-Act cycles were conducted to sustain this improvement. A persistent reduction in the unplanned extubation rate (0.58 per 100 patient-intubated days) began in February 2013. Causes included dislodgement during care and procedures and variation in the fixation of the endotracheal tube. The majority of events occurred in very low birth weight infants during the daytime shift.

Conclusions.—Unplanned extubations in the NICU can be reduced by education of staff and by implementing standard practices of care.

Sustainability of any practice change to improve quality is critically dependent on culture change within the NICU. We suggest that the benchmark for unplanned extubation should be a rate < 1 per 100 patient-intubated days.

▶ Inadvertent extubations are a problem in the neonatal intensive care unit (NICU) environment for myriad reasons: uncuffed endotracheal tubes, unrestrained patients, difficult stabilization, patient motion, a trend toward less sedation, and the high equipment-to-patient weight ratios, to name a few. In this quality improvement (QI) project, the objective was to reduce the number of unplanned extubations in a single center NICU. After a baseline period in which the background rate was determined, 5 cycles occurred in which potentially better practices were implemented. Each time, there was a reduction in the event rate, with the investigators achieving their goal of less than 1 unexpected extubation per 100 patient-intubated days.

In many ways, this QI project demonstrates what many others have shown: QI works. Purists can argue that these are historically controlled data, that most of the potentially better practices selected are not scientifically validated, and that, as a single-center experience, it may not be exportable. We heard the same arguments when standardized feeding protocols showed a reduction in the incidence of necrotizing enterocolitis, and yet they work.

It would be nice to have had more information about this project, such as staffing ratios, number of therapists per shift, measure of acuity, for example, to know whether the recommended benchmark is feasible in a unit with higher acuity or fewer staff, as well as the resources that were provided by the hospital to support the project.

Nevertheless, as this article aptly demonstrates, the key to the success of most QI projects is education, behavioral change, and reinforcement.

S. M. Donn, MD

Comparative effectiveness of surfactant preparations in premature infants

Trembath A, on behalf of the Best Pharmaceuticals for Children Act—Pediatric Trials Network (Case Western Reserve Univ, Cleveland, OH; et al)

J Pediatr 163:955-960, 2013

Objective.—To compare effectiveness of 3 surfactant preparations (beractant, calfactant, and poractant alfa) in premature infants for preventing 3 outcomes: (1) air leak syndromes; (2) death; and (3) bronchopulmonary dysplasia (BPD) or death (composite outcome).

Study Design.—We conducted a comparative effectiveness study of premature infants admitted to 322 neonatal intensive care units in the US from 2005-2010 who were treated with beractant, calfactant, or poractant alfa. We compared the incidence of air leak syndromes, death, and BPD or death, adjusting for gestational age (GA), antenatal steroids, discharge year, and small for GA status.

Results.—A total of 51 282 infants received surfactant; 40% received beractant, 30% calfactant, and 30% poractant alfa. Median birth weight was 1435 g (IQR 966-2065); median GA was 30 weeks (27-33). On adjusted analysis, we observed a similar risk of air leak syndromes (calfactant vs beractant OR = 1.17 [95% CI: 0.95, 1.43]; calfactant vs poractant OR = 1.23 [0.98, 1.56]; beractant vs poractant OR = 1.06 [0.87, 1.29]), death (calfactant vs beractant OR = 1.14 [0.93, 1.39]; calfactant vs poractant OR = 0.98 [0.78, 1.23]; beractant vs poractant OR = 0.86 [0.72, 1.04]), and BPD or death (calfactant vs beractant OR = 1.08 [0.93, 1.26]; calfactant vs poractant OR = 1.19 [1.00, 1.41]; beractant vs poractant OR = 1.10 [0.96, 1.27]).

Conclusions.—Beractant, calfactant, and poractant alfa demonstrated similar effectiveness in prevention of air leak syndromes, death, and BPD or death in premature infants when adjusted for site. Previously described differences in mortality between surfactants likely do not represent true differences in effectiveness but may relate to site variation in outcomes.

▶ As new surfactant replacement products have entered the market over the past 25 years, their manufacturers have jockeyed for market share by suggesting, if not quite outright claiming, that one product had some advantage or another over competing formulations. These conversations were not informed by much reliable data, as the available comparative studies were often flawed by small sample sizes, use of short-term outcome variables, weak subject selection or randomization methods, or retrospective study designs. Nonetheless, the perception that animal-derived preparations more rapidly improved lung compliance and lowered oxygen requirements led to their dominance in the market and disappearance of the synthetic product (Exosurf), which was the first surfactant to come to market. Evidence to guide selection among the 3 animal-derived surfactants has remained elusive, however, with mixed results reported in published comparisons. This work provides an answer to that question, and it is good news. Analyzing data from a large national clinical database, these authors report that they were unable to identify any significant differences in rates of air leak, death, or death or bronchopulmonary dysplasia among infants treated with beractant (Survanta), calfactant (Infasurf), or poractant alfa (Curosurf). Although the study was retrospective, the conclusions are strengthened by large sample sizes (> 15 000 in each group) and statistical rigor. The authors correctly suggest that this is likely to be the best evidence we will obtain, given the improbability of an adequately powered randomized trial. Those of us who have relied on a single product in our facilities for the past several years (who are undoubtedly in a large majority) can rest easy that we have not been inadvertently using an inferior product. As these authors note, these conclusions mean that the choice of surfactant preparation has to be based on factors other than these clinical results.

Entry of a new, fully synthetic surfactant, lucinactant (Surfaxin) into the market in the past 3 years has reopened this debate. Early results suggest that this product is equal in clinical effectiveness and potentially may have benefits (such as lower risk of inflammatory responses or transmission of infection), compared with animal-derived products.[1] A pharmacoeconomic analysis of 2 randomized comparative trials has suggested that lower rates of reintubation among babies treated with lucinactant may yield substantial cost savings.[2] Although it may be premature to conclude that we should universally adopt this new product, this work does provide an important reminder that choices among nominally therapeutically equivalent products require consideration of many other factors, including cost per dose, number of doses typically required, and effects on requirements for and costs of other care components during the hospitalization. Many years of postmarketing surveillance will likely be required to acquire an appreciation of more subtle outcome effects, such as neurodevelopmental consequences of hemodynamic instability during drug administration.

W. E. Benitz, MD

References

1. Jordan BK, Donn SM. Lucinactant for the prevention of respiratory distress syndrome in premature infants. *Expert Rev Clin Pharmacol.* 2013;6:115-121.
2. Guardia CG, Moya FR, Sinha S, Simmons PD, Segal R, Greenspan JS. A pharmacoeconomic analysis of in-hospital costs resulting from reintubation in preterm infants treated with lucinactant, beractant, or poractant alfa. *J Pediatr Pharmacol Ther.* 2012;17:220-227.

Surfactant Deficiency in Infants with Severe Acute Viral Bronchiolitis

Hartmann F, Fiori HH, Ramos Garcia PC, et al (Pontifícia Universidade Católica do Rio Grande do Sul (PUCRS), Porto Alegre, Brazil; et al)

J Pediatr 164:1432-1435, 2014

Objectives.—To evaluate surfactant content and function through the lamellar body count (LBC) and stable microbubble test (SMT) in mechanically ventilated infants with severe acute viral bronchiolitis.

Study Design.—Controlled cross-sectional study of 32 infants receiving mechanical ventilation: 16 with a diagnosis of acute viral bronchiolitis and 16 with normal lungs. Tracheal fluid was collected and LBC was performed in an automated cell counter. Samples were kept frozen and thawed for testing. At the time of analysis, samples were diluted in a dithiothreitol solution, vortexed for 10 seconds, and aspirated by the cell counter. SMT was performed using the Pattle technique.

Results.—In the bronchiolitis group, the median (IQR) LBC was significantly lower than in the control group: 130 000 (61 250-362 250) vs 518 000 (180 250-896 000) lamellar bodies/μL; $P = .003$. Median (IQR) SMT values were also significantly lower in the bronchiolitis group: 10 (2-13) vs 400 (261-615) microbubbles/mm^2; $P < .001$.

Conclusions.—Infants with acute viral bronchiolitis have reduced surfactant content and function. We speculate that these simple tests may be useful to identify infants with bronchiolitis who would benefit from surfactant replacement therapy.

▶ This study evaluated the surfactant status of 32 infants requiring mechanical ventilation. Half of them had acute viral bronchiolitis, and half had normal lungs. Surfactant quantity, estimated by the lamellar body count, and surfactant function, measured by the stable microbubble test, were compared from samples of aspirated tracheal fluid. Both quantity and function of surfactant were diminished in the group with acute viral bronchiolitis.

There are a couple of messages from this article. First, viral upper respiratory infections affect not only the airways but lung parenchyma as well. The effect of inflammation on surfactant inactivation has been well documented. Moreover, surfactant-protein A appears to enhance clearance of respiratory syncytial virus. Second, repletion of the surfactant pool through exogenous administration might benefit this population of infants and expand the indications for therapy.

Finally, the other implication here is that surfactant dysfunction is yet another aspect of acute viral respiratory infections, of which respiratory syncytial virus is the most common, and for which there is an effective immunoprophylactic agent. It seems that we ought to be increasing its use and not finding unsubstantiated reasons to limit it.

S. M. Donn, MD

A Randomized Controlled Trial of Two Nasal Continuous Positive Airway Pressure Levels after Extubation in Preterm Infants

Buzzella B, Claure N, D'Ugard C, et al (Univ of Miami Miller School of Medicine/Jackson Memorial Hosp, Miami, FL)
J Pediatr 164:46-51, 2014

Objective.—To compare extubation failure rate with two ranges of nasal continuous positive airway pressure (NCPAP) in oxygen dependent preterm infants.

Study Design.—Preterm infants of birth weight 500-1000 g and gestational age 23-30 weeks, extubated for the first time during the first 6 weeks while requiring fraction of inspired oxygen ≥ 0.25, were randomly assigned to a NCPAP range of 4-6 (low NCPAP) or 7-9 (high NCPAP) cmH_2O.

Results.—Infants were randomized to low (n = 47) or high NCPAP (n = 46) at day 16.3 ± 14.7 and 15.5 ± 12.4, respectively. Rates of extubation failure per criteria (24% vs 43%, P = .04, OR and 95% CI: 0.39 [0.16-0.96]) and re-intubation (17% vs 38%, P = .023, 0.33 [0.016-0.85]) within 96 hours were significantly lower in the high-compared with the low NCPAP group. This was mainly due to a strikingly lower failure rate in the 500-750 g birth weight strata. Duration of ventilation, bronchopulmonary dysplasia, or severe bronchopulmonary dysplasia did not differ significantly. No infant developed pneumothorax during 96 hours post-extubation.

Conclusions.—Extubation failure in preterm infants with residual lung disease was lower with NCPAP range of 7-9 compared with 4-6 cm H_2O. These findings suggest the need for higher distending pressure post-extubation in the more immature infants who are still oxygen dependent (Table 2).

► Since description of the application of continuous positive airway pressure (CPAP) for support of very low birth weight infants with respiratory distress syndrome by Gregory and colleagues in 1971, this technique has been a major component of the care of newborn infants with respiratory failure. Four decades of extensive use have provided an abundance of experience, leading to many beliefs about how, when, and for whom this treatment should be used. Although there is little doubt that many of those beliefs are correct, there is surprisingly little empirical evidence to guide optimal use of this essential technology. By addressing the question of how much distending pressure is needed to facilitate successful extubation in extremely low birth weight infants who have been supported with endotracheal positive pressure ventilation, this article helps address that void. The authors are careful to point out that these results should not be extrapolated to guidance of early ventilation strategies for such infants. By design, infants who were relatively well ($FiO_2 < 0.25$; 16% of enrolled infants) or with more prolonged ventilator dependency (not extubated until after 6 weeks of age; 20% of enrolled infants) were not randomized, so extension of these results to those groups would also be inappropriate.

TABLE 2.—Primary and Secondary End-Points During 96 hours Post-Extubation and Respiratory Outcomes

	All Infants 500-1000 g		BW Strata 500-750 g		751-1000 g	
	Low NCPAP (n = 47)	High NCPAP (n = 46)	Low NCPAP (n = 20)	High NCPAP (n = 22)	Low NCPAP (n = 27)	High NCPAP (n = 24)
Failed extubation per criteria within 96 h	20 (43)	11 (24)[‡]	14 (70)	6 (27)[†]	6 (22)	5 (21)
Re-intubation within 96 h	18 (38)	8 (17)[§*]	11 (55)	4 (18)[*]	7 (26)	4 (17)
Re-intubation within 7 d	24 (51)	14 (30)[¶*]	12 (60)	9 (41)	12 (44)	5 (21)
Total ventilator d	27 ± 20	22 ± 16	38 ± 20	31 ± 15	19 ± 17	13 ± 11
Total oxygen d	53 (29-127)	54 (28-103)	86 (43-203)	77 (38-137)	44 (21-83)	52 (18-102)
BPD	16 (34)	18 (39)	10 (50)	12 (55)	6 (22)	6 (25)
Severe BPD	10 (21)	8 (17)	8 (40)	5 (23)	2 (7)	3 (12)

Data are number (percent), mean ± SD or median (10th-90th percentile).
*$P < .05$ by Pearson χ^2.
†$P < .01$ by Pearson χ^2.
‡$P = .04$, common OR 0.39 and 95% CI: 0.16-0.96 by Mantel–Haenszel.
§$P = .023$, common OR 0.33 and 95% CI: 0.012-0.85 by Mantel–Haenszel.
¶$P = .034$, common OR 0.39 and 95% CI: 0.16-0.93 by Mantel–Haenszel.

The trial might also be criticized because the intervention was not masked, and decisions regarding readiness for extubation and need for reintubation were at the discretion of the treating clinicians. Nonetheless, the results show clinically and statistically significant differences between the low (4–6 cm H_2O) and high CPAP (7–9 cm H_2O) groups in rates of extubation failure within 96 hours and of reintubation within 96 hours or 7 days (see Table 2). (Extubation failure was defined as $PaCO_2 \geq 65$ mm Hg with an increase above baseline >15 mm Hg, $FiO_2 > 0.60$ with an increase of ≥0.20 above baseline, apnea or bradycardia episodes requiring reintubation, nasal breakdown requiring cessation of CPAP, or titration of CPAP outside the assigned range.) Although the analysis (presumably by Student *t* test, because the data are shown as mean ± SD) did not demonstrate a statistically significant difference in number of ventilator days between CPAP groups for either weight stratum or for the entire cohort, consistently fewer days of ventilation in both groups suggest that a more robust analysis (using nonparametric 2-way analysis of variance, for example) may have yielded a different result. No subjects developed air leak or signs of cardiovascular or gastrointestinal compromise with the higher level of CPAP, and rates of death and common complications of prematurity did not differ between groups. While we await confirmation of these observations, it seems prudent to provide a higher level of CPAP (7–9 cm H_2O) to facilitate extubation of 500 to 750 g infants with an FiO_2 requirement ≥0.25 in the first 6 weeks after birth.

W. E. Benitz, MD

Heliox for mechanically ventilated newborns with bronchopulmonary dysplasia

Szczapa T, Gadzinowski J, Moczko J, et al (Poznań Univ of Med Sciences, Poland)

Arch Dis Child Fetal Neonatal Ed 99:F128-F133, 2014

Objective.—We assessed the safety and studied the influence of short-term helium-oxygen (heliox) mechanical ventilation (MV) on respiratory function, gas exchange and oxygenation in infants with bronchopulmonary dysplasia (BPD) or at high risk for BPD.

Design.—A pilot, time-series study.

Setting.—Neonatal intensive care unit.

Patients.—Infants with severe BPD who required MV.

Interventions.—MV with helium–oxygen and air–oxygen mixtures.

Main Outcome Measures.—Respiratory parameters, acid–base balance, oxygenation and vital signs were recorded at five time points: initially during MV with air–oxygen, after 15 and 60 min of helium–oxygen MV, and 15 and 60 min after return to air–oxygen MV.

Results.—15 infants with BPD were enrolled. Helium–oxygen MV was well tolerated and was associated with a statistically significant increase in tidal volume, dynamic compliance and peak expiratory flow rate. An improvement in oxygenation and a decrease in fraction of inspired oxygen was also observed. During helium–oxygen MV there was a significant decrease in the oxygenation index and alveolar–arterial oxygen tension difference. The PaO_2/fraction of inspired oxygen (FiO_2) ratio increased significantly during helium–oxygen ventilation. A decrease in $PaCO_2$ and an increase in pH were also observed during helium–oxygen administration, however this was not statistically significant. After ventilation with helium–oxygen was discontinued, the infants' respiratory function and oxygenation deteriorated and supplemental oxygen requirements increased accordingly.

Conclusions.—Helium–oxygen MV is safe and resulted in improvement of respiratory function and oxygenation in infants with severe BPD requiring MV.

▶ In this small pilot study, Szczapa and colleagues evaluated the use of heliox, an 80:20 mixture of helium:oxygen on 15 infants with or at risk for bronchopulmonary dysplasia (BPD) who were ventilator-dependent. A quasi-experimental model was used, with each patient serving as his or her own control, and respiratory function, gas exchange, and oxygenation were the primary metrics analyzed. The rationale for using heliox was that its lower density, compared with a nitrogen-oxygen mixture, would reduce airway turbulence in narrowed airways and enhance gas diffusion in the alveoli.

The study population consisted of 15 infants requiring supplemental oxygen (mean of 0.54) and mechanical ventilation (average mean airway pressure of 9 cm H_2O, range of duration 28–70 days), and all had radiographs compatible with the diagnosis of BPD. Measurements were taken before a 1-hour exposure to heliox, at 15 and 60 minutes of heliox therapy, and at 15 and 60 minutes after heliox, while receiving oxygen-air. The heliox appeared to be well tolerated. There was a statistically significant increase in exhaled tidal volume and minute ventilation during heliox, there was an improvement in dynamic compliance, and the peak expiratory flow rate also improved with heliox. Heliox also enabled a significant reduction in the FiO_2. All of these changes reversed when the heliox was switched back to air-oxygen mixtures.

Although this pilot study does not allow for sweeping conclusions, it is a successful short-term feasibility trial with proof-of-concept support. There is a signal that heliox alters pulmonary mechanics and gas exchange, justifying a larger randomized controlled trial, although it will be difficult to conduct for a number of reasons, including blinding, standardization of equipment, and controlling for the myriad factors that contribute to the pathogenesis of BPD. Nevertheless, this was a well-performed pilot study that certainly suggests a role for heliox in BPD treatment. It will be up to us to define that role.

S. M. Donn, MD

Impact of early surfactant and inhaled nitric oxide therapies on outcomes in term/late preterm neonates with moderate hypoxic respiratory failure

Konduri GG, for the Neonatal Inhaled Nitric Oxide Study Group (Med College of Wisconsin, Milwaukee; Indiana Univ School of Medicine, Indianapolis; Stanford Univ, Palo Alto, CA; et al)

J Perinatol 33:944-949, 2013

Objective.—We conducted a *post-hoc* analysis of early inhaled nitric oxide (iNO)-randomized controlled trial data to identify associations pertinent to the management of moderate hypoxic respiratory failure in term/late preterm infants.

Study Design.—Univariate and multivariate logistic regression analyses were used to determine risk factors for the progression of respiratory failure and extracorporeal membrane oxygenation (ECMO)/death.

Result.—Among the 299 enrolled infants, oxygenation index (OI) <20 at enrollment (odds ratio 0.52, confidence interval (CI) 0.27 to 0.97) and surfactant use before randomization (odds ratio 0.47, CI 0.24 to 0.91) were associated with decreased ECMO/death rates. Early surfactant use for respiratory distress syndrome, perinatal aspiration syndrome and pneumonia/sepsis was associated with lower risk of ECMO/death ($P < 0.001$). Early iNO (OI 15 to 25) decreased the progression of respiratory failure to OI >30 ($P = 0.002$) and to composite outcome of OI >30 or ECMO/death ($P = 0.02$).

Conclusion.—This *post-hoc* analysis suggests that early use of surfactant and iNO in moderate respiratory failure is associated with improved outcomes.

▶ This post hoc analysis of data generated in an earlier trial of inhaled nitric oxide (iNO) for hypoxemic respiratory failure in term and late preterm infants has 2 interesting signals that could certainly be fertile future research paths. Although this is a diverse population with heterogeneous pathophysiology, there appears to be a benefit of initiating iNO earlier in the disease course. Although it is hard to ascertain mechanisms in a post hoc analysis, it makes sense to postulate that intercepting the cycle of pulmonary hypertension early might avoid the composite effects of inflammation, ventilator-induced lung injury, and surfactant inactivation or inhibition, with a very low risk for adverse effects. Second, surfactant repletion makes good sense in this situation. Multiple factors are capable of depleting the functional surfactant pool, including protein leak, inflammation, oxidative stress, and pulmonary hemorrhage. Restoring normal gas diffusion and lung mechanics might enable reduction in ventilatory support and improve oxygen uptake and reduction in ventilatory support, decreasing lung injury and perhaps improving cardiac performance. The challenge now is to design the right trials to test these hypotheses prospectively.

As an aside, it is time for us to find something better than the oxygenation index (OI) to express the degree of lung injury. The OI has never really been prospectively validated, and so much has changed since its initial application during the early extracorporeal membrane oxygenation trials of the 1980s. Moreover, because "mean airway pressure" on conventional ventilation is not the same as it is on high-frequency oscillatory ventilation, comparisons are next to impossible. Finally, it is a manipulatable metric in that once optimal lung inflation has been accomplished, further increases in mean airway pressure only result in hyperinflation without enhanced oxygenation, and the OI increases.

Maybe there's an industrious fellow or two out there looking for a project that might make a difference.

S. M. Donn, MD

Tracheomegaly in Infants with Severe Congenital Diaphragmatic Hernia Treated with Fetal Endoluminal Tracheal Occlusion

Zani A, Sellars M, Allen P, et al (King's College Hosp, London, UK; et al)

J Pediatr 164:1311-1315, 2014

Objective.—To measure and evaluate the effects of tracheal dimensions on survival and ventilation in a large series of infants with congenital diaphragmatic hernia (CDH) treated antenatally with fetal endoluminal tracheal occlusion (FETO).

Study Design.—Tracheal dimensions on chest radiograph (CR) were measured by 2 blinded radiologists. Survival, day 1 best oxygenation index and duration of ventilation, continuous positive airway pressure, and hospital stay were recorded. Survivors with a minimum 12-month follow-up were longitudinally compared for incidence of gastroesophageal reflux, chest infections, chest deformities, and hernia recurrence.

Results.—Seventy infants with CDH (41 who underwent FETO) were treated between 2004 and 2010. Hernia repair was performed in 26 infants without FETO (8 with patch repair) and 35 infants with FETO (26 with patch repair; $P = .0015$). Infants with FETO had a wider trachea than those without FETO at T1 ($P < .0001$) and between T1 and the carina ($P < .0001$). Tracheal diameter was similar in survivors and nonsurvivors in the FETO group. Tracheal size was not correlated with day 1 best oxygenation index in the FETO group ($R^2 = 0.17$) or the non-FETO group ($R^2 = 0.07$). There were no between-group differences in duration of mechanical ventilation ($P = .30$), continuous positive airway pressure ($P = .20$), or hospital stay ($P = .30$). In the longitudinal study, tracheal widths were larger on the last CR than on preoperative CR in patients without FETO (T1, $P = .02$; widest point, $P = .001$; carina, $P = .0001$), and for patients with FETO at the widest point ($P < .0001$) and at the carina ($P < .0001$), but not at T1 ($P = .12$). There were no differences in clinical variables between the FETO and non-FETO groups.

Conclusion.—FETO has a significant impact on tracheal size of infants with CDH; however, tracheal size does not affect survival or the requirement for early respiratory support.

▶ This study attempted to examine the impact of fetal endoluminal tracheal occlusion (FETO) for antenatally diagnosed congenital diaphragmatic hernia

(CDH) on the size of the trachea and its effect on mortality and ventilation. Infants who survived for at least 12 months were longitudinally followed for other complications.

FETO resulted in a larger tracheal diameter compared with infants with CDH not undergoing the same treatment. However, this did not have an effect on acute ventilatory status, as assessed by the best oxygenation index on day 1. Although there were no statistically significant differences, it would have been helpful to present more data, especially the proportion of infants in each group who received high frequency ventilation. Moreover, I wondered why the investigators chose the Oxygenation Index as the metric to assess ventilatory function. Tracheal size would be expected to affect airway resistance, and thus ventilation more than oxygenation, so some measure of carbon dioxide removal would be more meaningful.

In the longitudinal study, 38 patients (24 FETO, 14 non-FETO) were available for follow-up. Tracheal growth velocity was similar. There did not appear to be any significant differences in the incidence of the need for fundoplication for severe reflux, hospital admissions for severe chest infections, or chest wall deformities. What is worrisome, however, despite not reaching statistical significance (presumably from small numbers) was the rate of recurrence of the CDH, which was seen in 6 patients (30%) in the FETO group, but only 1 patient (8%) in the non-FETO group.

The jury is still out.

S. M. Donn, MD

Extracorporeal Life Support in Patients with Congenital Diaphragmatic Hernia: How Long Should We Treat?

Kays DW, Islam S, Richards DS, et al (Univ of Florida, Gainesville; Univ of Utah, Salt Lake City)

J Am Coll Surg 218:808-817, 2014

Background.—Congenital diaphragmatic hernia (CDH) is a frequently lethal birth defect and, despite advances, extracorporeal life support (ie, extracorporeal membrane oxygenation [ECMO]) is commonly required for severely affected patients. Published data suggest that CDH survival after 2 weeks on ECMO is poor. Many centers limit duration of ECMO support.

Study Design.—We conducted a single-institution retrospective review of 19 years of CDH patients treated with ECMO, designed to evaluate which factors affect survival and duration of ECMO and define how long patients should be supported.

Results.—Of two hundred and forty consecutive CDH patients without lethal associated anomalies, 96 were treated with ECMO and 72 (75%) survived. Eighty required a single run of ECMO and 65 survived (81%), 16 required a second ECMO run and 7 survived (44%). Of patients still on ECMO at 2 weeks, 56% survived, at 3 weeks 46% survived, and at 4 weeks, 43% of patients still on ECMO survived to discharge. After

5 weeks of ECMO, survival had dropped to 15%, and after 40 days of ECMO support there were no survivors. Apgar score at 1 minute, Apgar score at 5 minutes, and Congenital Diaphragmatic Hernia Study Group predicted survival all correlated with survival on ECMO, need for second ECMO, and duration of ECMO. Lung-to-head ratio also correlated with duration of ECMO. All survivors were discharged breathing spontaneously with no support other than nasal cannula oxygen if needed.

Conclusions.—In patients with severe CDH, improvement in pulmonary function sufficient to wean from ECMO can take 4 weeks or longer, and might require a second ECMO run. Pulmonary outcomes in these CDH patients can still be excellent, and the assignment of arbitrary ECMO treatment durations <4 weeks should be avoided.

▶ This article reported on a nearly 20-year experience of neonatal extracorporeal membrane oxygenation (ECMO) use in patients with congenital diaphragmatic hernia (CDH) unresponsive to conventional support and not accompanied by lethal anomalies. They attempted to determine if there should be a limit to the duration of extracorporeal support in these infants. Their sample size consisted of 240 consecutive CDH patients, of which, 96 were treated with ECMO and 72 (75%) survived to discharge. On this basis, the authors recommended not arbitrarily limiting the duration of ECMO therapy to less than 4 weeks.

Quite frankly, I found this report to be irresponsible. There is little we do to newborns that is more invasive than ECMO. If our goal is solely to discharge the baby from the neonatal intensive care unit alive, than ECMO has no limit. On the other hand, to make broad sweeping recommendations without examining the later outcomes and quality of survival—and there has been a 22-year interval to do so—clearly undermines the credibility of the recommendation. CDH is a devastating anomaly, which often affects multiple organs, not only the lung, but the heart and brain.

This really begs the question—Just because we can, should we?

S. M. Donn, MD

Fetal growth restriction and pulmonary hypertension in premature infants with bronchopulmonary dysplasia

Check J, Gotteiner N, Liu X, et al (Northwestern Univ Feinberg School of Medicine, Chicago, IL)

J Perinatol 33:553-557, 2013

Objective.—To identify the association between birth weight (BW)-for-gestational age (GA) and pulmonary hypertension (PHTN) at 36 weeks in infants with moderate-severe bronchopulmonary dysplasia (BPD).

Study Design.—In this retrospective cohort study, we followed 138 premature infants (≤28 weeks) with moderate and severe BPD (National Institutes of Health consensus definition) born at Prentice Women's Hospital between 2005 and 2009. BW percentiles were calculated using the Fenton growth curve for premature infants. PHTN was determined using a standardized algorithm of echocardiogram review at 36 weeks. Logistic regression was used to evaluate the associations between BW percentile subgroups and PHTN, taking into account antenatal and neonatal factors that were related to PHTN.

Result.—PHTN was associated with small BW-for-GA, ranging from thresholds of <10th to <25th percentile ($P<0.001$). These associations remained significant when comparing BW <25th percentile to the reference group (50 to 89th percentile); after adjustment for GA, gender, multiple gestation, race/ethnicity (odds ratio (OR) = 4.2; 95% confidence interval (CI) = 1.5, 12.1); and after further adjustment for maternal vascular disease, intrauterine infection, oligohydramnios and relevant postnatal factors (OR = 5.7; 95% CI = 1.5, 21.2). Longitudinal follow-up of this cohort showed a trend toward higher morbidity and death among PHTN infants with BW <25th percentile.

Conclusion.—BW-for-GA is an important predictor of PHTN in premature infants with moderate-severe BPD. Our findings contribute to the growing evidence supporting fetal mechanisms of later onset pulmonary vascular disease.

▶ After completion of 11 trials that enrolled nearly 3300 preterm infants with respiratory failure, the expected benefit of inhaled nitric oxide in that population has not been shown. An individual-subject meta-analysis[1] found no impact on death or chronic lung disease (as a combined outcome) or on severe neuroimaging abnormalities, either in the group in its entirety or in subgroups defined by several patient characteristics including birth weight, gestational age, oxygenation index, presence of patent ductus arteriosus, and signs of pulmonary hypertension. Consensus statements and review articles have concluded that inhaled nitric oxide cannot be recommended for routine treatment of respiratory failure in premature neonates, yet there remains a deep suspicion that there must be some subset of preterm infants who might benefit from use of that agent. For example, data from a small subset of subjects enrolled in the PiNO trial suggest a potential benefit for infants who have suspected pulmonary hypoplasia in association with premature rupture of membranes and oligohydramnios.[2]

This report takes a step back from consideration of therapy and attempts to identify factors that predict the presence of pulmonary hypertension in preterm infants with chronic lung disease. Among infants born at ≤28 weeks of gestation who had a persistent oxygen requirement at 36 weeks postmenstrual age, those with echocardiographic signs of pulmonary hypertension were smaller, less mature, and more likely to be black. In several multivariate risk adjustment models, low birth weight for gestational age (< 25th percentile) was also a significant predictor of increased risk for pulmonary hypertension. Among infants with pulmonary hypertension, those with birth weights less than the 25th percentile were more likely to die (5 of 22 vs 0 of 17), but this difference did not quite reach statistical significance ($P = .056$ by Fisher Exact test). It is unfortunate that mortality rates for infants with bronchopulmonary dysplasia (BPD) who did not have pulmonary hypertension were not reported, as that would allow the potentially more cogent comparison of mortality between small-for-gestational-age (SGA) infants with and without pulmonary hypertension. If all 20 small-for-dates infants without pulmonary hypertension at 36 weeks survived to discharge, pulmonary hypertension in SGA infants with BPD would have been a significant predictor of mortality ($P = .049$ by Fisher Exact test). Although these observations certainly must be considered preliminary, they suggest the hypothesis that SGA infants born at or before 28 weeks of gestation may constitute a particularly high-risk group that may benefit from inhaled nitric oxide therapy. This hypothesis is ripe for testing in a randomized, controlled trial.

W. E. Benitz, MD

References

1. Askie LM, Ballard RA, Cutter GR, et al. Inhaled nitric oxide in preterm infants: an individual-patient data meta-analysis of randomized trials. *Pediatrics.* 2011;128: 729-739.
2. Chock VY, Van Meurs KP, Hintz SR, et al. Inhaled nitric oxide for preterm premature rupture of membranes, oligohydramnios, and pulmonary hypoplasia. *Am J Perinatol.* 2009;26:317-322.

Variation in the Use of Diuretic Therapy for Infants With Bronchopulmonary Dysplasia

Slaughter JL, Stenger MR, Reagan PB (The Ohio State Univ College of Medicine and Nationwide Children's Hosp, Columbus; The Res Inst at Nationwide Children's Hosp, Columbus, OH)
Pediatrics 131:716-723, 2013

Objectives.—To determine (1) between-hospital variation in diuretic use for infants with bronchopulmonary dysplasia (BPD), including hospital-specific treatment frequency, treatment duration, and percentage of infants receiving short (≤5 consecutive days) versus longer (>5 days) courses, and to determine (2) demographic and clinical variables associated with diuretic administration.

Methods.—A retrospective cohort study was conducted with the use of the Pediatric Health Information System to determine between-hospital variation in diuretic utilization patterns (primary outcome) and variables associated with diuretic use among <29-week-gestation infants with evolving BPD at age 28 days who were discharged between January 2007 and June 2011.

Results.—During the 54-month study period, 1429 infants within 35 hospitals met the inclusion criteria for BPD at age 28 days, with 1222 (86%) receiving diuretic therapy for a median of 9 days (25th–75th percentile: 2–33 days). Short courses were administered to 1203 (83%) infants, and 570 (40%) infants received treatment for >5 consecutive days. Furosemide was the most widely prescribed diuretic (1218 infants; 85%), although chlorothiazide had the longest median duration of use (21 days; 25th–75th percentile: 8–46 days). The range of infants receiving a diuretic course of >5 days duration varied by hospital from 4% to 86%, with wide between-hospital variation even after adjustment for confounding variables.

Conclusions.—The frequency of diuretic administration to infants with BPD at US children's hospitals, as well as the specific diuretic regimen used, varies markedly by institution. Safety and effectiveness research of long-term diuretic therapy for BPD patients is needed to develop evidence based recommendations.

▶ This article reported the findings of a 4-year (2007–2011) retrospective cohort study evaluating the use of diuretics in infants with evolving bronchopulmonary dysplasia (BPD). Data were extracted from the Children's Hospital Association Pediatric Health Information System database. This database is assembled from 41 freestanding children's hospitals in the United States, representing 85% of such entities. The studied population comprised a total of 1429 admissions. Analysis of the data showed wide institutional differences in practices, including the specific agents used and the duration of therapy. This is hardly surprising, for as the authors indicate, there is little evidence of long-term effectiveness.

The use of diuretics to treat BPD is a long-standing practice in neonatology, handed down from one generation of neonatologists to the next. The basic tenet is that infants with BPD handle lung water poorly and that diuretic therapy may improve lung mechanics and gas exchange and enable the provision of more calories to improve nutrition and hence growth. Yet a closer look at the pathophysiology reveals a picture that can best be described as a dog chasing its tail. We administer a diuretic, and the baby diuresis. Nurses comment that the baby's urine output is up, and maybe he/she looks better. However, that urine also contains sodium, potassium, and calcium (some of which may be leached from bones and wind up in renal tubules, causing nephrolithiasis and nephrocalcinosis). We are wise to the salt and mineral loss, which we replete with supplementation, forcing us to do repetitive lab tests, and the repletion, in turn, causes fluid retention, which we treat with more diuretic.

When I see a practice that has variability this wide, I can only conclude that our depth of understanding is extremely shallow. We have little idea of what we are doing, and the chance to do harm may be substantial. This article strongly indicates the need to evaluate this practice through a large, randomized, multicenter trial and that we need to look beyond urine output and short-term respiratory improvement to assess both efficacy and safety. We are already 40 years late.

S. M. Donn, MD

Death or Neurodevelopmental Impairment at 18 to 22 Months Corrected Age in a Randomized Trial of Early Dexamethasone to Prevent Death or Chronic Lung Disease in Extremely Low Birth Weight Infants

Stark AR, on behalf of the Eunice Kennedy Shriver National Institute of Child Health and Human Development Neonatal Research Network (Vanderbilt Univ School of Medicine, Nashville, TN; et al)

J Pediatr 164:34-39.e2, 2014

Objective.—To evaluate the incidence of death or neurodevelopmental impairment (NDI) at 18-22 months corrected age in subjects enrolled in a trial of early dexamethasone treatment to prevent death or chronic lung disease in extremely low birth weight infants.

Study Design.—Evaluation of infants at 18-22 months corrected age included anthropomorphic measurements, a standard neurological examination, and the Bayley Scales of Infant Development-II, including the Mental Developmental Index and the Psychomotor Developmental Index. NDI was defined as moderate or severe cerebral palsy, Mental Developmental Index or Psychomotor Developmental Index <70, blindness, or hearing impairment.

Results.—Death or NDI at 18-22 months corrected age was similar in the dexamethasone and placebo groups (65% vs 66%, $P = .99$ among those with known outcome). The proportion of survivors with NDI was also similar, as were mean values for weight, length, and head circumference and the proportion of infants with poor growth (50% vs 41%, $P = .42$ for weight less than 10th percentile); 49% of infants in the placebo group received treatment with corticosteroid compared with 32% in the dexamethasone group ($P = .02$).

Conclusion.—The risk of death or NDI and rate of poor growth were high but similar in the dexamethasone and placebo groups. The lack of a discernible effect of early dexamethasone on neurodevelopmental outcome may be due to frequent clinical corticosteroid use in the placebo group.

▶ In the late 1990s, recognition that early postnatal use of corticosteroids is associated with an increased risk of intestinal perforation along with growing concerns about adverse effects of postnatal steroid exposure on long-term neurodevelopmental outcome dampened enthusiasm for use of dexamethasone for prevention or treatment of bronchopulmonary dysplasia (BPD). Despite issuance of consensus statements in 2002 and 2010 cautioning about these adverse effects and highlighting the weakness of evidence for long-term benefits of such treatments, the ambivalence of practitioners about the utility of this treatment is evident in our continuing use of dexamethasone as rescue therapy in nearly 10% of very low birth weight infants. This report provides reassurance that this practice may at least not be harmful, as long-term follow-up of infants enrolled in a large randomized trial did not show an increased risk of death or neurodevelopment, either separately or together, in subjects treated with a tapering regimen of dexamethasone (total dose, 7.64 mg/kg over 10 days beginning within 24 hours of birth). That trial was halted early because of an excess incidence of intestinal perforation in the treatment group, so these long-term results should not motivate adoption of that regimen. Furthermore, nearly half of the infants assigned to the placebo group received open-label steroid treatment, and those infants were substantially more likely to have abnormal neurologic findings at follow-up (41% vs 3%); this cross-contamination of the control group raises substantial doubts about the validity of that reassurance. The known adverse effects of early postnatal dexamethasone (intestinal perforation, in particular) remain sufficient to make the case that such treatment is harmful and does not merit further investigation. We do not yet know, however, whether early treatment with hydrocortisone or later selective treatment with either hydrocortisone or dexamethasone may offer some benefit. Three ongoing trials of hydrocortisone for prevention or treatment of evolving BPD may help answer these questions. There is much work to do before we can translate the widely shared anecdotal experience of marked improvement in severity of lung disease, often enabling extubation, in preterm infants treated with steroids into an evidence-based strategy for management of BPD.

W. E. Benitz, MD

Association between Postnatal Dexamethasone for Treatment of Bronchopulmonary Dysplasia and Brain Volumes at Adolescence in Infants Born Very Preterm

Cheong JLY, for the Victorian Infant Collaborative Study Group (Royal Women's Hosp, Melbourne, Victoria, Australia; et al)

J Pediatr 164:737-743.e1, 2014

Objectives.—To compare brain volumes in adolescents who were born extremely preterm (<28 weeks gestation) who had received postnatal dexamethasone, and to determine if there was a postnatal dexamethasone dose–response effect on brain volumes.

Study Design.—Geographical cohort study of extremely preterm adolescents born in 1991-1992 in Victoria, Australia. T1-weighted magnetic resonance imaging was performed at 18 years of age. Segmented and parcellated brain volumes were calculated using an automated segmentation method (FreeSurfer) and compared between groups, with and without adjustment for potential confounders. The relationships between total postnatal dexamethasone dose and brain volumes were explored using linear regression.

Results.—Of the 148 extremely preterm participants, 55 (37%) had received postnatal dexamethasone, with a cumulative mean dose of 7.7 mg/kg. Compared with participants who did not receive postnatal dexamethasone, those who did had smaller total brain tissue volumes (mean difference −3.6%, 95% CI [−7.0%, −0.3%], *P* value = .04) and smaller white matter, thalami, and basal ganglia volumes (all $P < .05$). There was a trend of smaller total brain and white matter volumes with increasing dose of postnatal dexamethasone (regression coefficient −7.7 [95% CI −16.2, 0.8] and −3.2 [−6.6, 0.2], respectively).

Conclusions.—Extremely preterm adolescents who received postnatal dexamethasone in the newborn period had smaller total brain tissue volumes than those who did not receive postnatal dexamethasone, particularly white matter, thalami, and basal ganglia. Vulnerability of brain tissues or structures associated with postnatal dexamethasone varies by structure and persists into adolescence.

► I echo the thoughts expressed by Kristi Watterberg in the editorial that accompanied this report.[1] The authors of this cohort study did a remarkable job of following a large group of children who had received postnatal dexamethasone as part of the treatment for bronchopulmonary dysplasia (BPD) to determine if there was a dose-response effect on the reduction of brain volume, as found on magnetic resonance imaging performed at 18 years of age. Compared with participants who had not received postnatal dexamethasone, the treated children had smaller total brain volumes and decreased white matter, thalamic, and basal ganglia volumes.

Although it may be next to impossible to control for all of the factors that could have contributed to these findings, this association is again a worrisome one, given the widespread use of steroid therapy in babies with BPD. Although it may be argued that the likelihood of steroid receipt—as well as the dose and duration of therapy—increases with severity of disease, and the sicker the baby the greater the risk of brain injury, we need to face the fact that the downside of steroid therapy is significant, and there is certainly a biological plausibility in the inhibitory effects that steroids play on alveolar growth. The short-term benefits in improving respiratory function often lead to repeated courses and difficulty in weaning many babies from steroid treatment, and the effects probably differ depending on which corticosteroid is used.

Nevertheless, this superb long-term cohort study sends a very powerful message, even if it does not prove a cause and effect relationship.

S. M. Donn, MD

Reference

1. Watterberg KL. Dexamethasone and the brain at age 18 years: randomize the first baby—and follow-up. *J Pediatr.* 2014;164:687-689.

Mesenchymal Stem Cells for Bronchopulmonary Dysplasia: Phase 1 Dose-Escalation Clinical Trial

Chang YS, Ahn SY, Yoo HS, et al (Sungkyunkwan Univ School of Medicine, Seoul, Korea; MEDIPOST Co Ltd, Seoul, Korea)

J Pediatr 164:966-972.e6, 2014

Objective.—To assess the safety and feasibility of allogeneic human umbilical cord blood (hUCB)-derived mesenchymal stem cell (MSC) transplantation in preterm infants.

Study Design.—In a phase I dose-escalation trial, we assessed the safety and feasibility of a single, intratracheal transplantation of hUCB-derived MSCs in preterm infants at high risk for bronchopulmonary dysplasia (BPD). The first 3 patients were given a low dose (1×10^7 cells/kg) of cells, and the next 6 patients were given a high dose (2×10^7 cells/kg). We compared their adverse outcomes, including BPD severity, with those of historical case-matched comparison group.

Results.—Intratracheal MSC transplantation was performed in 9 preterm infants, with a mean gestational age of 25.3 ± 0.9 weeks and a mean birth weight of 793 ± 127 g, at a mean of 10.4 ± 2.6 days after birth. The treatments were well tolerated, without serious adverse effects or dose-limiting toxicity attributable to the transplantation. Levels of interleukin-6, interleukin-8, matrix metalloproteinase-9, tumor necrosis factor α, and transforming growth factor $\beta 1$ in tracheal aspirates at day 7 were significantly reduced compared with those at baseline or at day 3 post-transplantation. BPD severity was lower in the transplant recipients, and rates of other adverse outcomes did not differ between the comparison group and transplant recipients.

Conclusion.—Intratracheal transplantation of allogeneic hUCB-derived MSCs in preterm infants is safe and feasible, and warrants a larger and controlled phase II study.

▶ In recent years, stem cell-based therapies have been the subject of active basic and translational research, with the hope of becoming a therapeutic breakthrough for many incurable diseases. In neonatology, bronchopulmonary dysplasia (BPD) and hypoxic-ischemic encephalopathy (HIE) are 2 diseases associated with lifelong consequences and no means to repair the injured organs. In search of novel approaches to these problems, stem cell therapies have been extensively tested in preclinical models of both BPD and HIE, with encouraging results. Mesenchymal stem cells (MSCs), in particular, have been tested in murine models of BPD and reported to attenuate alveolar and lung vascular injury. MSCs are also being widely used in clinical trials on adults and are particularly appealing because of their relatively simple isolation and production. In this study, Chang et al reported the results of the first phase I, dose-escalation trial of a single intratracheal administration of umbilical cord blood-derived MSCs to preterm infants. Nine infants at high risk for BPD (25.3 ± 0.9 weeks of gestational age, 10.4 ± 2.6 days old, still requiring ventilator support) were treated with either a low dose (n = 3) or a high dose (n = 6) of intratracheal MSCs. All infants tolerated the treatment well, without signs of cardiorespiratory compromise. BPD severity was lower in treated infants compared with historical matched controls, although this phase I study does not allow us to reach any conclusions regarding the efficacy of this intervention. Nevertheless, this first-of-its-kind study found that intratracheal administration of MSCs is feasible, well tolerated, and safe in the short term in extremely preterm neonates. Long-term follow-up of these infants is imperative, given the theoretical potential of MSCs to enhance tumor growth or lead to malignant transformation. Additional studies are needed to establish the efficacy of this intervention and to clarify issues related to mechanisms of action, safety, and dosing strategies.

M. Sola-Visner, MD

Late Outcomes of a Randomized Trial of High-Frequency Oscillation in Neonates

Zivanovic S, for the United Kingdom Oscillation Study Group (King's College London, UK; et al)

N Engl J Med 370:1121-1130, 2014

Background.—Results from an observational study involving neonates suggested that high-frequency oscillatory ventilation (HFOV), as compared with conventional ventilation, was associated with superior small-airway function at follow-up. Data from randomized trials are needed to confirm this finding.

Methods.—We studied 319 adolescents who had been born before 29 weeks of gestation and had been enrolled in a multicenter, randomized trial that compared HFOV with conventional ventilation immediately after birth. The trial involved 797 neonates, of whom 592 survived to hospital discharge. We compared follow-up data from adolescents who had been randomly assigned to HFOV with follow-up data from those who had been randomly assigned to conventional ventilation, with respect to lung function and respiratory health, health-related quality of life, and functional status, as assessed with the use of questionnaires completed when the participants were 11 to 14 years of age. The primary outcome was forced expiratory flow at 75% of the expired vital capacity (FEF_{75}).

Results.—The HFOV group had superior results on a test of small-airway function (z score for FEF_{75}, −0.97 with HFOV vs. −1.19 with conventional therapy; adjusted difference, 0.23 [95% confidence interval, 0.02 to 0.45]). There were significant differences in favor of HFOV in several other measures of respiratory function, including forced expiratory volume in 1 second, forced vital capacity, peak expiratory flow, diffusing capacity, and impulse-oscillometric findings. As compared with the conventional-therapy group, the HFOV group had significantly higher ratings from teachers in three of eight school subjects assessed, but there were no other significant differences in functional outcomes.

Conclusions.—In a randomized trial involving children who had been born extremely prematurely, those who had undergone HFOV, as compared with those who had received conventional ventilation, had superior lung function at 11 to 14 years of age, with no evidence of poorer functional outcomes.

▶ High-frequency oscillatory ventilation (HFOV) has been proposed as a means to reduce lung injury in preterm infants by providing a constant pressure to maintain lung volumes, while ventilating with very low tidal volumes. This approach has not been universally embraced, however, partly because of concerns from an early randomized trial comparing HFOV (using a low-volume strategy) with conventional ventilation (CV), in which infants in the HFOV group had a significantly higher incidence of grade 3/4 intraventricular hemorrhage and periventricular leukomalacia. Subsequent studies did not confirm those findings, but the risks and benefits of HFOV were inconsistent. The United Kingdom Oscillation Study (UKOS) was a multicenter, randomized trial in which very preterm infants were randomly assigned to receive either HFOV (using a high-volume strategy) or conventional ventilation within 1 hour after birth. In this article, Zivanovic et al reports on the outcomes of 319 surviving children from the UKOS study, at 11 to 14 years of age. The primary outcome was small airway function, assessed by measurement of forced expiratory flow at 75% of the expired vital capacity (FEF_{75}), but a battery of pulmonary function studies was performed. Behavioral outcomes, health-related quality of life, and academic achievement were assessed with questionnaires filled by children, parents, and teachers. Overall, children in the HFOV group had significantly better pulmonary function test results compared with the CV group. The overall differences were relatively small, but the percentage of children with FEF_{75} results below the 10th percentile was 37% in the HFOV compared with 47% in the CV group, a finding of likely clinical significance. Academically, the HFOV group was rated higher in 3 of 8 school subjects assessed. Overall, this study supports that the early use of HFOV in preterm neonates is associated with better results in tests of small airway function in teenage years compared with CV, without detrimental neurodevelopmental effects.

M. Sola-Visner, MD

Accurate Automated Apnea Analysis in Preterm Infants

Vergales BD, Paget-Brown AO, Lee H, et al (Univ of Virginia, Charlottesville; The College of William and Mary, Williamsburg, VA)
Am J Perinatol 31:157-162, 2014

Objective.—In 2006 the apnea of prematurity (AOP) consensus group identified inaccurate counting of apnea episodes as a major barrier to progress in AOP research. We compare nursing records of AOP to events detected by a clinically validated computer algorithm that detects apnea from standard bedside monitors.

Study Design.—Waveform, vital sign, and alarm data were collected continuously from all very low-birth-weight infants admitted over a 25-month period, analyzed for central apnea, bradycardia, and desaturation (ABD) events, and compared with nursing documentation collected from charts. Our algorithm defined apnea as > 10 seconds if accompanied by bradycardia and desaturation.

Results.—Of the 3,019 nurse-recorded events, only 68% had any algorithm-detected ABD event. Of the 5,275 algorithm-detected prolonged apnea events > 30 seconds, only 26% had nurse-recorded documentation within 1 hour. Monitor alarms sounded in only 74% of events of algorithm-detected prolonged apnea events > 10 seconds. There were 8,190,418 monitor alarms of any description throughout the neonatal intensive care unit during the 747 days analyzed, or one alarm every 2 to 3 minutes per nurse.

Conclusion.—An automated computer algorithm for continuous ABD quantitation is a far more reliable tool than the medical record to address the important research questions identified by the 2006 AOP consensus group.

▶ Impaired respiratory control and resultant apnea, bradycardia, and desaturation remain major areas of consternation in the neonatal intensive care unit and beyond. These events are percipients for both pharmacotherapy and ventilatory support, and their long-term consequences are unclear, hence the need to better characterize such events via computer algorithm, as done by Vergales and her colleagues at the University of Virginia.

The first observation that nursing observation underestimates these exceedingly frequent events is not surprising and has been previously documented by these investigators. More surprising is the reverse—namely, that in far more than 30% of nurse-recorded events, the computer algorithm did not find an apnea event of at least 10 seconds' duration. The likely explanation is that impedance-based respiratory monitoring failed to identify episodes of mixed or obstructive apnea with continuing chest wall motion in the absence of airflow.

Great strides have been made in documenting continuous heart rate and oxygen saturation levels in neonates over prolonged periods. This circumvents reliance on respiratory monitoring, even though immature respiratory control superimposed on a lung with decreased oxygen reserves is the major problem. However, it is important not to give up on noninvasive measurement of airflow and effective ventilation; several bioengineering groups are pursing this challenge. Such novel collaboration between clinical scientists and bioengineers is important if we are to advance in addressing the major outstanding issue: Do these episodes of apnea, bradycardia, and saturation matter?

R. J. Martin, MD
J. M. Di Fiore, BSEE

Application of Transcutaneous Carbon Dioxide Tension Monitoring with Low Electrode Temperatures in Premature Infants in the Early Postnatal Period

Hirata K, Nishihara M, Oshima Y, et al (Osaka Med Ctr and Res Inst for Maternal and Child Health, Japan)
Am J Perinatol 31:435-439, 2014

Objective.—The aim of this article is to evaluate the accuracy, precision, and safety of transcutaneous carbon dioxide tension ($TcPCO_2$) monitoring at different electrode temperatures in preterm infants in the early postnatal period.

Study Design.—A total of 26 neonates with a median birth weight of 974 g (432–1,694 g) and gestational age of 28.0 weeks (26.1–31.3 weeks) were studied in the first 5 days of life. A total of 252 simultaneous pairs ($TcPCO_2$ and arterial carbon dioxide tension [$PaCO_2$]) were analyzed at 38, 39, and 40°C at 26 and 27 weeks, and at 38, 39, 40, and 42°C at 28 to 31 weeks.

Results.—The mean difference of $TcPCO_2$ and $PaCO_2$ (bias) increased from 3.93 mm Hg at 42°C to 5.64 mm Hg at 40°C, 6.58 mm Hg at 39°C, and 6.07 mm Hg at 38°C. Standard deviation (SD) of the bias increased from 4.17 mm Hg at 42°C to 4.76 mm Hg at 40°C, 5.29 mm Hg at 39°C, and 5.07 mm Hg at 38°C. Adverse skin lesions were not observed.

Conclusion.—$TcPCO_2$ measurements are the most accurate and precise at an electrode temperature of 42°C. However, in premature babies, monitoring at 38, 39, and 40°C is possible provided a bias correction of 6 mm Hg and SD of 5 mm Hg are applied.

▶ Although transcutaneous measurements of oxygen ($TcPO_2$) and carbon dioxide ($TcPCO_2$) tensions have been around for decades, their popularity has waxed and waned. The simplicity and reliability of pulse oximetry all but replaced $TcPO_2$, and the cost, labor intensiveness, and variable reliability, as well as the emergence of end-tidal CO_2 monitoring, resulted in the decline of $TcPCO_2$ monitoring for many years.

Recent observations of the importance of not only absolute PCO_2 tensions but also the rapidity of change have placed new importance on $TcPCO_2$ monitoring. This is especially important when a baby is switched from conventional to high-frequency ventilation, where PCO_2 can drop dramatically.

Some of the reluctance in using $TcPCO_2$ in very preterm babies has been the worry about skin burns because of the high temperature to which the electrode is heated. In this observational study, the investigators demonstrated reasonable reliability of the device at lower temperatures. Although the scatter is wider, there is still a reasonable correlation. Moreover, the value of the device as a trend monitor makes it invaluable in many clinical situations in which arterial blood gas sampling is not possible.

S. M. Donn, MD

Test–retest reliability of the infant car-seat challenge

Davis NL, Gregory ML, Rhein L (Univ of Maryland Hosp for Children, Baltimore; Beth Israel Deaconess Med Ctr, Boston, MA; Boston Children's Hosp, MA)

J Perinatol 34:54-58, 2014

Objective.—To evaluate how a single infant car-seat challenge (ICSC) predicts subsequent respiratory physiology in premature infants.

Study Design.—Prospective observational study of infants born at <37 weeks gestational age. Subjects underwent three ICSCs and we evaluated clinical characteristics, pass rate, and predictive value of a single ICSC pass.

Result.—Completed three ICSCs on 60 subjects. Seven failed initial ICSC (11.7%). Those who failed had lower birth weights. Of the 53 that initially passed, 47 passed two subsequent tests (89%). Those who passed an initial test and failed a subsequent test had lower weights at each ICSC.

Conclusion.—Our results indicate that passing an ICSC is highly predictive of passing subsequent ICSCs. Lower weights at birth and at the time of ICSC were associated with increased risk of failure. We recommend including low birth weight as an inclusion criterion for ICSCs.

▶ Since 1991, the American Academy of Pediatrics has recommended performance of an infant car-seat challenge (ICSC) test on preterm infants before discharge from the hospital. That recommendation is based on observations that preterm infants and, to a lesser extent, term infants, have more episodes of airway obstruction and oxygen desaturation after extended periods of being upright in an infant car seat coupled with concern that those additional episodes of respiratory instability may lead to neurodevelopmental compromise. It has also been surmised that airway compromise caused by neck flexion during sleep while upright in a car seat may place infants at an increased risk of sudden infant death. The evidence supporting several links in these putative chains of causation is remarkably scant, however. The criteria for "failure" of an ICSC have never been clearly defined. In this report, the authors defined failure as any desaturation to less than 90% for more than 10 seconds; apnea for greater than 20 seconds; an episode of bradycardia to less than 80 beats per minute; or any worrisome alteration in vital signs, work of breathing, or respiratory distress confirmed by a physician or nurse practitioner. Infants who had no such events during a 90-minute period of monitoring in a car seat were very likely (89%) to pass subsequent tests. The predictive value of such abnormalities was much lower; however, more than half of the infants who failed the first test passed a subsequent test performed within 96 hours. The authors suggest that this may reflect improving respiratory control with advancing maturity, but the observation raises some doubt about even the short-term predictive value of a failed ICSC. Although there are a few case reports of apparent life-threatening events and sudden deaths of infants in car seats, we do not know whether being in a car seat increases the risk of these events, or, if so, by how much. Most importantly, no evidence directly correlates ICSC findings with either sudden death or neurodevelopmental outcome, so it is not clear what we should be looking for or what we may be preventing by those maneuvers. These questions are ripe for systematic study, perhaps through inclusion of detailed information about ICSC findings in searchable form in the electronic medical record to enable correlation with later events. Until such data are available, this standard practice will remain at the margins of evidence-based medicine. This investigation of the reproducibility of ICSC testing is a strong start toward remediation of that condition.

W. E. Benitz, MD

Two-Year Outcomes of a Randomized Controlled Trial of Inhaled Nitric Oxide in Premature Infants

Durrmeyer X, for the European Union Nitric Oxide Study Group (Centre Hospitalier Intercommunal de Créteil, France; et al)
Pediatrics 132:e695-e703, 2013

Background and Objectives.—The European Union Nitric Oxide trial was designed to assess the potential benefits of inhaled nitric oxide (iNO) compared with placebo in infants with respiratory failure. This follow-up study evaluated respiratory, neurodevelopmental, and other outcomes for infants entered into the European Union Nitric Oxide trial to age 2 years.

Methods.—In a multicenter, randomized, double-blind study, preterm infants born at <29 weeks' gestation with moderate respiratory failure were allocated to receive iNO (5 ppm) or placebo for 7 to 21 days. Subjects underwent assessments at 1 and 2 years corrected for prematurity.

Results.—At 36 weeks' postmenstrual age, 696 of 792 infants were alive; 4 in the iNO arm subsequently died before age 2 years compared with 7 in the control arm. We evaluated 95% of the survivors at 12 months and 90% at 2 years. In the iNO arm, 244 of 363 (67.2%) infants had survived without disability at age 2 years compared with 270 of 374 (72.2%) who received placebo ($P = .094$). Mean (SD) cognitive composite scores (Bayley Scales of Infant and Toddler Development, third edition) were 94 (13) in the iNO group and 95 (14) in the placebo group; in the iNO group, 19% scored <85 and 9.5% developed cerebral palsy compared with 13.3% and 9%, respectively. There were no significant differences in hospitalizations overall or due to respiratory illness in use of home oxygen therapy or respiratory medications, in growth, or in other health outcomes.

Conclusions.—At 2 years of age, low-dose (5 ppm) iNO started early (<24 hours after birth) for a median of 20 days did not affect neurodevelopmental or other health outcomes.

▶ Demonstration that inhaled nitric oxide (iNO) is protective against physiologic and histopathologic manifestations of bronchopulmonary dysplasia (BPD) in experimental animals led to more than a dozen randomized controlled trials of iNO for prevention of BPD in preterm human infants. Although these trials yielded tantalizing glimpses of beneficial effects, those often came through post-hoc subgroup analyses, no consistent pattern of short-term advantages has become apparent, and only a single trial found a statistically significant reduction in the rate of death or BPD. Although heterogeneity of trial designs makes pooling of data across these trials largely inappropriate, consistently negative results from different trial designs also suggest that failure to show benefits is not merely an artifact of an infelicitous choice of study population, enrollment criteria, timing, dose, or duration of treatment. However, these disappointing results were offset by suggestions of potential neurodevelopmental benefits. As late follow-up data have accrued, that possibility has not been realized. This report confirms the absence of late pulmonary or neurosensory benefits among subjects enrolled in yet another study, the European Union Nitric Oxide trial. These results are similar to those reported from other large clinical trials, which also found no improvement in outcomes at 2 to 5 years (depending on the study).[1-4] Accordingly, the main conclusion of the National Institutes of Health Consensus Conference—that inhaled nitric oxide is not indicated for management of preterm infants with respiratory failure—remains valid, unless re-evaluations of study subjects at school age provide evidence that compels revision. For now, at least, efforts to reduce the burdens of chronic lung disease and neurodevelopmental impairments in preterm infants will have to pursue other avenues.

W. E. Benitz, MD

References

1. Hintz SR, Van Meurs KP, Perritt R, et al. Neurodevelopmental outcomes of premature infants with severe respiratory failure enrolled in a randomized controlled trial of inhaled nitric oxide. *J Pediatr.* 2007;151:16-22.
2. Huddy CL, Bennett CC, Hardy P, et al. The INNOVO multicentre randomised controlled trial: neonatal ventilation with inhaled nitric oxide versus ventilatory support without nitric oxide for severe respiratory failure in preterm infants: follow up at 4-5 years. *Arch Dis Child Fetal Neonatal Ed.* 2008;93:F430-F435.
3. Watson RS, Clermont G, Kinsella JP, et al. Clinical and economic effects of iNO in premature newborns with respiratory failure at 1 year. *Pediatrics.* 2009;124: 1333-1343.
4. Walsh MC, Hibbs AM, Martin CR, et al. Two-year neurodevelopmental outcomes of ventilated preterm infants treated with inhaled nitric oxide. *J Pediatr.* 2010;156: 556-561.e1.

8 Central Nervous System and Special Senses

Intraventricular Hemorrhage and Neurodevelopmental Outcomes in Extreme Preterm Infants

Bolisetty S, on behalf of the New South Wales and Australian Capital Territory Neonatal Intensive Care Units' Data Collection (Royal Hosp for Women, Sydney, Australia; et al)

Pediatrics 133:55-62, 2014

Objective.—Not many large studies have reported the true impact of lower-grade intraventricular hemorrhages in preterm infants. We studied the neurodevelopmental outcomes of extremely preterm infants in relation to the severity of intraventricular hemorrhage.

Methods.—A regional cohort study of infants born at 23 to 28 weeks' gestation and admitted to a NICU between 1998 and 2004. Primary outcome measure was moderate to severe neurosensory impairment at 2 to 3 years' corrected age defined as developmental delay (developmental quotient >2 SD below the mean), cerebral palsy, bilateral deafness, or bilateral blindness.

Results.—Of the 1472 survivors assessed, infants with grade III–IV intraventricular hemorrhage (IVH; $n = 93$) had higher rates of developmental delay (17.5%), cerebral palsy (30%), deafness (8.6%), and blindness (2.2%). Grade I–II IVH infants ($n = 336$) also had increased rates of neurosensory impairment (22% vs 12.1%), developmental delay (7.8% vs 3.4%), cerebral palsy (10.4% vs 6.5%), and deafness (6.0% vs 2.3%) compared with the no IVH group ($n = 1043$). After exclusion of 40 infants with late ultrasound findings (periventricular leukomalacia, porencephaly, ventricular enlargement), isolated grade I–II IVH ($n = 296$) had increased rates of moderate-severe neurosensory impairment (18.6% vs 12.1%). Isolated grade I–II IVH was also independently associated with a higher risk of neurosensory impairment (adjusted odds ratio 1.73, 95% confidence interval 1.22–2.46).

Conclusions.—Grade I–II IVH, even with no documented white matter injury or other late ultrasound abnormalities, is associated with adverse neurodevelopmental outcomes in extremely preterm infants.

▶ Grade III and IV intraventricular hemorrhage (IVH), cystic periventricular leukomalacia, and late ventriculomegaly are recognized predictors of adverse neurodevelopmental sequelae in preterm infants, but less is known about the impact of Grade I and II IVH. In the above retrospective regional cohort study, the authors analyzed prospectively collected data from all 10 tertiary care neonatal intensive care units (NICUs) in New South Wales and the Australian Capital Territory. All 2701 infants between 23 and 28 weeks' gestation admitted to the NICUs between 1998 and 2004 were assessed for study eligibility. Infants with major congenital anomalies and those who died before first cranial ultrasound were excluded. A standard cranial ultrasound protocol using the Papile classification was followed. Ultrasound interpretation was based on the reports of radiologists and/or neonatologists at time of hospitalization. Infants received a standardized neurodevelopmental assessment and a review of the medical record between ages 2 and 3, corrected for prematurity. Moderate neurosensory impairment was defined as development between 2 and 3 standard deviations below the mean, moderate cerebral palsy, or deafness. Severe impairment was defined as development 3 standard deviations below the mean, severe cerebral palsy, or bilateral blindness.

Multivariate analysis was conducted using logistic regression models and adjusted for significant clinical characteristics. Of 2414 infants initially enrolled in the study, 1472 survivors were assessed. Analyses were performed to determine the relationship between the study groups (no IVH, grade I–II IVH, grade III–IV IVH) and neurodevelopmental outcome; 62.2% of the infants with grade III–IV IVH died before their 2- to 3-year assessment, compared with 15.7% of the infants with grade I–II IVH and 11% of the infants with no IVH. Surviving infants lost to follow-up before the age 2- to 3-year assessment tended to be healthier on many initial measures, such as a higher birth weight, absence of systemic infection, and less need for home oxygen compared with those who completed the age 2- to 3-year assessments.

Pregnancy-induced hypertension, antenatally detected intrauterine growth restriction, cesarean delivery, and antenatal steroids were protective against IVH. Male gender, low Apgar scores at birth, and delivery outside a tertiary care center were associated with a higher risk of grade III–IV IVH. Major morbidities including chronic lung disease, postnatal steroid therapy, patent ductus arteriosus, necrotizing enterocolitis, sepsis, and severe retinopathy of prematurity were significantly associated with IVH of any grade. Pneumothorax was associated with grade III–IV IVH. Higher rates of moderate-severe neurosensory impairment were seen with increasing grades of IVH. The impairment rates for no-IVH infants was 12.1%; for grade I–II IVH, 22%; and for grade III–IV IVH, 43%. When periventricular leukomalacia, porencephalic cyst, and ventricular dilatation were excluded, isolated grade I–II IVH resulted in an 18.6% rate of impairment. The adjusted odds ratios for moderate-severe impairment were 1.61 (95% confidence interval 1.14–2.28) for infants with grade I–II IVH and

3.81 (95% confidence interval 2.30–6.30) for infants with grade III–IV IVH, compared with infants with no IVH. Small for gestational age, male gender, periventricular leukomalacia, chronic lung disease, and retinopathy of prematurity independently predicted significant adverse outcomes.

A limitation of the study is that ultrasound does not easily identify white matter injury, which may contribute to adverse outcomes in the grade I–II IVH group. Nonetheless, this well-designed study adds to the growing number of studies from different populations reporting similarly concerning developmental outcomes among infants with isolated low grades of IVH. This article suggests that a cautious approach toward long-term developmental outcomes may be indicated when counseling families of infants with grade I–II IVH. Long-term follow-up and screening for adverse neurodevelopmental outcomes is indicated for this population.

C. A. Buysse, MD

Risk Factors for Intraventricular Hemorrhage in Term Asphyxiated Newborns Treated With Hypothermia

Al Yazidi G, Srour M, Wintermark P (McGill Univ, Montreal, Quebec, Canada)

Pediatr Neurol 50:630-635, 2014

Background.—Intraventricular hemorrhage is rare in term newborns. Severe asphyxia is recognized as one of the risk factors of intraventricular hemorrhage in these newborns. Therapeutic hypothermia, which is the only available treatment for the limitation of brain injury in term asphyxiated newborns, may cause fluctuations of cerebral blood flow, possibly placing the newborn more at risk for intraventricular hemorrhage. The literature regarding the incidence of intraventricular hemorrhage in the context of neonatal hypoxic-ischemic encephalopathy and hypothermia is sparse.

Methods.—We present a clinical observation and review the literature regarding the risk factors for intraventricular hemorrhage in term asphyxiated newborns treated with hypothermia.

Results.—We describe the clinical course of a term newborn with severe hypoxic-ischemic encephalopathy who developed significant intraventricular hemorrhage during the rewarming period after the 72-hour hypothermia.

Conclusion.—This newborn presented several risk factors for intraventricular hemorrhage, including severe asphyxia, hemodynamic instability, hemostasis disturbances, instrument delivery, venous sinus thrombosis, and hypoglycemia. Hypothermia and rewarming also may have contributed by causing fluctuations in cerebral blood flow.

▶ Sometimes case reports and anecdotes can be instructional. Not this one. The authors present the case of a full-term newborn who was asphyxiated at birth, underwent neuroprotective cooling, and was diagnosed with an intraventricular hemorrhage (IVH). Using this case, they summarized a list of risk factors for IVH in full-term newborns. OK, but what's new?

More concerning was the decision to subject this baby to cooling. This was a growth-restricted infant with a 24-hour history of decreased movement and a nonreassuring fetal heart rate pattern. The cord pH of 7.15 is not terribly abnormal and would not qualify the infant for cooling in any of the published large clinical trials. Intrauterine growth restriction is also a risk factor for IVH. Was he initially polycythemic or thrombocytopenic? Could this baby have sustained a prenatal stroke, and could his difficult transition be an effect rather than a cause? The timing of the hemorrhage is a presumption. It does not appear that daily neuroimaging was performed.

It is also troublesome that cooling was chosen as a culprit. In all of the clinical trials, the incidence of coagulopathy and other systemic complications was no different between cooled and control groups. Maybe all of the fluid boluses and pressors were equally or even more contributory.

I wonder if this would have been accepted if submitted to a neonatal journal.

S. M. Donn, MD

Can neurophysiological assessment improve timing of intervention in posthaemorrhagic ventricular dilatation?

Klebermass-Schrehof K, Rona Z, Waldhör T, et al (Med Univ of Vienna, Austria; et al)

Arch Dis Child Fetal Neonatal Ed 98:F291-F297, 2013

Objective.—Intraventricular haemorrhage is still the most common cause of brain lesion in preterm infants and development of a posthaemorrhagic ventricular dilatation (PHVD) can lead to additional neurological sequelae. Flash visual evoked potentials (fVEP) and amplitude-integrated electroencephalography (aEEG) are non-invasive neurophysiological monitoring tools. The aim of the study was to evaluate fVEPs and aEEGs in preterm infants with progressive PHVD prior to and after neurosurgical intervention for cerebrospinal fluid removal and to correlate the findings with severity of ventricular dilatation.

Design.—fVEPs and aEEGs were performed weekly in infants with developing PHVD. As soon as the ventricular index reached the 97th percentile recordings were performed twice a week.

Methods.—17 patients admitted to the neonatal intensive care unit of the Medical University of Vienna who developed progressive PHVD were evaluated using fVEP and aEEG until and after reduction of intracranial pressure by placement of an external ventricular drainage.

Results.—In all 17 cases (100%) wave latencies of fVEP increased above normal range and aEEG showed increased suppression in 13 patients (76%) with increasing ventricular dilatation. Both methods showed normalisation of patterns mostly within a week of successful therapeutic intervention (mean 8.5 days). Both changes in fVEP latencies and aEEG background patterns were detected before clinical signs of elevated intracranial pressure occurred. In only 10 patients (58.8%) ventricular width exceeded the 97th percentile + 4 mm.

Conclusions.—fVEP and aEEG are useful additional tools for the evaluation of preterm infants with progressive PHVD.

► Clear criteria identifying whether to intervene in posthemorrhagic hydrocephalus, the optimal timing of intervention, and what procedure to perform have not been well established, hence these topics often evoke lively debate among neonatologists, neurologists, and neurosurgeons. The investigators conducting this study of 17 infants with progressive posthemorrhagic ventricular dilatation admitted to the neonatal intensive care unit of the Medical University of Vienna assessed amplitude-integrated electroencephalography (aEEG) flash visual-evoked potentials (fVEP). Although imaging showed, in just 59% of the infants, ventricular widths beyond the 97th percentile + 4 mm, the scientists that found 76% of infants exhibited a suppressed pattern on aEEG, and all exhibited increased fVEP wave latencies. Although further study clearly is needed, these data suggest that aEEG and fVEP might be useful tools to provide objective noninvasive measures that can easily be followed sequentially to assess at least short-term functional brain effects of ventricular dilatation. The accompanying editorial by Linda deVries[1] outlines well the challenges facing clinicians caring for babies with posthemorrhagic ventricular dilatation.

L. J. Van Marter, MD, MPH

Reference

1. deVries LS, Brouwer AJ, Groenendaal F. Posthaemorrhagic ventricular dilatation: when should we intervene? *Arch Dis Child Fetal Neonatal Ed.* 2013;98:F284-F285.

Cerebral desaturations in preterm infants: a crossover trial on influence of oxygen saturation target range

Schmid MB, Hopfner RJ, Lenhof S, et al (Univ Med Ctr, Ulm, Germany)

Arch Dis Child Fetal Neonatal Ed 98:F392-F398, 2013

Objective.—To test the hypothesis that a higher pulsoximetric arterial oxygen saturation (SpO_2) target range is associated with reduced cerebral tissue oxygen desaturations from baseline during events of hypoxaemia or bradycardia.

Design.—Randomised crossover trial.

Setting.—Single tertiary care neonatal intensive care unit.

Patients.—Sixteen preterm infants with severe intermittent hypoxaemia or bradycardia.

Interventions.—SpO_2 target was set to 80—92% and 85—96% for 4 h each in random sequence. On a subsequent day, the target sequence was reversed and the study was repeated.

Main Outcome Measures.—We simultaneously recorded cerebral tissue oxygen saturation (cerebral StO_2), SpO_2 and heart rate. Cerebral StO_2 was measured by near infrared spectroscopy. The primary outcome was the cumulative cerebral StO_2 desaturation score representing the area below a cerebral StO_2 baseline value before onset of each hypoxaemic or bradycardic event.

Results.—During low SpO_2 target range the median (IQR) cumulative cerebral StO_2 desaturation score was higher (27384 (15825–37396) vs 18103 (6964–32946), $p = 0.011$) and the mean ($\pm$SD) number of events was higher (29.1 ($\pm$15.3) vs 21.1 ($\pm$11.4), $p = 0.001$). More time was spent with SpO_2 below 80% (57.2 ($\pm$24.8) min vs 34.0 ($\pm$29.6) min, $p = 0.006$). Total time of hyperoxaemia (defined as SpO_2 $\geq$97% and $\geq$99%, respectively) and total time with cerebral StO_2 <60% and <55% were similar.

Conclusions.—A lower SpO_2 target range was associated with a greater cumulative cerebral StO_2 desaturation score, caused by more frequent SpO_2 desaturations. However, time at very low cerebral StO_2 was not affected. Episodes of hyperoxaemia were not reduced.

▶ Thanks to the SUPPORT[1] and BOOST II[2] studies, neonatologists now appreciate the increased mortality risk associated with assigning preterm babies to a lower oxygen saturation (SpO_2) target. There exists, however, little information regarding the implications of oxygen saturation targets on brain oxygenation and later neurodevelopment. Schmidt and colleagues' clever study provides a window into this aspect. The investigators enrolled 16 preterm infants in a randomized crossover study of the impact of SpO_2 target ranges on cerebral oxygenation. The investigators found that the lower SpO_2 target range was linked with more frequent cerebral desaturations as well as episodes of arterial hypoxemia. Surprisingly, the lower SpO_2 target range was not associated with fewer periods of hyperoxemia. It is clear that further work is needed to define SpO_2 levels associated with optimal cerebral oxygenation and to understand the effects of cerebral oxygen desaturation on later growth and development.

L. J. Van Marter, MD, MPH

References

1. SUPPORT Study Group of the Eunice Kennedy Shriver NICHD Neonatal Research Network, Carlo WA, Finer NN, Walsh MC, et al. Target ranges of oxygen saturation in extremely preterm infants. *N Engl J Med.* 2010;362:1959-1969.
2. The BOOST II United Kingdom, Australia, and New Zealand Collaborative Groups, Stenson BJ, Tarnow-Mordi WO, Darlow BA. Oxygen saturation and outcomes in preterm infants. *N Engl J Med.* 2013;368:2094-2104.

Neuroimaging in the Evaluation of Neonatal Encephalopathy

Barnette AR, Horbar JD, Soll RF, et al (St Francis Med Ctr, Cape Girardeau, MO; Univ of Vermont, Burlington; et al)
Pediatrics 133:e1508-e1517, 2014

Background and Objective.—Computed tomography (CT) is still used for neuroimaging of infants with known or suspected neurologic disorders. Alternative neuroimaging options that do not expose the immature brain to radiation include MRI and cranial ultrasound. We aim to characterize and compare the use and findings of neuroimaging modalities, especially CT, in infants with neonatal encephalopathy.

Methods.—The Vermont Oxford Network Neonatal Encephalopathy Registry enrolled 4171 infants ($\geq$36 weeks' gestation or treated with therapeutic hypothermia) between 2006 and 2010 who were diagnosed with encephalopathy in the first 3 days of life. Demographic, perinatal, and medical conditions were recorded, along with treatments, comorbidities, and outcomes. The modality, timing, and results of neuroimaging were also collected.

Results.—CT scans were performed on 933 of 4107 (22.7%) infants, and 100 of 921 (10.9%) of those received multiple CT scans. Compared with MRI, CT provided less detailed evaluation of cerebral injury in areas of prognostic significance, but was more sensitive than cranial ultrasound for hemorrhage and deep brain structural abnormalities.

Conclusions.—CT is commonly used for neuroimaging in newborn infants with neonatal encephalopathy despite concerns over potential harm from radiation exposure. The diagnostic performance of CT is inferior to MRI in identifying neonatal brain injury. Our data suggest that using cranial ultrasound for screening, followed by MRI would be more appropriate than CT at any stage to evaluate infants with neonatal encephalopathy.

▶ This study of infants reported to the Vermont Oxford Network Neonatal Encephalopathy Registry describes utilization rates and diagnostic findings among various imaging techniques applied to the large international group of registrants. Among 4171 infants, computed tomography (CT) was performed on 23%; 49% had ultrasound (US) examinations, and 65% underwent magnetic resonance imaging (MRI). Sixteen percent underwent no neuroimaging, 85% of whom survived. The diagnostic information gleaned by MRI was found to be superior to that of CT. In view of concern regarding exposure of the developing brain to radiation and the low performance of CT, the authors recommend use of US and MRI and avoidance of CT for babies experiencing neonatal encephalopathy. Two of the greatest obstacles to MRI have been the time required in the scanner and the perception that sedation is required. As the authors note, these should no longer represent barriers: the advent of scanners that now acquire images much more quickly and the demonstrated safety of unsedated MRI[1] underscore the feasibility of the recommendations.

L. J. Van Marter, MD, MPH

Reference

1. Mathur AM, Neil JJ, McKinstry RC, Inder TE. Transport, monitoring, and successful brain MR imaging in unsedated neonates. *Pediatr Radiol.* 2008;38:260-264.

Neuroimaging in the Evaluation of Neonatal Encephalopathy

Barnette AR, Horbar JD, Soll RF, et al (St Francis Med Ctr, Cape Girardeau, MO; Univ of Vermont, Burlington; et al)

Pediatrics 133:e1508-e1517, 2014

Background and Objective.—Computed tomography (CT) is still used for neuroimaging of infants with known or suspected neurologic disorders. Alternative neuroimaging options that do not expose the immature brain to radiation include MRI and cranial ultrasound. We aim to characterize and compare the use and findings of neuroimaging modalities, especially CT, in infants with neonatal encephalopathy.

Methods.—The Vermont Oxford Network Neonatal Encephalopathy Registry enrolled 4171 infants (≥36 weeks' gestation or treated with therapeutic hypothermia) between 2006 and 2010 who were diagnosed with encephalopathy in the first 3 days of life. Demographic, perinatal, and medical conditions were recorded, along with treatments, comorbidities, and outcomes. The modality, timing, and results of neuroimaging were also collected.

Results.—CT scans were performed on 933 of 4107 (22.7%) infants, and 100 of 921 (10.9%) of those received multiple CT scans. Compared with MRI, CT provided less detailed evaluation of cerebral injury in areas of prognostic significance, but was more sensitive than cranial ultrasound for hemorrhage and deep brain structural abnormalities.

Conclusions.—CT is commonly used for neuroimaging in newborn infants with neonatal encephalopathy despite concerns over potential harm from radiation exposure. The diagnostic performance of CT is inferior to MRI in identifying neonatal brain injury. Our data suggest that using cranial ultrasound for screening, followed by MRI would be more appropriate than CT at any stage to evaluate infants with neonatal encephalopathy.

► For entry into the Vermont Oxford Neonatal Encephalopathy Registry. As an example, a near-term or term infant with a 5-minute Apgar score of ≤3 would qualify for entry. The majority of infants in this report were admitted to the registry because of seizures within the first 72 hours after birth (57.4%). Nearly half of the infants had a 5-minute Apgar score of ≤3 (49.6%); however, it is not possible from the data presented to determine how many were encephalopathic. Overall, approximately 38% of the registry infants received therapeutic hypothermia.

In the abstract, the authors note that computed tomography (CT) scans were performed on 22.7% of the infants. What is not evident is that the percent of infants who had at least 1 CT decreased steadily from 36.2% in 2006 to 15.2% in 2010. Given the adverse publicity surrounding the high doses of radiation that may be associated with the acquisition of CT, most likely the percentage has continued to decrease.

Finally, in the Conclusions section of the abstract, the authors state that their data suggest that using cranial ultrasound for screening followed by magnetic resonance imaging (MRI) would be more appropriate than CT at any stage to evaluate infants with neonatal encephalopathy. In fact, data presented in the article indicate that for infants who had multiple types of neuroimaging performed on the same day, cranial ultrasound was less sensitive than either CT or MRI for all hemorrhages and abnormalities. When CT and MRI obtained on the same day were compared, both images detected hemorrhages and brainstem injury equally well, but MRI was superior in detecting deep nuclear gray matter and cerebellar injury. These data raise questions regarding the utility of head ultrasound in this group of infants. In addition, before MRI can be promoted as the diagnostic imaging of choice, several issues need to be resolved, including lack of interpretation expertise, the length of acquisition time, and, in many instances, the need for sedation. In the interim, judicious use of CT may be warranted.

L. A. Papile, MD

Xenon Ventilation During Therapeutic Hypothermia in Neonatal Encephalopathy: A Feasibility Study

Dingley J, Tooley J, Liu X, et al (Swansea Univ, UK; Univ of Bristol, UK; et al)
Pediatrics 133:809-818, 2014

Background and Objectives.—Therapeutic hypothermia has become standard of care in newborns with moderate and severe neonatal encephalopathy; however, additional interventions are needed. In experimental models, breathing xenon gas during cooling offers long-term additive neuroprotection. This is the first xenon feasibility study in cooled infants. Xenon is expensive, requiring a closed-circuit delivery system.

Methods.—Cooled newborns with neonatal encephalopathy were eligible for this single-arm, dose-escalation study if clinically stable, under 18 hours of age and requiring less than 35% oxygen. Xenon duration increased stepwise from 3 to 18 hours in 14 subjects; 1 received 25% xenon and 13 received 50%. Respiratory, cardiovascular, neurologic (ie, amplitude-integrated EEG, seizures), and inflammatory (C-reactive protein) effects were examined. The effects of starting or stopping xenon rapidly or slowly were studied. Three matched control subjects per xenon treated subject were selected from our cooling database. Follow-up was at 18 months using mental developmental and physical developmental indexes of the Bayley Scales of Infant Development II.

Results.—No adverse respiratory or cardiovascular effects, including post-extubation stridor, were seen. Xenon increased sedation and suppressed seizures and background electroencephalographic activity. Seizures sometimes occurred during rapid weaning of xenon but not during slow weaning. C-reactive protein levels were similar between groups. Hourly xenon consumption was 0.52 L. Three died, and 7 of 11 survivors had mental and physical developmental index scores ≥70 at follow-up.

Conclusions.—Breathing 50% xenon for up to 18 hours with 72 hours of cooling was feasible, with no adverse effects seen with 18 months' follow-up.

► In this feasibility trial, inhalational xenon was added to inspiratory gases during mechanical ventilation of a group of babies undergoing neuroprotective hypothermia. Xenon appeared to act synergistically with cooling to improve neuroprotection. The experience also led to the observation that too rapid weaning of xenon may lead to seizure recurrence, perhaps by loss of *N*-methyl-D-aspartate receptor inhibition.

As the authors aptly described, hypoxic-ischemic brain injury results in the initiation of the neurotoxic cascade. Further improvements in neuroprotection may well depend on interrupting the cascade at multiple points, and xenon appears to be able to do this. Will we see a large, multicenter randomized, controlled trial? There may be significant obstacles. Xenon is expensive, must be scavenged, and cannot be used in infants requiring high concentrations of oxygen. Because persistent pulmonary hypertension and pulmonary dysfunction (shock lung) frequently accompany hypoxic-ischemic brain injury, the population of infants available to study may be extremely limited. Nevertheless, this study was a good start.

S. M. Donn, MD

Predictive value of the amplitude integrated EEG in infants with hypoxic ischaemic encephalopathy: data from a randomised trial of therapeutic hypothermia

Azzopardi D, on behalf of the TOBY study group (Hammersmith Hosp, London, UK)

Arch Dis Child Fetal Neonatal Ed 99:F80-F82, 2014

The amplitude integrated EEG (aEEG) is reputed to be one of the best predictors of neurological outcome following hypoxic ischaemic encephalopathy in term newborns and was used to select infants into trials of neuroprotection with hypothermia, but its predictive value and the effect of moderate hypothermia on the aEEG have not previously been examined in a randomised study. The positive predictive value (PPV) of the aEEG recorded within 6 h of birth for death or disability at 18 months of age was determined in 314 infants born after 35 weeks gestation who were randomised to receive standard care with or without cooling for 72 h. The aEEG was classified according to voltage and by pattern. The PPV of a severely abnormal aEEG assessed by the voltage and pattern methods was 0.63 and 0.59 respectively in non-cooled infants and 0.55 and 0.51 in cooled infants ($p > 0.05$). Although the differences in PPV between cooled and non-cooled groups were not significant, they are consistent with observational studies showing a lower PPV in infants treated with hypothermia, probably due to a neuroprotective effect of cooling.

▶ Amplitude-integrated electroencephalography (aEEG) was first applied to asphyxiated neonates nearly 3 decades ago with the goal of finding an accurate tool to predict outcomes. Early reports suggested that an abnormal aEEG has a good positive predictive value (PPV) for adverse outcome, between 0.73 and 1.00.[1] Armed with these encouraging results, some trials of therapeutic hypothermia used abnormal aEEG as a criterion for patient selection.

In this report, the TOBY Study group analyzed their prerandomization tracings to assess the PPV of aEEG in the context of a randomized controlled trial (RCT) of whole-body hypothermia. Despite multiple classification methods, the authors found much lower PPVs than suggested by data from the precooling era, ranging from 0.23 in cooled infants with a moderately abnormal tracing up to 0.71 in the noncooled group with a severely abnormal aEEG. Cooling was associated with lower predictive value, although this was not statistically significant. Strengths of this study are that the aEEGs were performed in the context of an RCT, and the vast majority of infants were recruited from within the United Kingdom, thereby reducing effects of practice variation.

These results are similar to those from the National Institute of Child Health and Human Development (NICHD) aEEG study, which reported reduced predictive capacity of aEEG, even in noncooled infants (0.62).[2] They differ from the CoolCap trial, which examined infants enrolled in the trial along with pretrial noncooled infants and posttrial infants who were cooled and found very good PPV in noncooled infants.[3] Importantly, that study showed lower PPVs for cooled infants, particularly in the first 24 hours after birth. How do we reconcile these results? Given that the TOBY and NICHD studies were performed chronologically later, the infants randomized to noncooling in those trials may have benefited from improvements in clinical management, resulting in a lower rate of the primary outcome. Artifact detection and overall familiarity with aEEG technology has also improved in recent years, with the potential for reduced misclassification bias.

From the robust body of literature of aEEG in the precooling era, we know that later assessments are better than earlier recordings and time to recovery of a normal background pattern and sleep-wake cycles are important predictors of outcome.[4-6] In short, the TOBY study confirms that an early "snapshot" aEEG does not afford the opportunity to assess these important variables and provide the predictive accuracy desired by clinicians. Rather than discarding aEEG as a predictive tool in HIE, future studies should instead focus on trends in aEEG variables over time, particularly now that cooling is the standard of care and decisions such as withdrawal of care often takes place after a period of assessment for evolution in clinical status and aEEG recovery.[7]

A. S. Davis, MD, MS

References

1. Spitzmiller RE, Phillips T, Meinzen-Derr J, Hoath SB. Amplitude-integrated EEG is useful in predicting neurodevelopmental outcome in full-term infants with hypoxic-ischemic encephalopathy: a meta-analysis. *J Child Neurol.* 2007;22:1069-1078.
2. Shankaran S, Pappas A, McDonald SA, et al. Predictive value of an early amplitude integrated electroencephalogram and neurologic examination. *Pediatrics.* 2011;128:e112-e120.
3. Thoresen M, Hellström-Westas L, Liu X, de Vries LS. Effect of hypothermia on amplitude-integrated electroencephalogram in infants with asphyxia. *Pediatrics.* 2010;126:e131-e139.
4. Toet MC, Hellstrom-Westas L, Groenendaal F, Eken P, de Vries LS. Amplitude integrated EEG 3 and 6 hours after birth in full term neonates with hypoxic-ischaemic encephalopathy. *Arch Dis Child Fetal Neonatal Ed.* 1999;81:F19-F23.

5. van Rooij LG, Toet MC, Osredkar D, van Huffelen AC, Groenendaal F, de Vries LS. Recovery of amplitude integrated electroencephalographic background patterns within 24 hours of perinatal asphyxia. *Arch Dis Child Fetal Neonatal Ed.* 2005;90:F245-F251.
6. Osredkar D, Toet MC, van Rooij LG, van Huffelen AC, Groenendaal F, de Vries LS. Sleep-wake cycling on amplitude-integrated electroencephalography in term newborns with hypoxic-ischemic encephalopathy. *Pediatrics.* 2005;115: 327-332.
7. Massaro AN, Tsuchida T, Kadom N, et al. aEEG evolution during therapeutic hypothermia and prediction of NICU outcome in encephalopathic neonates. *Neonatology.* 2012;102:197-202.

Acute neonatal encephalopathy and seizures recurrence: A combined aEEG/EEG study

Mastrangelo M, Fiocchi I, Fontana P, et al (V. Buzzi Hosp, Milan, Italy; et al)
Seizure 22:703-707, 2013

Purpose.—To evaluate amplitude-integrated EEG (aEEG) in comparison with conventional (cEEG) for the identification of electrographic seizures in neonates with acute neonatal encephalopathies.

Methods.—Thirty-one conventional cEEG/aEEG long-term recordings from twenty-eight newborns were reviewed in order to assess the electrographic seizure detection rate and recurrence in newborns. Two paediatric neurologists and one neonatologist, blinded to the raw full array cEEG, were asked to mark any events suspected to be an electrographic seizures on aEEG. They were asked to decide if the displayed aEEG trace showed the pattern of a single seizure (SS), repetitive seizures (RS) or status epilepticus (SE). Their ability to recognize electrographic seizures on aEEG was compared to seizures identified on full array cEEG.

Results.—25 of the 31 long-term cEEGs recordings showed electrographic seizures. The two paediatric neurologists and the neonatologist identified SE in 100% of the reviewed traces using aEEG alone while they identified 49.4% and 37.5% of electrographic seizures using aEEG alone. Overall, the correct identification ranged from 23.5% to 30.7% for SS and 66% for RS. The inter-observer agreement (*k*) for the identification of SE for the two paediatric neurologists and the neonatologist was 1.0. Overall the inter-observer agreement (*k*) for the detection of SS, RS and SE of the two paediatric neurologists was 0.91.

Conclusions.—In our study the observers identified SE in 100% of the reviewed traces using raw aEEG alone, thus aEEG might represent a useful tool to detect SE in the setting of NICU. SS may not be reliably identified using aEEG alone. Simultaneous recording of the raw cEEG/aEEG provides a good level of sensitivity for the detection of neonatal electrographic seizures.

▶ This study attempted to assess the reliability of amplitude-integrated electroencephalography (aEEG) at diagnosing electrical seizures in encephalopathic newborns. It used the conventional EEG as the gold standard. The aEEG tracings were interpreted by 2 pediatric neurologists and 1 neonatologist. Twenty-eight babies underwent 31 comparative studies over a 3-year period. There was a 100% concordance of the interpreters when infants were in electrical status, but the aEEG diagnosis of single seizures and repetitive seizures fell to 49% and 38% of those seen on the conventional EEG.

The aEEG (cerebral function monitor) is becoming more widely used in neonatal intensive care units across the world. Its utility is enhanced by easy availability, ease of use, and a relatively short learning curve. However, correct interpretation requires proper lead placement, recognition of artifact, and the training and experience of the reader. As these investigators have correctly suggested, the aEEG should be considered a screening tool, with abnormal results confirmed by a properly performed conventional EEG. Furthermore, the diagnosis of convulsive activity requires observation of not only the aEEG compressed signal but also the raw EEG signal.

The validity of the aEEG as a prognostic tool has yet to be established. Although it was required for enrollment in several of the randomized cooling trials, we have questioned whether a "normal" or "mildly abnormal" tracing should be a basis for exclusion from hypothermic neuroprotection.[1] Clearly, more work is needed.

S. M. Donn, MD

Reference

1. Sarkar S, Barks JD, Donn SM. Should amplitude-integrated electroencephalography be used to identify infants suitable for hypothermic neuroprotection? *J Perinatol.* 2008;28:117-122.

Factors Associated with Permanent Hearing Impairment in Infants Treated with Therapeutic Hypothermia

Smit E, Liu X, Gill H, et al (Univ of Bristol, UK)

J Pediatr 163:995-1000, 2013

Objective.—To define the incidence of hearing impairment, document plasma gentamicin concentrations, and identify factors associated with permanent hearing impairment in infants subjected to therapeutic hypothermia for moderate or severe neonatal encephalopathy.

Study Design.—Data were collected prospectively in a regional center providing therapeutic hypothermia. Cooled infants at ≥36 weeks gestation with moderate or severe neonatal encephalopathy were analyzed if a full dataset was available (n = 108), including clinical variables and gentamicin trough levels. Infants with hearing impairment were identified, and survivors were followed up with neurodevelopmental evaluation at age 18 months. Stepwise logistic regression identified factors associated with hearing impairment.

Results.—Nine infants died, and among the survivors, 10.1% developed a permanent hearing impairment. The trough gentamicin level was above the recommended cutoff of 2 mg/L in 37% of the infants in the entire cohort and in 90% of the infants with hearing impairment. Logistic regression analysis identified high trough gentamicin level, low cord pH, and hypoglycemia (<46.8 mg/dL) in the first postnatal hour as significantly associated with hearing impairment. The need for inotropic support was close to significant ($P = .055$).

Conclusion.—Hearing impairment was a common finding among cooled infants. Plasma gentamicin levels were commonly >2 mg/L. Based on these findings, we propose changes in gentamicin dosing interval and trough level monitoring to minimize the risk of potentially toxic levels in cooled newborns.

▶ The standard gentamicin dosing for term a newborn infant is 4 to 5 mg/kg every 24 hours, with trough plasma gentamicin levels routinely checked before the administration of the third or fourth dose. If there is a concern for altered renal function, trough levels are frequently checked after the second dose. A previous retrospective study by these authors showed trough levels of gentamicin exceeding the recommended level of 2 mg/L in 36% of cooled infants using the standard dosing regimen.[1]

In this observational study, clinical and outcome data were collected prospectively for 136 infants who received therapeutic hypothermia for moderate to severe neonatal encephalopathy and met the original entry criteria for the CoolCap trial. A full data set was available for 79% of the infants cooled during the study period. At the time of discharge to home, 9 infants were identified with hearing loss and an additional hearing impaired infant was identified at a year of age. Eight of the infants with hearing impairment required amplification with a hearing aid, and 2 had cochlear implants. For each cooled infant with hearing impairment, 2 cooled infants without hearing impairment were matched for asphyxial severity based on cord blood pH, 10-minute Apgar score, and anticonvulsant and inotrope use to ensure that significant differences between the hearing-impaired and normal-hearing groups were not likely related to more severe neonatal encephalopathy.

Based on their findings, the investigators recommend an initial dose of 4 mg/kg of gentamicin for infants undergoing cooling for neonatal encephalopathy and that a subsequent dose not be given until the trough level drops below 2 mg/L. In a concurrent pharmacokinetic study Frymoyer, et al[2] showed that a gentamicin dose of 4 to 5 mg/kg at a 36-hour dosing interval is predicted to achieve target peak and trough concentrations in more than 90% of encephalopathic infants undergoing cooling.

L. A. Papile, MD

References

1. Liu X, Borooah M, Stone J, Chakkarapani E, Thoresen M. Serum gentamicin concentrations in encephalopathic infants are not affected by therapeutic hypothermia. *Pediatrics*. 2009;124:310-315.
2. Frymoyer A, Meng L, Bonifacio SL, Verotta D, Guglielmo BJ. Gentamicin pharmacokinetics and dosing in neonates with hypoxic ischemic encephalopathy receiving hypothermia. *Pharmacotherapy*. 2013;33:718-726.

Anticonvulsant effect of xenon on neonatal asphyxial seizures

Azzopardi D, Robertson NJ, Kapetanakis A, et al (King's College London, UK; Univ College London, UK; et al)

Arch Dis Child Fetal Neonatal Ed 98:F437-F439, 2013

Xenon, a monoatomic gas with very high tissue solubility, is a noncompetitive inhibitor of N-methyl-D-aspartate (NMDA) glutamate receptor, has antiapoptotic effects and is neuroprotective following hypoxic ischaemic injury in animals. Xenon may be expected to have anticonvulsant effects through glutamate receptor blockade, but this has not previously been demonstrated clinically. We examined seizure activity on the real time and amplitude integrated EEG records of 14 full-term infants with perinatal asphyxial encephalopathy treated within 12 h of birth with 30% inhaled xenon for 24 h combined with 72 h of moderate systemic hypothermia. Seizures were identified on 5 of 14 infants. Seizures stopped during xenon therapy but recurred within a few minutes of withdrawing xenon and stopped again after xenon was restarted. Our data show that subanaesthetic levels of xenon may have an anticonvulsant effect. Inhaled xenon may be a valuable new therapy in this hard-to-treat population.

▶ In animal models of hypoxic ischemic brain injury, xenon gas has been shown to be neuroprotective.[1] However, xenon cannot be synthesized but needs to be fractionally distilled from liquid oxygen. Because of its low abundance in the atmosphere, the cost of distilled xenon is extremely high, precluding its widespread use as a therapeutic agent. The recent development of a closed-circulatory system, enabling the reuse of xenon gas and mechanical replenishment of oxygen has made its clinical use more feasible.[2]

This report is an observational study from an ongoing randomized neuroprotection trial, TOBY-XE, in which inhaled xenon is being used as an adjuvant neuroprotective therapy to induced hypothermia. Selection criteria for the trial are similar to those of the previous TOBY hypothermia trial: gestational age between 36 and 43 weeks, evidence of asphyxia at birth, and the presence of moderate or severe encephalopathy and an abnormal amplitude-integrated EEG. In addition, treatment with systemic hypothermia must be initiated within 6 hours of birth.

The authors' observation of a paucity of seizures during xenon therapy and their recurrence upon discontinuing xenon suggests that the neuroprotection afforded by xenon includes anticonvulsant effects, in addition to its antiapoptotic effects. If xenon therapy proves to be effective in mitigating brain damage from both hypoxia-ischemia and seizure activity, xenon therapy certainly could be worth its high cost.

L. A. Papile, MD

References

1. Ma D, Hossain M, Chow A, et al. Xenon and hypothermia combine to provide neuroprotection from neonatal asphyxia. *Ann Neurol.* 2005;58:182-193.

2. Faulkner SD, Downie NA, Mercer CJ, Kerr SA, Sanders RD, Robertson NJ. A xenon recirculating ventilator for the newborn piglet: developing clinical applications of xenon for neonates. *Eur J Anaesthesiol.* 2012;29:577-585.

Moderate and Late Preterm Birth: Effect on Brain Size and Maturation at Term-Equivalent Age

Walsh JM, Doyle LW, Anderson PJ, et al (Royal Women's Hosp, Parkville, Victoria, Australia; Univ of Melbourne, Australia)
Radiology 2014 [Epub ahead of print]

Purpose.—To compare the size of multiple brain structures, maturation in terms of both brain myelination and gyral development, and evidence of brain injury between moderate and late preterm (MLPT) and term-born infants at term-equivalent age.

Materials and Methods.—The study was approved by the human research ethics committees of the participating hospitals, and informed parental consent was obtained for all infants. One hundred ninety-nine MLPT and 50 term-born infants underwent 3-T magnetic resonance (MR) imaging brain examinations at 38-44 weeks of corrected gestational age. T1- and T2-weighted MR images were compared between groups for size of multiple cerebral structures, degree of myelination in the posterior limb of the internal capsule, gyral maturation, signal intensity abnormalities, and presence of cysts by a single assessor who was blinded to the gestational group and perinatal course of the infants. Group differences were compared by using linear regression for continuous variables and logistic regression for categorical variables, and interrater and intrarater reliability was assessed by using intraclass correlation coefficients.

Results.—Compared with those in the term-born control group, measurements of brain biparietal diameter, corpus callosum, basal ganglia and thalami, and cerebellum were smaller in infants in the MLPT group (all $P \leq .01$), while extracerebral space was larger ($P < .0001$). Myelination of the posterior limb of the internal capsule was less developed, and gyral maturation was delayed in the MLPT group (both $P < .001$). Signal intensity abnormalities and cysts were uncommon in both groups, with 13 (6.5%) MLPT infants and one (2%) term infant having abnormalities. Inter- and intrarater reliability was good for most measures, with intraclass correlation coefficients generally greater than 0.68.

Conclusion.—MLPT birth is associated with smaller brain size, less-developed myelination of the posterior limb of the internal capsule, and more immature gyral folding than those associated with full-term birth. These brain changes may form the basis of some of the long-term neurodevelopmental deficits observed in MLPT children.

▶ Recent years have brought widespread recognition that late preterm birth is far from risk-free. It is increasingly appreciated that a variety of adverse neurodevelopmental outcomes are among the hazards of late preterm birth. In this valuable study, Walsh and colleagues evaluated neuroimaging findings between 2 groups: 199 moderate and late preterm infants and 50 term-born infants. The infants underwent 3-T magnetic resonance imaging brain examinations at 38 to 44 weeks of corrected gestational age, and the images were reviewed by a single reviewer blinded to the infants' gestational ages and hospital courses. The study found smaller brain size, less developed myelination of the posterior limb of the internal capsule, and more immature gyral folding among the moderate and late preterm infants compared with their term counterparts. These data provide a structural basis for some of the observed neurodevelopmental deficits observed among moderate and late preterm infants. What remains unanswered is whether postnatal interventions can be identified that could lead to enhanced brain growth and development among infants in whom such abnormalities are identified.

L. J. Van Marter, MD, MPH

Association between Postnatal Dexamethasone for Treatment of Bronchopulmonary Dysplasia and Brain Volumes at Adolescence in Infants Born Very Preterm

Cheong JL, for the Victorian Infant Collaborative Study Group (Royal Women's Hosp, Victoria, Australia; et al)

J Pediatr 164:737-743, 2014

Objectives.—To compare brain volumes in adolescents who were born extremely preterm (<28 weeks gestation) who had received postnatal dexamethasone, and to determine if there was a postnatal dexamethasone dose–response effect on brain volumes.

Study Design.—Geographical cohort study of extremely preterm adolescents born in 1991-1992 in Victoria, Australia. T1-weighted magnetic resonance imaging was performed at 18 years of age. Segmented and parcellated brain volumes were calculated using an automated segmentation method (FreeSurfer) and compared between groups, with and without adjustment for potential confounders. The relationships between total postnatal dexamethasone dose and brain volumes were explored using linear regression.

Results.—Of the 148 extremely preterm participants, 55 (37%) had received postnatal dexamethasone, with a cumulative mean dose of 7.7 mg/kg. Compared with participants who did not receive postnatal dexamethasone, those who did had smaller total brain tissue volumes (mean difference −3.6%, 95% CI [−7.0%, −0.3%], P value = .04) and smaller white matter, thalami, and basal ganglia volumes (all $P < .05$). There was a trend of smaller total brain and white matter volumes with increasing dose of postnatal dexamethasone (regression coefficient −7.7 [95% CI −16.2, 0.8] and −3.2 [−6.6, 0.2], respectively).

Conclusions.—Extremely preterm adolescents who received postnatal dexamethasone in the newborn period had smaller total brain tissue volumes than those who did not receive postnatal dexamethasone, particularly white matter, thalami, and basal ganglia. Vulnerability of brain tissues or structures associated with postnatal dexamethasone varies by structure and persists into adolescence.

▶ Although the conclusions in this abstract are accurate, they need to be qualified. The data presented were abstracted from a cohort study and, as the title of the article states, represent an association between postnatal dexamethasone therapy and decreased brain volumes in adolescence, not a causal relationship. As was emphasized in the accompanying editorial comment, sorting out the effects of prematurity and its attendant complications from the effects of a specific therapeutic intervention can only be done in a randomized clinical trial.[1] This is especially true for the use of postnatal dexamethasone, because the therapy is inextricably linked to the diagnosis of bronchopulmonary dysplasia which, in itself, is associated with a reduction in brain volumes.[2,3] In addition, the fact that there was essentially no difference in the volumes of the hippocampus or cerebellum, the 2 regions of the brain most susceptible to dexamethasone neurotoxicity in experimental studies, suggests that there were factors other than postnatal dexamethasone therapy that caused the observed difference in brain volumes. Finally, without neuropsychological correlates, it is difficult to know if there are any consequences to having a diminished brain volume.

L. A. Papile, MD

References

1. Watterberg K. Dexamethasone and the brain at age 18 years: randomize the first baby-follow-up. *J Pediatr.* 2014;164:687-689.
2. Uno H, Eisele S, Sakai A, et al. Neurotoxicity of glucocorticoids in the primate brain. *Horm Behav.* 1994;28:336-348.
3. Noguchi KK, Walls KC, Wozniak DF, Olney JW, Roth KA, Farber NB. Acute neonatal glucocorticoid exposure produces selective and rapid cerebellar neural progenitor cell apoptotic death. *Cell Death Differ.* 2008;15:1582-1592.

Association between Postnatal Dexamethasone for Treatment of Bronchopulmonary Dysplasia and Brain Volumes at Adolescence in Infants Born Very Preterm

Cheong JLY, for the Victorian Infant Collaborative Study Group (Royal Women's Hosp, Melbourne, Victoria, Australia; et al)

J Pediatr 164:737-743.e1, 2014

Objectives.—To compare brain volumes in adolescents who were born extremely preterm (<28 weeks gestation) who had received postnatal dexamethasone, and to determine if there was a postnatal dexamethasone dose–response effect on brain volumes.

Study Design.—Geographical cohort study of extremely preterm adolescents born in 1991-1992 in Victoria, Australia. T1-weighted magnetic resonance imaging was performed at 18 years of age. Segmented and parcellated brain volumes were calculated using an automated segmentation method (FreeSurfer) and compared between groups, with and without adjustment for potential confounders. The relationships between total postnatal dexamethasone dose and brain volumes were explored using linear regression.

Results.—Of the 148 extremely preterm participants, 55 (37%) had received postnatal dexamethasone, with a cumulative mean dose of 7.7 mg/kg. Compared with participants who did not receive postnatal dexamethasone, those who did had smaller total brain tissue volumes (mean difference −3.6%, 95% CI [−7.0%, −0.3%], *P* value = .04) and smaller white matter, thalami, and basal ganglia volumes (all $P < .05$). There was a trend of smaller total brain and white matter volumes with increasing dose of postnatal dexamethasone (regression coefficient −7.7 [95% CI −16.2, 0.8] and −3.2 [−6.6, 0.2], respectively).

Conclusions.—Extremely preterm adolescents who received postnatal dexamethasone in the newborn period had smaller total brain tissue volumes than those who did not receive postnatal dexamethasone, particularly white matter, thalami, and basal ganglia. Vulnerability of brain tissues or structures associated with postnatal dexamethasone varies by structure and persists into adolescence.

▶ Traditionally, we have become accustomed to 2- to 3-year follow-up with a concluding statement that "continued follow-up is planned and/or required." It is thus both refreshing and very informative to see the truly long-term outcomes of a cohort of preterm infants exposed to postnatal steroid therapy during their sojourn in the neonatal intensive care unit. In view of the adverse short-term outcomes with postnatal steroids, including hypertension, hyperglycemia/diabetes, cerebral palsy, and bowel perforation in addition to growth cessation when receiving corticosteroids, devastating long-term consequences may have been anticipated.

Cheong et al did observe that individuals born extremely preterm have smaller brain volumes than term-born controls at age 18 years. Indeed, high-dose postnatal dexamethasone treatment for bronchopulmonary dysplasia (BPD) was associated with decreased brain volumes on magnetic resonance imaging (MRI) scan at 18 years of age, specifically total brain tissue, cortical white matter, thalamus, and basal ganglia nuclei. However, there were no significant differences in the hippocampus or cerebellum, areas of the brain with very high concentrations of glucocorticoid receptors. These findings replicate those of prior reports.[1-4]

Cheong et al highlight the difficulty of attributing the MRI findings to the corticosteroids, particularly in a nonrandomized trial, as smaller brain volumes are a characteristic of preterm babies who have not received steroids, but the findings are exaggerated in the steroid-treated group. Furthermore, other studies have linked postnatal corticosteroids to adverse long-term growth, smaller head circumferences, and poorer neurodevelopmental outcome, reinforcing the possibility that these long-term brain differences may, in part, be caused by the steroids.[5,6]

"That this therapy was one of many contributing factors is underscored by the authors' finding that the strength of the association between dexamethasone therapy and decreased brain volumes was weakened when other factors (gestational age, sex, small for gestational age status, BPD, major brain injury) were added to the model."[7]

The long-term follow-up of all patients enrolled in interventional trials during the neonatal period are time consuming and expensive but essential, and the results more than justify the costs.

A. A. Fanaroff, MD, FRCPE

References

1. Cheong JL, Anderson PJ, Roberts G, et al. Contribution of brain size to IQ and educational underperformance in extremely preterm adolescents. *PLoS One.* 2013;8:e77475.
2. de Kieviet JF, Zoetebier L, van Elburg RM, Vermeulen RJ, Oosterlaan J. Brain development of very preterm and very low-birthweight children in childhood and adolescence: a meta-analysis. *Dev Med Child Neurol.* 2012;54:313-323.
3. Lax ID, Duerden EG, Lin SY, et al. Neuroanatomical consequences of very preterm birth in middle childhood. *Brain Struct Funct.* 2013;218:575-585.
4. Yeh TF, Lin YJ, Lin HC, et al. Outcomes at school age after postnatal dexamethasone therapy for lung disease of prematurity. *N Engl J Med.* 2004;350:1304-1313.
5. Doyle LW, Ehrenkranz RA, Halliday HL. Dexamethasone treatment after the first week of life for bronchopulmonary dysplasia in preterm infants: a systematic review. *Neonatology.* 2010;98:289-296.
6. ter Wolbeek M, de Sonneville LM, de Vries WB, et al. Early life intervention with glucocorticoids has negative effects on motor development and neuropsychological function in 14–17 year-old adolescents. *Psychoneuroendocrinology.* 2013; 38:975-986.
7. Watterberg KL. Dexamethasone and the brain at age 18 years: randomize the first baby—and follow-up. *J Pediatr.* 2014;164:687-689.

Human milk feeding prevents retinopathy of prematurity (ROP) in preterm VLBW neonates

Manzoni P, on behalf of the Italian Task Force for the study and prevention of Neonatal Fungal Infections; the Italian Society of Neonatology (S. Anna Hosp, Torino, Italy; et al)
Early Hum Dev 89:S64-S68, 2013

Background.—Retinopathy of prematurity (ROP) is a multifactorial disease, but little is known about its relationships with neonatal nutritional policies. Human, maternal milk is the best possible nutritional option for all premature infants, including those at high risk for severe complications of prematurity, such as ROP.

Objective.—This is a secondary analysis of data collected during two multicenter RCTs performed consecutively (years 2004 through 2008) by a network of eleven tertiary NICUs in Italy. The two trials aimed at assessing effectiveness of fluconazole prophylaxis (Manzoni et al., N Engl J Med 2007 Jun 14;356(24):2483–95), and of bovine lactoferrin supplementation (Manzoni et al., JAMA 2009 Oct 7;302(13):1421–8), in prevention of invasive fungal infection, and of late-onset sepsis in

VLBW infants, respectively. We tested the hypothesis that exclusive feeding with fresh maternal milk may prevent ROP of any stage – as defined by the ETROP study – in VLBW neonates, compared to formula feeding.

Methods.—We analyzed the database from both trials. Systematic screening for detection of ROP was part of the protocol of both studies. The definition of threshold ROP was as defined by the ETROP study. Univariate analysis was performed to look for significant associations between ROP and several possible associated factors, and among them, the type of milk feeding (maternal milk or formula for preterms). When an association was indicated by $p < 0.05$, multiple logistic regression was used to determine the factors significantly associated with ROP.

Results.—In both trials combined, 314 infants received exclusively human maternal milk (group A), and 184 a preterm formula because their mothers were not expected to breastfeed. The clinical, demographical and management characteristics of the neonates did not differ between the two groups, particularly related to the presence of the known risk factors for ROP. Overall, ROP incidence (any stage) was significantly lower in infants fed maternal milk (11 of 314; 3.5%) as compared to formula-fed neonates (29 of 184; 15.8%) (RR 0.14; 95% CI 0.12–0.62; $p = 0.004$). The same occurred for threshold ROP (1.3% vs. 12.3%, respectively; RR 0.19; 95% CI 0.05–0.69; $p = 0.009$).

At multivariate logistic regression controlling for potentially confounding factors that were significantly associated to ROP (any stage) at univariate analysis (birth weight, gestational age, days on supplemental oxygen, systemic fungal infection, outborn, hyperglycaemia), type of milk feeding retained significance, human maternal milk being protective with $p = 0.01$.

Conclusions.—Exclusive human, maternal milk feeding since birth may prevent ROP of any stage in VLBW infants in the NICU.

▶ The title is an overstatement of the data presented in this article. At best, the data suggest an association between exclusive use of maternal milk and a decrease in the frequency of retinopathy of prematurity (ROP).

As stated in the abstract, this study is a secondary analysis of data from 2 randomized clinical trials. A total of 808 very low birth weight infants were enrolled in the 2 trials, of which 498 are included in this study. Infants who received mixed (maternal + formula and/or banked human milk) feeding or did not attain a maternal milk intake of > 50 mL/kg/day were excluded. Although it is true that multivariate analysis showed exclusive use of formula feeding was significantly associated with a higher incidence of ROP, it was not the only risk factor, as the following data indicate.

	Odds Ratio	95% CI	*P* value
Hyperglycemia	9.88	0.01–0.47	0.006
Gestational Age	7.29	0.03–0.85	0.01
Exclusive formula feeding	6.65	1.02–4.98	0.01
Birth weight	0.25	1.00–1.02	0.04

In the introduction, the authors note that human milk feeding has been speculated to be protective toward ROP but state that this is controversial because the data have been derived from observational retrospective studies or from secondary analysis of RCTs having other primary endpoints. Because this study is more of the same, all that can be said is the possibility that maternal milk feeding may prevent/mitigate ROP is intriguing.

L. A. Papile, MD

Ophthalmologic Outcome at 30 Months' Corrected Age of a Prospective Swedish Cohort of Children Born Before 27 Weeks of Gestation: The Extremely Preterm Infants in Sweden Study

Holmström GE, Källen K, Hellström A, et al (Uppsala Univ, Sweden; Lund Univ, Sweden; Univ of Gothenburg, Sweden; et al)

JAMA Ophthalmol 132:182-189, 2014

Importance.—Follow-up at 30 months' corrected age reveals eye and visual problems in one-third of children born extremely prematurely (<27 weeks' gestation).

Objective.—To investigate the ophthalmologic outcome of extremely preterm children at 30 months' corrected age.

Design, Setting, and Participants.—A prospective, population-based follow-up study (Extremely Preterm Infants in Sweden Study [EXPRESS]) was conducted in Sweden. The population included extremely preterm infants (<27 weeks' gestation) born in Sweden between 2004 and 2007, of whom 491 survived until age 2.5 years. Screening for retinopathy of prematurity (ROP) was performed in the neonatal period. At 30 months' corrected age, an ophthalmologic assessment was performed in 411 of 491 children (83.7%).

Main Outcomes and Measures.—Visual acuity, manifest strabismus, and refractive errors were evaluated.

Results.—Visual impairment was identified in 3.1% of the children, and 1.0% were blind. Refractive errors, defined as myopia less than −3 diopters (D), hypermetropia greater than +3 D, astigmatism 2 D or more, and/or anisometropia 2 D or more, were found in 25.6% of the children, and 14.1% had manifest strabismus. There were significant associations between visual impairment and treated ROP ($P = .02$), cognitive disability ($P < .001$), and birth weight ($P = .02$). Multiple regression analyses revealed significant associations between strabismus and treated ROP ($P < .001$), cognitive disability ($P < .01$), and cerebral palsy ($P = .02$). Refractive errors were significantly correlated with severity of ROP (right eye, $P < .001$; left eye, $P < .01$). Children who had been treated for ROP had the highest frequency (69.0%) of eye and visual abnormalities.

Conclusions and Relevance.—One-third of the extremely prematurely born children in this study had some kind of eye or visual problems, such as visual impairment, strabismus, or major refractive error. Despite being born extremely preterm, the present cohort has a similar prevalence of blindness and visual impairment as in previous Swedish cohorts of children born less prematurely.

► The EXPRESS study[1,2] has yielded and will continue to yield important data from a population-based observational cohort in Sweden. Population-based cohorts certainly trump regional or single-center cohorts. The original intent was to be proactive with regard to the care of extremely preterm and low birth weight infants. The investigators had recognized their self-fulfilling prophecy that if no efforts were expended on these infants, they would inevitably die. They aimed initially to determine the 1-year survival in all infants born before 27 gestational weeks during 2004–2007. The incidence of extreme prematurity was 3.3 per 1000 live births, about one-third of the rate in the United States. There were 707 liveborn and 304 stillbirths born to 887 mothers in 904 deliveries (102 multiple births) in all obstetric and neonatal units in Sweden from April 1, 2004, to March 31, 2007. Overall mortality was 45% between 22 and 26 weeks' gestation (ranging from 93% at 22 weeks to 24% at 26 weeks). Lower risk of infant death was associated with tocolytic treatment antenatal corticosteroids, surfactant treatment, and birth at a level III hospital. Among 1-year survivors, 45% had no major neonatal morbidity. Having completed their initial task, they are now diligently following this rich cohort to determine the morbidity and have already published the neurodevelopmental problems.[3] Impressively for the publication on the visual outcomes, they have been able to capture 95% of the original cohort. The eye findings are impressive with one-third of the infants having some visual disturbance. To no one's surprise babies that had treatment for retinopathy have significantly more visual impairment.

It is encouraging that in this very sick cohort, only 1% of the children are blind, and 3% have major visual impairment. Strabismus is a major issue. More babies with cerebral palsy had visual findings. Unfortunately, the cohort did not all have brain scans, so it is impossible to separate the ocular from the neurologic causes of strabismus.

A. A. Fanaroff, MD, FRCPE

References

1. Fellman V, Hellström-Westas L, Norman M, et al; EXPRESS Group. One-year survival of extremely preterm infants after active perinatal care in Sweden. *JAMA*. 2009;301:2225-2233.
2. EXPRESS Group. Incidence of and risk factors for neonatal morbidity after active perinatal care: extremely preterm infants study in Sweden (EXPRESS). *Acta Paediatr.* 2010;99:978-992.
3. Serenius F, Kallen K, Blennow M, et al; EXPRESS Group. Neurodevelopmental outcome in extremely preterm infants at 2.5 years after active perinatal care in Sweden. *JAMA*. 2013;309:1810-1820.

Neonatal stroke: a review of the current evidence on epidemiology, pathogenesis, diagnostics and therapeutic options
van der Aa NE, Benders MJNL, Groenendaal F, et al (Univ Med Ctr Utrecht, The Netherlands)
Acta Paediatr 103:356-364, 2014

Neonatal stroke, including perinatal arterial ischaemic stroke and cerebral sinovenous thrombosis, remains a serious problem in the neonate. This article reviews the current evidence on epidemiology, pathogenesis, diagnostics and therapeutic options.

Conclusion.—Although our understanding of the underlying mechanisms and possible risk factors has improved, little progress has been made towards therapeutic options. Considering the high incidence of neurological sequelae, the need for therapeutic options is high and should be the focus of future research.

▶ Interests and expertise of neonatologists and neurologists converge in efforts to understand the pathogenesis and improve the treatment and outcome of neonatal strokes. This thorough review highlights current understanding and major gaps in knowledge regarding perinatal arterial ischemic stroke (PAIS) and cerebral sinovenous thrombosis (CSVT). The authors address 5 themes: risk factors and mechanisms, diagnostic modalities, prognosis, acute therapy options (in particular the roles of hypothermia and anticoagulation), and approaches that could enhance recovery (neurotrophins and novel rehabilitation strategies). Overall, the authors provide a straightforward comprehensive overview of these topics. Several points merit consideration and commentary.

Neuroimaging is the primary modality for diagnosis of neonatal stroke. A critical issue for clinicians is the selection of most sensitive/specific/cost-effective modalities; there is little comparative data, and institutions vary substantially in access to resources and clinical expertise. For PAIS, the appropriate imaging modality, as the authors indicate, may differ across centers; it is likely that few sites share the expertise of the authors in application of cranial ultrasound scan for evaluation of cerebral parenchymal injury. There is growing concern regarding potential risk of radiation exposure, and the role of computed tomography for nonemergent neonatal and infant brain imaging is waning. There is consensus that diffusion-weighted magnetic resonance imaging (MRI) is the most informative modality for delineation of acute PAIS; the authors also highlight the utility of diffusion-weighted MRI (in particular signal abnormality at the level of the cerebral peduncle, reflecting degeneration of descending corticospinal tracts) for prediction of hemiplegic cerebral palsy. They comment on magnetic resonance angiography (MRA) as an indicator of asymmetric carotid blood flow; however, the utility MRA in this setting remains uncertain, and reduced blood flow could reflect reduced metabolic demand in areas of infarction. In the discussion of neurodiagnostic imaging for CSVT, the authors' illustrative magnetic resonance venograms (MRVs) are noncontrast studies; they acknowledge that noncontrast studies may be more subject to artifacts related to slow flow but do not explain their rationale for favoring noncontrast studies.

The authors support the utility of evaluation of protein-based assays of coagulation status for both PAIS and CSVT "shortly after diagnosis." Thrombophilias are identifiable risk factors for neonatal stroke, and coagulation assays are often obtained in this setting. Yet, stroke recurrence is rare, the cost of testing is high, results are often difficult to interpret, and typically the findings do not affect treatment decisions. Anticoagulant protein levels are physiologically lower (mean values for all < 50%) in normal healthy term or preterm infants compared with adult levels, until 6 months of age, and acquired deficiency states are common because of underlying medical conditions or consumption of coagulation proteins at the time of an acute thrombotic event. Low protein C or S levels in the neonatal period typically prompt repetition of functional assays later in infancy to confirm or refute a diagnosis of inherited deficiencies. Thus, it could be argued that the clinical utility of these assays is uncertain.

The authors cite very broad ranges of outcome for both PAIS and CSVT, and the factors that contribute to diverse outcomes not well understood. The authors allude briefly to "differences in the redirection of care" as potentially influencing variation in outcomes reported from different centers. This complex issue is a frequent topic of informal discussion but is rarely included in formal review articles. Establishing a framework for how to systematically collect and report information about clinical decision making in neonates at high risk for poor neurologic outcome remains an important challenge for the field.

The Future Directions section is thoughtful and well balanced. The authors highlight the complexities inherent in studying these disorders and identify priorities for future collaborative research.

S. M. Donn, MD

Alterations in Brain Structure and Neurodevelopmental Outcome in Preterm Infants Hospitalized in Different Neonatal Intensive Care Unit Environments

Pineda RG, Neil J, Dierker D, et al (Washington Univ School of Medicine, St Louis, MO)

J Pediatr 164:52-60.e2, 2014

Objective.—To evaluate associations between neonatal intensive care unit (NICU) room type (open ward and private room) and medical outcomes; neurobehavior, electrophysiology, and brain structure at hospital discharge; and developmental outcomes at 2 years of age.

Study Design.—In this prospective longitudinal cohort study, we enrolled 136 preterm infants born <30 weeks gestation from an urban, 75-bed level III NICU from 2007-2010. Upon admission, each participant was assigned to a bedspace in an open ward or private room within the same hospital, based on space and staffing availability, where they remained for the duration of hospitalization. The primary outcome was developmental performance at 2 years of age (n = 86 infants returned for testing, which was 83% of survivors) measured using the Bayley Scales of Infant and Toddler Development, 3rd Edition. Secondary outcomes were: (1) medical factors throughout the hospitalization; (2) neurobehavior; and (3) cerebral injury and maturation (determined by magnetic resonance imaging and electroencephalography).

Results.—At term equivalent age, infants in private rooms were characterized by a diminution of normal hemispheric asymmetry and a trend toward having lower amplitude integrated electroencephalography cerebral maturation scores ($P=.02$; $\beta=-0.52$ [CI −0.95, −0.10]). At age 2 years, infants from private rooms had lower language scores ($P=.006$; $\beta=-8.3$ [CI −14.2, −2.4]) and a trend toward lower motor scores ($P=.02$; $\beta=-6.3$ [CI −11.7, −0.99]), which persisted after adjustment for potential confounders.

Conclusion.—These findings raise concerns that highlight the need for further research into the potential adverse effects of different amounts of sensory exposure in the NICU environment.

▶ Could the chaotic, bright, and noisy environment of the typical open-bay, multibed neonatal intensive care unit (NICU) actually be good for babies? This report suggests that the answer to this question may be "yes"! This unexpected and counterintuitive result raises concerns about the current trend to single patient rooms as NICUs are rebuilt or replaced. There are reasons for caution in a rush to judgment. Although the room assignments were pseudorandom, infants assigned to private rooms were significantly more likely than those in open wards to have Medicaid insurance coverage (79% vs 52%, $P=.004$); analyses were adjusted to account for that difference. To account for multiple comparisons, the authors adopted a cutoff of $P < .01$ to define strong relationships; given that at least 15 intergroup comparisons were performed, however, a more conservative cutoff would have been $P < .003$, at which the most significant observed difference would have been only marginally so. High proportions of Medicaid insurance (67%), non-Caucasian race (50%), and multiple gestation (34%) as well as low parental visitation rates (described in a prior report) may compromise extrapolation to units that do not share those characteristics. Nonetheless, the observed differences in language scores and brain structure should not be casually dismissed. Although these observations must be confirmed in other settings, they imply that the longstanding impetus to reduce overstimulation of preterm infants in our nurseries may have finally reached the tipping point at which less sensory input results in understimulation and developmental compromise. It is intriguing that differences in language scores were greatest among infants with moderate-to-severe brain injury (grade III–IV intraventricular hemorrhage, cystic periventricular leukomalacia, or cerebellar hemorrhage). In those infants, language scores were higher by 18.6 (95% confidence interval [CI], 9.2 to 28; $P=.0002$) for those in open wards compared with those in private rooms. Among infants without moderate-to-severe brain injury, however, language scores did not differ between those environments (mean difference, 4.2; 95% CI, −1 to 9.4; $P=.1$). This suggests a target group for studying focused interventions to ensure provision of appropriate sensory stimulation—light, sound, touch, taste, odor, and social interaction—to optimize developmental outcomes. As privacy and infection control concerns drive the transition to private rooms in our units, the answers to these questions will assume increasing importance and countermeasures to prevent social and sensory isolation are likely to be necessary.

W. E. Benitz, MD

9 Gastrointestinal Health and Nutrition

Gut microbiota in preterm infants: assessment and relevance to health and disease

Berrington JE, Stewart CJ, Embleton ND, et al (Newcastle upon Tyne Hosps NHS Foundation Trust, UK; Univ of Northumbria, Newcastle upon Tyne, UK)

Arch Dis Child Fetal Neonatal Ed 98:F286-F290, 2013

Background.—In preterm infants the establishment of the gut microbiota influences the development of morbid conditions such as late-onset sepsis (LOS) and necrotizing enterocolitis (NEC), which cause significant mortality. Changes in the intestinal barrier appear to contribute to both of these conditions, with gut microbiota playing key roles in developing barrier function, integrity, and mucosal and systemic immune function. Improved understanding of the microbiota of infants in neonatal intensive care units and of the relationship to current care practices may permit the establishment of healthier gut microbiota patterns and reduce problems.

Preterm Factors Associated with Microbiota.—Delivery mode and care can affect the makeup of the gut microbiota. Vaginally delivered term infants acquire gut microbiota from maternal exposures and the environment, whereas preterm infants delivered by caesarean section can have microbiota altered by the presence of antenatal and postnatal antibiotics, infection control measures, minimal exposure to maternal flora, less exposure to breast milk, and the effects of other medications. Although proof of these impacts is lacking, changes in microbiota in preterm compared to term infants appear to affect the development of NEC and LOS through a complex process. Most studies show that preterm microbiota exhibit more limited diversity, a more unstable profile, and delayed acquisition of "adult" profiles compared to term microbiota. However, neither standard cultures nor molecular approaches have shown a single microbial cause for NEC.

Interventions Associated with Altered Microbiota.—The effects of interventions that manipulate the microbiota tend to be complex, multidimensional, and nonlinear in causality. It is unclear whether maternal antibiotics can affect infant microbiota, but elective caesarean section may lead to a less than healthy microbiota profile. Postnatally, breast milk contains immunonutrients and growth factors that promote a bifidobacteria-dominant microbiota in healthy infants, but not in preterm infants. Oral antibiotics such as vancomycin or gentamicin produce a dominance of staphylococci in the preterm gut.. Antibiotics have not demonstrated any effect on colonization with bifidobacteria.

Among the deliberate interventions undertaken to manipulate preterm gut microbiota are the uses of prebiotics and other nutrients, probiotics, and lactoferrin. Prebiotics, which promote colonization with probiotics and are often short-chain carbohydrates, are added to some formulas to increase bifidobacterial counts in stools of preterm infants. A serendipitous increase in *Lactobacillus* species accompanies their use in preterm infants. Probiotics reduce the incidence of NEC but do not affect LOS. Some neonatal units routinely administer probiotics, which are well-tolerated and appear safe, although studies of large numbers of infants are needed to confirm this. Bovine lactoferrin (BLF) supplementation is associated with reduced LOS in very low birth weight infants. Lactoferrin enhances the cell proliferation of enterocytes and aids tight endothelial cell junctions, but in low doses can also stimulate the differentiation of enterocytes and the expression of intestinal digestive enzymes. Free radical activity is suppressed when iron is added to milk. BLF is bacteriostatic, inhibits growth by sequestering iron, and binds to lipopolysaccharide on the cell surface of enteropathogens, inhibiting surface expressed virulence factors. It also inhibits viral attachment and replication and is fungicidal. However, its effect on the microbiota is not yet known.

Conclusions.—Studies indicate the intestinal microbial community in preterm infants may be significantly associated with NEC and LOS, among other diseases. Although these investigations are not sufficiently large and have limitations that affect their applicability and insights into the mechanisms at work, it appears that alterations of the microbiota occur in preterm compared to term infants. Molecular studies of gut microbiota of preterm and term infants are needed to translate the basic scientific data into improved approaches to care and better outcomes.

► Recent work highlights the potential role of the human microbiome in health and disease. This concise but comprehensive review article outlines methodologies for assessing gut microbiota, their relationship to neonatal conditions, and factors that influence or can be used to manipulate the neonatal microbiome. It is a worthwhile read for all in the field of newborn health.

L. J. Van Marter, MD, MPH

Intestinal epithelial cell apoptosis and loss of barrier function in the setting of altered microbiota with enteral nutrient deprivation

Demehri FR, Barrett M, Ralls MW, et al (Univ of Michigan Health System, Ann Arbor)

Front Cell Infect Microbiol 3:105, 2013

Total parenteral nutrition (TPN), a commonly used treatment for patients who cannot receive enteral nutrition, is associated with significant septic complications due in part to a loss of epithelial barrier function (EBF). While the underlying mechanisms of TPN-related epithelial changes are poorly understood, a mouse model of TPN-dependence has helped identify several contributing factors. Enteral deprivation leads to a shift in intestinal microbiota to predominantly Gram-negative Proteobacteria. This is associated with an increase in expression of proinflammatory cytokines within the mucosa, including interferon-γ and tumor necrosis factor-α. A concomitant loss of epithelial growth factors leads to a decrease in epithelial cell proliferation and increased apoptosis. The resulting loss of epithelial tight junction proteins contributes to EBF dysfunction. These mechanisms identify potential strategies of protecting against TPN-related complications, such as modification of luminal bacteria, blockade of proinflammatory cytokines, or growth factor replacement (Figs 3 and 4).

▶ This review is fascinating because of the perspective it provides on the intestinal microbial ecology under the influence of total parenteral nutrition versus

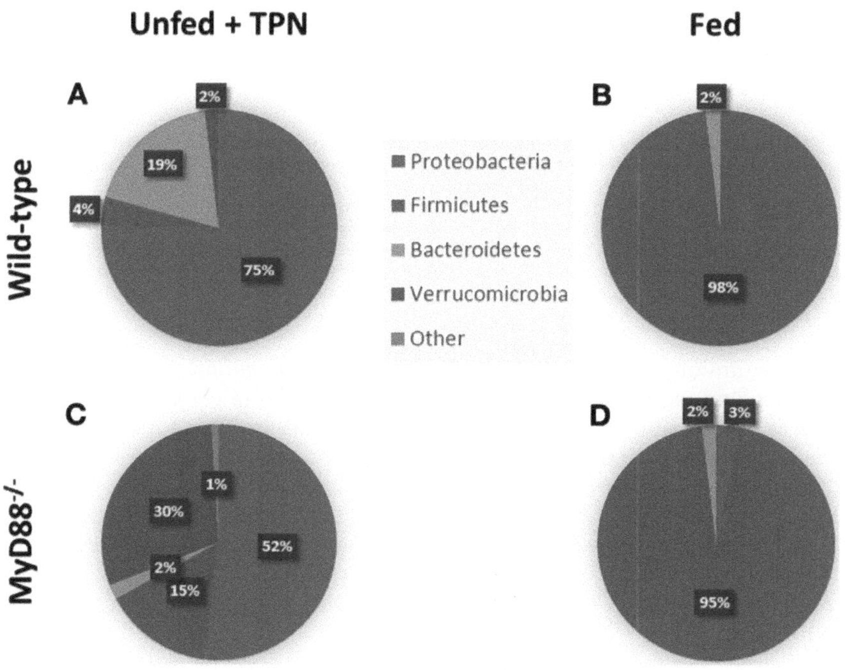

FIGURE 3.—Phylum-level changes in intestinal microbiota with TPN. Enteric bacteria from TPN-dependent mice (**A**) demonstrate a relative increase in Proteobacteria and Bacteroidetes vs. fed mice (**B**), where Firmicutes dominates.MyD88$^{-/-}$ mice, with defective TLR signaling, demonstrate an additional expansion of Verrucomicrobia with TPN-dependence (**C**) vs. fed controls (**D**). Akkermansia species predominate among the Verrucomicrobia. Adapted from Miyasaka et al. (2013). (Reprinted from Demehri FR, Barrett M, Ralls MW, et al. Intestinal epithelial cell apoptosis and loss of barrier function in the setting of altered microbiota with enteral nutrient deprivation. *Front Cell Infect Microbiol.* 2013;3:105.)

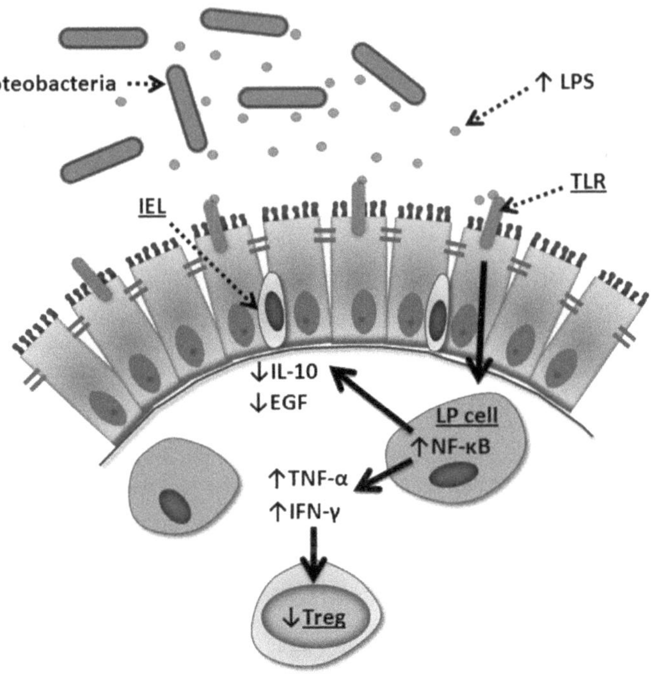

FIGURE 4.—Summary of TPN-induced epithelial signaling changes. Lack of enteral nutrition leads to a change in luminal microbiota where Gram-negative Proteobacteria dominate. Lipopolysaccharide (LPS) derived from these bacteria signal laminapropria (LP) cells via Toll-like receptors (TLR), leading to increased NF-κB transcription. This creates a pro-inflammatory state within creased TNF-α and IFN-γ, loss of T_{reg} cells, and decreased intraepithelial lymphocyte (IEL)-derived IL-10 and EGF. These changes lead to break down of tight junctions, loss of epithelial barrier function, bacterial translocation, and sepsis. (Reprinted from Demehri FR, Barrett M, Ralls MW, et al. Intestinal epithelial cell apoptosis and loss of barrier function in the setting of altered microbiota with enteral nutrient deprivation. *Front Cell Infect Microbiol.* 2013;3:105.)

enteral nutrition and the mechanisms of the complications that occur under these feeding regimens. Although this article primarily refers to studies in animals, it is of major interest in terms of clinical care in the neonatal intensive care unit where there is a reluctance to use the enteral route for feeding preterm infants, largely for fear of necrotizing enterocolitis (NEC).

Over the past few years, with the advent of the Human Microbiome Project, several investigators have begun to use microbial DNA-based sequencing technologies to identify taxa of bacteria present in the feces as a reflection of intestinal bacterial content in preterm infants.[1-4] One interesting finding in these studies is the predominance of the Proteobacteria phylum before the development of NEC in the cases compared with the controls. This review discusses studies that have shown this same phylum to predominate in animals nourished with total parenteral nutrition compared to enteral nutrition (Fig 3). It also presents a hypothesis on how this phylum, which comprises many Gram-negative pathogens with high levels of lipopolysaccharide in their cell walls, may induce intestinal inflammation and barrier breakdown on subsequent systemic inflammation (Fig 4).

These are intriguing relationships and underline the benefits of enteral versus parenteral nutrition.

J. Neu, MD

References

1. Mai V, Young CM, Ukhanova M, et al. Fecal microbiota in premature infants prior to necrotizing enterocolitis. *PLoS One*. 2011;6:e20647.
2. Torrazza RM, Neu J. The altered gut microbiome and necrotizing enterocolitis. *Clin Perinatol*. 2013;40:93-108.
3. Wang Y, Hoenig JD, Malin KJ, et al. 16S rRNA gene-based analysis of fecal microbiota from preterm infants with and without necrotizing enterocolitis. *ISME J*. 2009;3:944-954.
4. Morrow AL, Lagomarcino AJ, Schibler KR, et al. Early microbial and metabolomic signatures predict later onset of necrotizing enterocolitis in preterm infants. *Microbiome*. 2013;1:13.

Three Main Factors Define Changes in Fecal Microbiota Associated With Feeding Modality in Infants

Gomez-Llorente C, Plaza-Diaz J, Aguilera M, et al (Univ of Granada, Armilla; et al)

J Pediatr Gastroenterol Nutr 57:461-466, 2013

Objectives.—There are many differences in the fecal infant microbiota associated with various feeding methods. The aim of this study was to examine the major differences in the fecal microbiota of breast-fed (BF) and formula-fed (FF) infants and to describe the principal bacterial components that would explain the variability in the predominant bacterial families and genus clusters.

Methods.—Fecal samples from 58 infants, 31 of whom were exclusively BF and 27 of whom were exclusively FF with a standard formula in agreement with the European Society for Pediatric Gastroenterology, Hepatology, and Nutrition recommendations, were analyzed by fluorescent in situ hybridization combined with flow cytometry. Principal component analysis was used to maximize the information gained for the predominant bacterial families and genus clusters using a minimal number of bacterial groups.

Results.—The predominant detected group was *Bifidobacterium*, followed by Enterobacteriaceae and *Bacteroides* in both BF and FF infants. The *Lactobacillus* group was the only independent variable associated with FF infants. We also found that 3 principal components were sufficient to describe the association between the bacterial group, genus, and species studied in BF and FF infants; however, these components differed between BF and FF infants. For the former, the 3 factors found were *Bifidobacterium*/Enterobacteriaceae, *Lactobacillus/Bacteroides*, and *Clostridium coccoides/Atopobium*; for the latter, *Bifidobacterium*/Enterobacteriaceae, *Bacteroides* and *C coccoides* were observed.

Conclusions.—There is a clear clustering of components of infant microbiota based on the feeding method.

▶ Previous studies have evaluated the microbes in the feces of infants who were breast fed versus formula fed and have found some differences. However, with the advent of the Human Microbiome Project, the use of culture-based techniques appears to be of limited utility when one considers that about 70% of the microbes in the human intestine cannot be cultured. This study evaluates bacteria in the feces of 58 infants, 31 of whom were exclusively breast fed and 27 of whom were exclusively fed with commercial formula. The fecal samples were collected from healthy infants at approximately 12 weeks of age. Analysis of the microbes consisted of fluorescent in situ hybridization flow cytometry, limited to the use of primers for only 10 bacterial genus and species.

The results showed the Bifidobacteria genus highest among the microbes that were evaluated. There also appeared to be a clustering of the microbial associations into 3 principal components. However, it is somewhat disappointing that this work does not really add to our understanding of the microbial ecology of babies who are breast fed versus formula fed, as up-to-date metagenomic technologies were not used that would actually enable evaluation of the hundreds of microbial taxa expected to be present in the feces of the babies at this developmental stage. In addition to the paucity of actual taxonomic information, there is no hint about the functional differences incurred in the intestines of these infants because of the differences in microbes resulting from breast versus formula feeding.

Although the intent of the study is to address a very important topic, the study itself falls short and does not to add much to our knowledge of the differences in the intestinal microbial ecology of breast-fed versus formula-fed infants.

J. Neu, MD

Milk oligosaccharide sialyl(α2,3)lactose activates intestinal CD11c⁺ cells through TLR4

Kurakevich E, Hennet T, Hausmann M, et al (Univ of Zürich, Switzerland; Univ Hosp Zürich, Switzerland)

Proc Natl Acad Sci U S A 110:17444-17449, 2013

Breast milk oligosaccharides shape the intestinal environment by affecting mucosal immunity and bacterial colonization. To clarify the role of milk oligosaccharide sialyl(α2,3)lactose (3SL) in intestinal physiology and disease, we investigated colitis development in *Il10*$^{-/-}$ mice exposed to normal or 3SL-deficient milk during lactation. Onset and progression of intestinal inflammation were delayed in *Il10*$^{-/-}$ mice deficient for the α2,3 sialyltransferase 4 (ST3GAL4) responsible for 3SL biosynthesis. The proinflammatory role of 3SL was confirmed by showing that oral supplementation of newborn *Il10*$^{-/-}$;*St3gal4*$^{-/-}$ mice with 3SL increased colitis severity. Conversely, fostering of newborn *Il10*$^{-/-}$ mice to lactating *St3gal4*$^{-/-}$ mothers reduced colitis severity. 3SL directly stimulated mesenteric lymph node CD11c$^+$ dendritic cells and induced production of cytokines required for expansion of T_H1 and T_H17 T cells. The stimulatory effect of 3SL was attenuated in Tlr4- deficient CD11c$^+$ cells, demonstrating that 3SL induces inflammation through Toll-like receptor 4 (TLR4) signaling. Thus, 3SL directly modulates mucosal immunity, which increases susceptibility to colitis.

▶ There are certain carbohydrate molecules in our diets that intestinal microbes will use for their personal functions. For example, certain commensal bacteria in the gastrointestinal tract will use carbohydrates, sometimes termed *prebiotics*, for potentially useful purposes in the gastrointestinal tract. Other carbohydrates, such as the oligosaccharides found in high quantities in human milk, are also thought to have beneficial effects on the commensal microorganisms residing in an infant's intestine. The precise mechanism of these human milk oligosaccharides' interactions with the gut microbiota and host is not fully understood. They are thought to be provided as a metabolic substrate for bacteria, and these bacteria then use them for beneficial host microbial interactions.

This report discusses a certain milk oligosaccharide called *Sialyl (α2, 3) lactose* (3SL) and its role in intestinal physiology. The investigators used interleukin 10 (IL-10) knockout mice exposed to 3SL-deficient milk and found that the inflammation normally seen in these animals was delayed by the deficiency of the 3SL. Conversely, if they gave 3SL by oral supplementation to these animals, this stimulated the colitis. They found that this stimulation was through a certain type of the dendritic cell called the CD11c$^+$, and it induced the production of proinflammatory cytokines.

These results are somewhat surprising to me in that oligosaccharides found in human milk are considered to be protective and potentially antiinflammatory. However, this 3SL was found to be proinflammatory. The experiments suggested that this proinflammatory effect was not via stimulation of microbial expansion but rather directly on the CD11c$^+$ dendritic cell. Why is this important? For one thing, it appears that the adaptive immune system requires training, and a small amount of stimulation in the gastrointestinal tract of the very early newborn infant is thought to be potentially beneficial. The authors suggest that the proinflammatory action of this 3SL may actually serve to train the gastrointestinal tract for future contact with potentially pathogenic micro-organisms when this effect will be needed for protection. It appears we have a lot to learn about these oligosaccharides and their interaction with the microbiota and the host.

J. Neu, MD

Effects of Different Complementary Feeding Regimens on Iron Status and Enteric Microbiota in Breastfed Infants

Krebs NF, Sherlock LG, Westcott J, et al (Univ of Colorado School of Medicine, Aurora; et al)

J Pediatr 163:416-423.e4, 2013

Objective.—To compare iron status in breastfed infants randomized to groups receiving complementary feeding regimens that provided iron from fortified infant cereals or meats, and to examine the development of the enteric microbiota in these groups.

Study Design.—Forty-five exclusively breastfed 5-month-old infants were randomized to 1 of 3 feeding groups (FGs)—commercially available pureed meats, iron- and zinc-fortified infant cereals, or iron-only fortified infant cereals—as the first and primary complementary food through 9-10 months of age. Dietary iron was determined by monthly 3-day diet records. Iron status was assessed at the end of the study by measurements of hemoglobin, serum ferritin, and soluble transferrin receptor levels. In a subsample of 14 infants, enteric microbiota were profiled in monthly stool samples (5-9 months) by 16S ribosomal RNA gene pyrosequencing.

Results.—Infants in the 2 cereal FGs had 2- to 3-fold greater daily iron intakes versus the meat FG ($P < .0001$). More than one-quarter (27%) of the infants had a low serum ferritin level, and 36% were mildly anemic, with no significant differences by FG; more infants in the meat FG had a high soluble transferrin receptor value ($P = .03$). Sequence analysis identified differences by time and FG in the abundances of several bacterial groups, including significantly more abundant butyrate-producing *Clostridium* group XIVa in the meat FG ($P = .01$).

Conclusion.—A high percentage of healthy infants who were breastfed-only were iron-deficient, and complementary feeding, including iron exposure, influenced the development of the enteric microbiota. If these findings are confirmed, then reconsideration of strategies to both meet infants' iron requirements and optimize the developing microbiome may be warranted.

▶ This article is fascinating from the perspective that it provides very important pilot information about infants who are breastfed and then randomly assigned to feeding groups that contained iron- and zinc-fortified infant cereals, iron-only-fortified infant cereal, or pureed meats through the first 9 to 10 months of age. In this study, dietary iron was determined by diet records, and iron status was assessed by measurements of hemoglobin, serum ferritin, and soluble transferrin receptor levels. They also did enteric microbiome profiling using monthly stool samples and 16S ribosomal RNA sequencing. The infants in the 2 fortified cereal groups received considerably more iron than those babies in the meat-supplemented group. Despite this, the hemoglobin levels were very similar in the 3 groups. The iron-fortified cereal groups tended to have higher serum ferritins. Microbiota analysis using 16S Pyrosequencing suggested interesting differences in the bacterial phyla classifications. Although the numbers were very small, the meat-fed group had lower numbers of Bacteroidetes and higher Firmicutes.

When evaluating the microbiota on a subphylum level, the meat-fed group had higher quantities of *Clostridium* XIBa, a microbe that is highly associated with butyrate production. Why is this important? Butyrate is a major fuel for colonic epithelium and has major effects on interepithelial tight junctions as well as development of the immune system. One could speculate that the greater quantity of butyrate-producing bacteria could result in better health outcomes.

This study is interesting from the perspective that it offers some interesting preliminary data that needs to be followed up with larger studies. It shows that dietary factors such as meat feeding vs cereal feeding as well as quantity of iron supplemented in primarily breast milk-fed babies can result in a significant variability in the intestinal microbiome. Because the early microbiome has a major effect on subsequent development of the immune system, these results need to be seriously evaluated in a larger cohort of patients. It may have significant relevance in terms of subsequent development of various diseases related to the developing immune system, including autoimmune diseases, allergies, and asthma.

J. Neu, MD

Fecal S100A12: Identifying Intestinal Distress in Very-Low-Birth-Weight Infants

Däbritz J, Foell D, Wirth S, et al (Murdoch Children's Res Inst, Parkville, Australia; Univ Children's Hosp Münster, Germany; Helios Klinikum Wuppertal, Germany)

J Pediatr Gastroenterol Nutr 57:204-210, 2013

Objectives.—The aim of the study was to determine whether longitudinal measurements of fecal S100A12, a damage-associated molecular pattern protein, which is released from neutrophils or monocytes under stress, can detect very-low-birth-weight (VLBW) infants at risk for intestinal distress apart from necrotizing enterocolitis.

Methods.—This prospective study included 46 VLBW infants with intestinal distress and 49 reference patients. Meconium and stool samples were collected prospectively on alternate days for 4 weeks, and fecal S100A12 was measured by enzyme-linked immunosorbent assay.

Results.—Gestational age and weight at birth were significantly lower in patients with intestinal distress when compared to unaffected reference infants. Median levels of fecal S100A12 were significantly higher in patients with intestinal distress at onset of disease and before compared with unaffected reference infants. Median levels of fecal S100A12 declined steadily to baseline levels within 2 weeks after disease onset. The ideal cut-off value for identifying patients with intestinal distress within 7 days before disease onset was 60 μg/kg (sensitivity 0.73; specificity 0.55).

Conclusions.—Fecal S100A12 levels are increased in VLBW infants with intestinal distress; however, the potential for S100A12 as an early

biomarker is largely limited by overlaps between values of infants with intestinal distress and the reference population.

▶ Approximately 1 year before the publication of this report, the same authors published a report in the *Journal of Pediatrics*[1] in which they assessed stool samples and measured the inflammatory marker protein S100A12, which is released from neutrophils or monocytes under stress. They found that this marker was often increased 1 to 2 weeks before the clinical onset of necrotizing enterocolitis compared with control infants. The authors suggested that the pathophysiology of necrotizing enterocolitis may include a prolonged period of inflammation before clinical diagnosis and that it may be used as a biomarker but has limitations based on large overlaps between values for infants who developed necrotizing enterocolitis compared with control infants.

In this study, the authors aimed to determine whether longitudinal measurements of fecal S100A12 could detect very low birth weight infants at risk for intestinal distress apart from necrotizing enterocolitis. They found that fecal S100A12 levels were increased in very low birth weight infants with intestinal distress; however, as with necrotizing enterocolitis, the potential for S100A12 as an early biomarker was again limited by overlaps between values of infants with intestinal distress and the reference population.

The design of this study is one that involves clumping a large number of outcome variables into the term *intestinal distress*. The control group consisted of infants without any signs and symptoms of intestinal distress. The intestinal distress group, on the other hand, included infants with decreased intestinal motility as defined by a decrease in feeding judged by the clinicians caring for the babies, meconium plug syndrome, suspected stage I necrotizing enterocolitis, intestinal perforation, impaired intestinal blood circulation, and intestinal distress of unknown origin. Many of these results are highly subjective and prone to error. For example, how does one diagnose stage 1 necrotizing enterocolitis objectively? Feedings are often decreased for reasons not related directly to the intestine, again making this a very subjective outcome.

The results showed a difference in gestational age between the intestinal distress and control groups of 2 weeks, with the intestinal distress group having a mean of 27 weeks whereas the control group was 29 weeks of gestation. Thus, intestinal distress appeared to segregate to the less mature group as would be expected. The sensitivity and specificity is varied depending on what outcome measures were evaluated and were not higher than 73% and 55%, respectively. The receiver operating characteristic (ROC) curves showed areas of .68 before the onset of the disease, again, as with the sensitivity and specificity, not usually considered to be very good. When a time course analysis was done, it was found that there was no difference in S100A12 levels in distressed vs control babies at 24 to 27 weeks of gestation, but there were some differences at 28 to 31 weeks of gestation and 32 to 37 weeks of gestation. However, the baseline S100A812 level in the control infants was higher in the most immature babies, suggesting that the greater degree of immaturity actually was associated with higher S100A12 levels. This may have been a function of the in utero conditions in these infants that were most immature compared with the more mature infants.

Of interest is that the authors studied meconium plug syndrome. How could a baby meconium plug syndrome be analyzed with prior fecal sampling, as meconium plug syndrome appears by definition to be inspissated meconium, that is, the infant's first stool? Another question that arises is whether there was common use of enemas or other stimulators of stooling in these infants in the 5 neonatal intensive care units involved in the study. This was not mentioned in the report and could have an effect on the results as indicated.

Although fecal S100A12 may be a reasonable marker of intestinal distress and inflammation, its use according to the studies by this group on necrotizing enterocolitis and intestinal distress does not appear to be ready for any kind of routine use.

J. Neu, MD

Reference

1. Dabritz J, Jenke A, Wirth S, Foell D. Fecal phagocyte-specific S100A12 for diagnosing necrotizing enterocolitis. *J Pediatr.* 2012;161:1059-1064.

Secretory antibodies in breast milk promote long-term intestinal homeostasis by regulating the gut microbiota and host gene expression

Rogier EW, Frantz AL, Bruno MEC, et al (Univ of Kentucky, Lexington)

Proc Natl Acad Sci U S A 111:3074-3079, 2014

Maintenance of intestinal homeostasis requires a healthy relationship between the commensal gut microbiota and the host immune system. Breast milk supplies the first source of antigen-specific immune protection in the gastrointestinal tract of suckling mammals, in the form of secretory IgA (SIgA). SIgA is transported across glandular and mucosal epithelial cells into external secretions by the polymeric Ig receptor (pIgR). Here, a breeding scheme with polymeric Ig receptor-sufficient and -deficient mice was used to study the effects of breast milk-derived SIgA on development of the gut microbiota and host intestinal immunity. Early exposure to maternal SIgA prevented the translocation of aerobic bacteria from the neonatal gut into draining lymph nodes, including the opportunistic pathogen *Ochrobactrum anthropi*. By the age of weaning, mice that received maternal SIgA in breast milk had a significantly different gut microbiota from mice that did not receive SIgA, and these differences were magnified when the mice reached adulthood. Early exposure to SIgA in breast milk resulted in a pattern of intestinal epithelial cell gene expression in adult mice that differed from that of mice that were not exposed to passive SIgA, including genes associated with intestinal inflammatory diseases in humans. Maternal SIgA was also found to ameliorate colonic damage caused by the epithelial-disrupting agent dextran sulfate sodium. These findings reveal unique mechanisms through which SIgA in breast milk

may promote lifelong intestinal homeostasis, and provide additional evidence for the benefits of breastfeeding.

▶ It has long been known that babies who are breast fed may incur lifelong health benefits, but the mechanisms for these benefits have not been rigorously investigated. In this study, the effect of secretory IgA (SIgA) in breast milk and endogenous SIgA derived from the intestinal mucosa was investigated using a genetically modified mouse model deficient in the receptor for the SIgA and a breeding scheme that allowed for the evaluation of the differential effects of milk-derived SIgA and intestinal-derived SIgA in the offspring during different stages of development. The former source of SIgA (breast milk) provides an immediate source of this highly bioactive agent right after birth, whereas the SIgA derived from the intestine is a component of the adaptive immune response and takes time to develop.

In this study, genetically manipulated animals that have the capability to produce SIgA in their milk or in their intestines were evaluated. This study aimed to determine if early exposure to breast milk SIgA will result in responses in the intestine of the infant that will alter the funçtional expression of the developing intestine and the microbial ecology of the gastrointestinal tract, which, in turn, affects the immune responses and homeostatic mechanisms and protective mechanisms in the intestine of the developing animal.

In this study, early exposure to maternal SIgA from the breast milk promoted intestinal barrier function and altered the microbial ecology of the gastrointestinal tract against the development of certain Proteobacteria and Firmicute microorganisms that may induce greater inflammatory potential to the gastrointestinal tract than other microbes. Failure to receive SIgA in breast milk resulted in significantly increased translocation of aerobic bacteria into the mesenteric lymph nodes. The authors propose that early exposure to the passive SIgA in breast milk protects the neonates against invasion of potential pathogens across the epithelial barrier into the draining lymphatics.

Even more dramatic than those findings of decreased bacterial translocation with the SIgA, the differences in the microbiota of the offspring of the dams that provided SIgA versus those that did not were not only apparent at the time of weaning but increased as the mice aged after weaning. This finding supports the concept that both passive and active SIgA shape the composition of the gut microbiota throughout the individual's lifespan. This is important in that some of the microbes such as the Proteobacteria are commonly associated with exacerbations of the inflammation in older individuals with inflammatory bowel disease. Furthermore, these bacteria have been seen in higher quantities relative to other intestinal bacteria before the development of necrotizing enterocolitis in premature babies.

These studies are important in that they show some mechanisms through which SIgA in breast milk may serve to promote intestinal homeostasis, prevent microbial translocation, prevent damage, and promote in the microbiota, which may serve to be beneficial for individuals during their lifetime. Although it may be a bit of a leap to extrapolate these findings to humans, they serve as an excellent start to support the concept of the relationship between early SIgA exposure from breast milk and later health outcomes.

J. Neu, MD

Epigenetic Effects of Human Breast Milk

Verduci E, Banderali G, Barberi S, et al (Univ of Milan, Italy)
Nutrients 6:1711-1724, 2014

A current aim of nutrigenetics is to personalize nutritional practices according to genetic variations that influence the way of digestion and metabolism of nutrients introduced with the diet. Nutritional epigenetics concerns knowledge about the effects of nutrients on gene expression. Nutrition in early life or in critical periods of development, may have a role in modulating gene expression, and, therefore, have later effects on health. Human breast milk is well-known for its ability in preventing several acute and chronic diseases. Indeed, breastfed children may have lower risk of neonatal necrotizing enterocolitis, infectious diseases, and also of non-communicable diseases, such as obesity and related-disorders. Beneficial effects of human breast milk on health may be associated in part with its peculiar components, possible also via epigenetic processes. This paper discusses about presumed epigenetic effects of human breast milk and components. While evidence suggests that a direct relationship may exist of some components of human breast milk with epigenetic changes, the mechanisms involved are still unclear. Studies have to be conducted to clarify the actual role of human breast milk on genetic expression, in particular when linked to the risk of non-communicable diseases, to potentially benefit the infant's health and his later life (Table 1).

▶ The epigenetic effects of the components of human breast milk remain understudied. The term "epigenetics" refers to processes that induce heritable changes in gene expression without altering the gene sequence. These epigenetic processes include DNA methylation and histone modifications, which act on our DNA transcription mechanisms in a manner analogous to volume and tone modulation in a stereophonic music system. There are critical life-cycle periods such as embryonic, fetal, and early infancy stages in which nutritional epigenetics are being found to play a significant role in subsequent health and disease.

This review focuses on the epigenetic effects of breast milk and breastfeeding. Furthermore, it suggests that not only the nutritional components of breast milk but also the effects of these components on the infant microbiota may result in epigenetic effects. Some of the effects of breast milk on subsequent health include decreased prevalence of necrotizing enterocolitis, obesity, diabetes, and infectious diseases. For all of these, the expression of epigenetically modifiable target genes need to be involved. Table 1 provides some of the human milk components that are involved with the prevention of certain diseases and the epigenetically modifiable genes for which expressions are altered

TABLE 1.—Epigenetic Effect of Human Breast Milk Components on the Child's Health Outcomes

Human Milk Component	Prevention of	Gene (Expression)
Lactoferrin	NEC Disorders of immune system	NF-kB (reduced)[a]
Prostaglandin J	Obesity and related-disorders	PPARγ (increased)[b]
LCPUFA *n*-3	NAFLD	Liver lipogenic and cholesterol byosynthesis enzymes (reduced)[a]
	Progression of NAFLD	PPAR α and γ (increased)[b]
	High blood total cholesterol in adulthood	HMGCoA reductase (reduced)[a]
Cholesterol content	High blood total cholesterol in adulthood	HMGCoA reductase (reduced)[b]
Undigestible oligosaccharides	Gut dysbiosis and related alterations (NEC, infectious diseases, disorders of immune system, obesity and linked disorders)	Action on expression of different genes (e.g., NF-κB)[b]

[a]proved *in vitro* and/or animals.
[b]hypothesized in humans.

via the human milk components. This review points to particular epigenetic targets that require further study for our understanding to better promote health and to prevent these diseases.

J. Neu, MD

A Pacifier-Activated Music Player With Mother's Voice Improves Oral Feeding in Preterm Infants

Chorna OD, Slaughter JC, Wang L, et al (Vanderbilt Kennedy Ctr, Nashville, TN; Vanderbilt Univ, Nashville, TN; Vanderbilt Univ School of Medicine, Nashville, TN)
Pediatrics 133:462-468, 2014

Objectives.—We conducted a randomized trial to test the hypothesis that mother's voice played through a pacifier-activated music player (PAM) during nonnutritive sucking would improve the development of sucking ability and promote more effective oral feeding in preterm infants.

Methods.—Preterm infants between 34 0/7 and 35 6/7 weeks' postmenstrual age, including those with brain injury, who were taking at least half their feedings enterally and less than half orally, were randomly assigned to receive 5 daily 15-minute sessions of either PAM with mother's recorded voice or no PAM, along with routine nonnutritive sucking and maternal care in both groups. Assignment was masked to the clinical team.

Results.—Ninety-four infants (46 and 48 in the PAM intervention and control groups, respectively) completed the study. The intervention

TABLE 3.—Hospitalization Outcomes

Measure	Intervention, $n = 46$	Control, $n = 48$	P
Time to full oral feeds, d	31 (17–54)	38 (24–69)	.04
Length of hospital stay, d	41 (25–69)	50 (31–86)	.07
Discharge weight, g	2000 (1892–2228)	1990 (1902–2120)	.62

Values are median (interquartile range).
All P determined by using GEE linear regression controlling for twins.

group had significantly increased oral feeding rate (2.0 vs 0.9 mL/min, $P < .001$), oral volume intake (91.1 vs 48.1 mL/kg/d, $P = .001$), oral feeds/day (6.5 vs 4.0, $P < .001$), and faster time-to-full oral feedings (31 vs 38 d, $P = .04$) compared with controls. Weight gain and cortisol levels during the 5-day protocol were not different between groups. Average hospital stays were 20% shorter in the PAM group, but the difference was not significant ($P = .07$).

Conclusions.—A PAM using mother's voice improves oral feeding skills in preterm infants without adverse effects on hormonal stress or growth (Table 3).

▶ Many neonatal intensive care units are now using the single-room approach. As mentioned by the authors of this article, this design has been shown to be disadvantageous in certain situations in which the development of the infants is actually delayed because of the lack of stimulation. Other studies have also shown that music therapy may improve outcomes. In this study, a device that the authors call a pacifier-activated music player that uses a lullaby sung by the mother was evaluated to determine whether this would result in improved feeding in infants from 34 to 37 weeks' postmenstrual age. Babies with proven white-matter damage were included in the study. The table shows the outcome differences in terms of time to full oral feeds and length of hospitalization. There was a significant difference in time to full oral feeds of about 7 days with the lullaby group taking less time to full oral feeds, as well as a trend toward a lesser hospital stay by about 9 days ($P = .07$). The salivary cortisol levels did not differ between the 2 groups, but as the authors acknowledge, these were difficult to collect and analyze, thus blunting the validity of the results. Nevertheless, this seems to be a safe and innocuous technique to shorten the time to full enteral feedings and perhaps even shorten hospital stays (the number of infants in this study was not sufficient to test this). Whether the lullaby sung by another mother, the father, or even compared to Mozart, was not evaluated.

J. Neu, MD

A Pacifier-Activated Music Player With Mother's Voice Improves Oral Feeding in Preterm Infants

Chorna OD, Slaughter JC, Wang L, et al (Vanderbilt Kennedy Ctr, Nashville, TN; Vanderbilt Univ, Nashville, TN; Vanderbilt Univ School of Medicine, Nashville, TN)

Pediatrics 133:462-468, 2014

Objectives.—We conducted a randomized trial to test the hypothesis that mother's voice played through a pacifier-activated music player (PAM) during nonnutritive sucking would improve the development of sucking ability and promote more effective oral feeding in preterm infants.

Methods.—Preterm infants between 34 0/7 and 35 6/7 weeks' postmenstrual age, including those with brain injury, who were taking at least half their feedings enterally and less than half orally, were randomly assigned to receive 5 daily 15-minute sessions of either PAM with mother's recorded voice or no PAM, along with routine nonnutritive sucking and maternal care in both groups. Assignment was masked to the clinical team.

Results.—Ninety-four infants (46 and 48 in the PAM intervention and control groups, respectively) completed the study. The intervention group had significantly increased oral feeding rate (2.0 vs 0.9 mL/min, $P < .001$), oral volume intake (91.1 vs 48.1 mL/kg/d, $P = .001$), oral feeds/ day (6.5 vs 4.0, $P < .001$), and faster time-to-full oral feedings (31 vs 38 d, $P = .04$) compared with controls. Weight gain and cortisol levels during the 5-day protocol were not different between groups. Average hospital stays were 20% shorter in the PAM group, but the difference was not significant ($P = .07$).

Conclusions.—A PAM using mother's voice improves oral feeding skills in preterm infants without adverse effects on hormonal stress or growth.

▶ In 2005, Pinelli et al[1] did a Cochrane Review examining nonnutritive sucking (NNS) that included 21 studies, 15 of which were randomized controlled trials. NNS was found to decrease significantly the length of hospital stay in preterm infants. The review did not reveal a consistent benefit of NNS with respect to other major clinical variables (weight gain, energy intake, heart rate, oxygen saturation, intestinal transit time, age at full oral feeds, and behavioral state). The review identified other positive clinical outcomes of NNS: transition from tube to bottle feeds and better bottle-feeding performance. No negative outcomes were reported in any of the studies. Indeed, NNS is used extensively in the neonatal intensive care unit.

In 2010, Krueger et al[2] reported that systematically exposing preterm infants (before 34 weeks' gestation) to their mother's voice resulted in less feeding intolerance and quicker transition to full enteral feeding.

Chorna et al from Vanderbilt have completed a novel study by integrating a sensor into a routinely used pacifier and delivering a predetermined timed interval of auditory stimulus, in the form of the mother's voice, to preterm babies on detection of a suck that meets a preset pressure threshold. The subjects were late preterm infants and included some babies with significant white matter injury.

The results were very encouraging in that all aspects of feeding were enhanced. They demonstrated that a pacifier-activated music player (PAM) using the mother's voice resulted in faster achievement of full oral feedings compared with NNS with a standard pacifier and random exposure to mother's voice. They commented, "To our knowledge, this is the first demonstration of mother's voice used with a PAM to promote oral feeding skills. Involving mothers through music therapy to teach essential developmental skills to their infant promotes family-centered care in the NICU." They further speculated that the use of recorded maternal voice might compensate for lack of appropriate auditory stimulation in single—patient rooms, which have been associated with neurodevelopmental delays.[3] The technology appears to be simple, and hopefully the results will be validated and introduced into more nurseries. I congratulate the authors on a well-conducted novel trial, with meaningful clinically relevant outcomes.

A. A. Fanaroff, MD, FRCPE

References

1. Pinelli J, Symington A. Non-nutritive sucking for promoting physiologic stability and nutrition in preterm infants. *Cochrane Database Syst Rev.* 2005;(4):CD001071.
2. Krueger C, Parker L, Chiu SH, Theriaque D. Maternal voice and short-term outcomes in preterm infants. *Dev Psychobiol.* 2010;52:205-212.
3. Pineda RG, Neil J, Dierker D, et al. Alterations in brain structure and neurodevelopmental outcome in preterm infants hospitalized in different neonatal intensive care unit environments. *J Pediatr.* 2014;164:52-60.e2.

Randomized Trial of Exclusive Human Milk versus Preterm Formula Diets in Extremely Premature Infants

Cristofalo EA, Schanler RJ, Blanco CL, et al (Johns Hopkins School of Medicine, Baltimore, MD; Cohen Children's Med Ctr of New York, New Hyde Park; Univ of Texas Health Science Ctr, San Antonio; et al)

J Pediatr 163:1592-1595.e1, 2013

Objective.—To compare the duration of parenteral nutrition, growth, and morbidity in extremely premature infants fed exclusive diets of either bovine milk–based preterm formula (BOV) or donor human milk and human milk-based human milk fortifier (HUM), in a randomized trial of formula vs human milk.

Study Design.—Multicenter randomized controlled trial. The authors studied extremely preterm infants whose mothers did not provide their milk. Infants were fed either BOV or an exclusive human milk diet of pasteurized donor human milk and HUM. The major outcome was duration of parenteral nutrition. Secondary outcomes were growth, respiratory support, and necrotizing enterocolitis (NEC).

Results.—Birth weight (983 vs 996 g) and gestational age (27.5 vs 27.7 wk), in BOV and HUM, respectively, were similar. There was a significant difference in median parenteral nutrition days: 36 vs 27, in BOV vs HUM, respectively ($P = .04$). The incidence of NEC in BOV was 21% (5 cases) vs 3% in HUM (1 case), $P = .08$; surgical NEC was significantly higher in BOV (4 cases) than HUM (0 cases), $P = .04$.

Conclusions.—In extremely preterm infants given exclusive diets of preterm formula vs human milk, there was a significantly greater duration of parenteral nutrition and higher rate of surgical NEC in infants receiving preterm formula. This trial supports the use of an exclusive human milk diet to nourish extremely preterm infants in the neonatal intensive care unit.

▶ A reduction in necrotizing enterocolitis (NEC), both medical and surgical, was reported more than 20 years ago among infants who received only human milk when compared with infants less than or equal to 1850 grams birth weight who received all bovine-milk-based formula.[1] Those infants receiving a mixture of formula and human milk had an intermediate level of protection. This study preceded the use of powdered fortifiers for preterm milk. Feeding extremely low birth weight infants unfortified human milk would place them at risk for protein and mineral insufficiency associated with poor growth and metabolic bone disease, respectively.[1] This study included 926 infants, with approximately 220 in the same gestational age range as Cristofalo et al, who showed a higher rate of surgical NEC among 7 participating units and 53 patients between 500 and 1250 grams birth weight when fed preterm formula versus exclusive human milk and human-milk-based fortifier.[2]

The patients included those whose mothers did not provide their milk. Many of these women had factors (eg, illicit drug use) that might be associated with a greater risk of NEC for their infants. This study was powered for the primary outcome of duration of parenteral nutrition as a surrogate for feeding tolerance and neonatal morbidity. Infants fed the exclusive human milk diet required fewer days of parenteral nutrition (27 vs 36, respectively) versus the formula fed infants. However, 5 of 24 infants developed NEC in the Bovine group (21%) versus 1 of 19 infants in the exclusively human milk fed group (3%). Because of the small numbers, this was not statistically significant, but surgical NEC 17% in bovine group versus 0% in the exclusive human milk fed group was statistically significant.[2]

The authors agree that this is a small population. The rate of NEC in the bovine group is remarkable. NEC risk varies, but in large data sets, the risk range is around 7% among those of <1500 g birth weight. For example, the Neonatal Research Network of the National Institute of Child Health and Human Development over a 5-year period for truly extreme premature infants (weighing 501–750 grams at birth), the incidence was 11%, whereas those weighing 1251 to 1500 g, the incidence was 3%.[3] The Lactoferrin studies from Manzoni and colleagues, including a probiotic plus lactoferrin arm, 472 infants were studied, and 259 controls with approximate gestational age of 29 weeks had a 5.4% incidence of NEC.[4]

Infants of the Cristofalo study in the exclusive human milk feeding group grew statistically significantly slower in length from return to birth weight to end of study (0.84 cm/week vs 1.12 cm/week, respectively) and gained 2 grams per day less than the bovine group. This could easily be addressed with adjustments in fortification. Feeding tolerance measured by time to full enteral feedings was no different between the groups. Are these feeding tolerance observations also related to small sample size?

We are beginning to see important studies suggesting strategies for prevention of NEC through diet and agents affecting the microbiome of extremely preterm infants. This "inflammatory dysbiosis" must certainly be at the core of NEC and its prevention. The next step is for companies, health research institutes, and regulatory authorities to allow the testing of specific new products in conjunction with promotion of human milk feeding strategies to lead us to the best strategies to prevent NEC.

D. H. Adamkin, MD

References

1. Lucas A, Cole TJ. Breast milk and neonatal necrotising enterocolitis. *Lancet.* 1990;336:1519-1523.
2. Cristofalo EA, Schanler RJ, Blanco C, et al. Randomized trial of exclusive human milk versus preterm formula diets in extremely premature infants. *J Pediatr.* 2013; 163:1592-1595.e1.
3. Fanaroff AA, Stoll BJ, Wright LL, et al. Trends in neonatal morbidity and mortality for very low birthweight infants. *Am J Obstet Gynecol.* 2007;196: 147.e1-147.e8.
4. Manzoni P, Rinaldi M, Meyer M, et al. Bovine lactoferrin supplementation for prevention of necrotizing enterocolitis in preterm very-low-birth-weight neonates: a randomized trial. *Early Hum Dev.* 2011;87:S92.

Randomized Trial of Exclusive Human Milk versus Preterm Formula Diets in Extremely Premature Infants

Cristofalo EA, Schanler RJ, Blanco CL, et al (Johns Hopkins School of Medicine, Baltimore, MD; Cohen Children's Med Ctr of New York, New Hyde Park; Univ of Texas Health Science Ctr, San Antonio; et al)
J Pediatr 163:1592-1595.e1, 2013

Objective.—To compare the duration of parenteral nutrition, growth, and morbidity in extremely premature infants fed exclusive diets of either bovine milk-based preterm formula (BOV) or donor human milk and human milk-based human milk fortifier (HUM), in a randomized trial of formula vs human milk.

Study Design.—Multicenter randomized controlled trial. The authors studied extremely preterm infants whose mothers did not provide their milk. Infants were fed either BOV or an exclusive human milk diet of pasteurized donor human milk and HUM. The major outcome was duration of parenteral nutrition. Secondary outcomes were growth, respiratory support, and necrotizing enterocolitis (NEC).

Results.—Birth weight (983 vs 996 g) and gestational age (27.5 vs 27.7 wk), in BOV and HUM, respectively, were similar. There was a significant difference in median parenteral nutrition days: 36 vs 27, in BOV vs HUM, respectively ($P = .04$). The incidence of NEC in BOV was 21% (5 cases) vs 3% in HUM (1 case), $P = .08$; surgical NEC was significantly higher in BOV (4 cases) than HUM (0 cases), $P = .04$.

Conclusions.—In extremely preterm infants given exclusive diets of preterm formula vs human milk, there was a significantly greater duration of parenteral nutrition and higher rate of surgical NEC in infants receiving preterm formula. This trial supports the use of an exclusive human milk diet to nourish extremely preterm infants in the neonatal intensive care unit.

▶ The benefits of using mother's own milk rather than formula for feeding preterm infants are widely appreciated and supported by an extensive body of empiric evidence. Evidence that similar benefits accrue from use of donor human milk for preterm infants whose mothers are unable to provide their own milk, in contrast, is comparatively scant, consisting of only a single randomized trial in the most recent decade and a few trials published more than 30 years ago. In the most recent prior study, the authors found that "infants fed donor milk [fortified with bovine-based human milk fortifier] had similar rates of LOS, NEC, and other infection-related events, compared with infants fed preterm formula" and concluded that "donor milk offered no observed short-term advantage over formula for feeding of extremely premature infants."[1] This study comparing donor milk (fortified with a supplement prepared from human milk) with preterm formula reaches different conclusions. Infants randomly assigned to donor milk feedings had a shorter duration of parenteral nutrition and a lower rate of surgical necrotizing enterocolitis. There are several reasons why these observations should be applied with caution, however. Although the observed difference in surgical necrotizing enterocolitis (NEC) rates achieved statistical significance, it was the only one of several reported outcomes that did so, and no correction for multiple comparisons was applied. The estimated number needed to treat with donor milk feedings to prevent 1 case of surgical NEC is 6, but the confidence interval on that estimate is likely very wide. The donor milk used in this trial is a commercially prepared, standardized product prepared from human milk pooled from many donors, so its characteristics may not be representative of single-donor milk aliquots available from human milk banks. Finally, the high rate of late-onset sepsis in the study enrollees (66% overall, compared with less than 15% among comparable babies in the CPQCC Network) suggests that either the enrolled infants or their environment of care may not be representative of those items in other nurseries. These observations, therefore, provide only indirect, and relatively weak, support for an evidence-based mandate for "enhanced lactation support in the neonatal intensive care unit as well as an imperative to establish more human milk banks." Although those goals appear to be laudable, they are somewhat contradictory, as success with the former may obviate need for the latter. Strong evidence to guide these policy choices may be forthcoming from ongoing trials, such as the donor milk trial currently in progress in the NICHD Neonatal Research Network.

W. E. Benitz, MD

Reference

1. Schanler RJ, Lau C, Hurst NM, Smith EO. Randomized trial of donor human milk versus preterm formula as substitutes for mothers' own milk in the feeding of extremely premature infants. *Pediatrics*. 2005;116:400-406.

Effect of Fortifiers and Additional Protein on the Osmolarity of Human Milk: Is It Still Safe for the Premature Infant?

Kreissl A, Zwiauer V, Repa A, et al (Med Univ of Vienna, Austria)

J Pediatr Gastroenterol Nutr 57:432-437, 2013

Objectives.—The present guidelines of the American Academy of Pediatrics recommend that osmolarity not exceed 450 mOsm/kg (or approximately an osmolarity of 400 mOsm/L) for breast milk or infant formulae, to minimize the risk factors for necrotizing enterocolitis. A commercial protein supplement has been developed to meet special protein requirements (4.0–4.5 $g \cdot kg^{-1} \cdot day^{-1}$) of infants with a birth weight <1000 g. Because its effect on osmolarity has not been systematically studied, we characterized the effects of fortification on the osmolarity of human milk (HM).

Methods.—Osmolarity of fresh and processed HM was measured at baseline, after fortification with a commercial HM fortifier and after further supplementation with additional protein increasing in 0.5-g steps up to 4.0 g. Measurements were performed immediately after adding fortifier and/or protein and after 24 hours. In addition, changes in osmolarity were determined after adding therapeutic additives such as iron, multivitamin supplement, and calcium-phosphorus capsules.

Results.—Native HM samples ($n = 84$) had 297 mOsm/L, (median; 95% confidence interval 295–299 mOsm/L). Adding HM fortifier increased osmolarity up to 436 mOsm/L (95% confidence interval 431–441 mOsm/L). Additional protein supplementation increased osmolarity by 23.5 mOsm/L per 0.5-g step, up to a maximum of 605 mOsm/L. Pasteurization decreased osmolarity by 20–30 mOsm/L ($P < 0.001$), and storage for 24 hours slightly increased osmolarity (by 11.5 mOsm/L $P = 0.0002$). Therapeutic additives increased osmolarity up to 868 mOsm/L.

Conclusions.—Adding HM fortifier and additional protein to HM increased osmolarity to >400 mOsm/L and therefore above the recommended threshold. Because of the excessive increase in osmolarity combinations of HM + fortifier and additional protein should not be applied together with multivitamins or other additives (Table 3).

▶ The authors report an interesting relationship between additions to infant feeding and osmolarity that has actually been known for several years. But in this report, there is a nice quantitative description of the effects of incremental additives on human milk osmolarity that is clearly relevant to what we are feeding to preterm infants in the neonatal intensive care unit. Currently, the American Academy of Pediatrics recommends that osmolality cut off in infant formulas be 450 mOsm/kg, which approximates an osmolarity of 400 mOsm/L. In this study, with the addition of a protein hydrolysate that is commercially available in Europe, the osmolarity increased by approximately 130 mOsm/L from approximately 300 to 436. When additional protein was supplemented to levels of intake required for optimization of growth in very preterm infants, the osmolarity continued to increase in a stepwise manner. Finally, adding calcium and phosphorus supplements as well as multivitamin preparations increased the osmolarity to nearly 900 mOsm/L in some of the specimens (Table 3).

Although the evidence for a causal relationship between osmolarity of feedings and necrotizing enterocolitis in the literature is somewhat weak, this should still be of concern to the clinicians caring for these babies. It is known that gastrografin contrast medium with an osmolality of nearly 700 is associated with an increase in necrotizing enterocolitis (NEC). Furthermore, some of the older

TABLE 3.—Increase in Osmolarity of Human Milk, after Addition of Different Supplements

	Median Range, mOsm/L			
	Iron Supplement, n = 11	Ca/P Supplement, n = 11	Multivitamin Supplement, n = 11	All 3, n = 11
HM + HMF	453 432–495	453 432–495	453 432–495	453 432–495
HM + HMF + ADD	441 432–495	527 487–661	609 572–658	719 565–869
HM + HMF + ADD + 0.5 g P^+	481 453–518	531 476–554	632 584–665	675 559–762
HM + HMF + ADD + 1.0 g P^+	505 473–541	521 509–589	647 596–687	710 604–773
HM + HMF + ADD + 1.5 g P^+	534 506–555	559 525–601	668 613–755	720 641–769
HM + HMF + ADD + 2.0 g P^+	548 525–599	588 559–626	708 675–763	756 648–773
HM + HMF + ADD + 2.5 g P^+	582 529–598	621 563–736	729 675–768	773 690–961
HM + HMF + ADD + 3.0 g P^+	593 595–550	635 594–697	735 706–795	777 688–838
HM + HMF + ADD + 3.5 g P^+	620 567–751	633 600–703	769 717–819	796 690–858
HM + HMF + ADD + 4.0 g P^+	646.5 605–778	663 587–772	849 733–942	868 830–922

Human milk (HM) with human milk fortifier (HMF = Aptamil FMS 4.3%) and additional protein (P^+ = Aptamil Protein$^+$) mixtures in combination with therapeutic additives (ADD) (iron supplement [Ferrum Hausman], Ca/P supplement [Prescription Charitee Berlin], multivitamin supplement [Multibionta]) were added to HM. Data are presented as median and the range. *P* values reflecting Mann-Whitney *U* test are provided for information only.

studies, as reviewed by the authors of this report and Pearson et al,[1] although not rigorous evaluations of the relationship between NEC and osmolarity, should still be taken into account. Neonatologists should be aware of the osmolarity of compounds that they are adding to human milk and formula. Especially important are the multivitamin preparations that have as their carrier high osmolarity solutions such as glycerol.

Although this report strongly suggests that because of the excessive increase in osmolarity, with combinations of the human milk plus fortifier protein plus multivitamins and other additives, these should not be applied together. However, even though this is stated, being able to do this in practice will be a real challenge if we attempt to provide adequate protein, minerals, and multivitamins to these infants who need them.

J. Neu, MD

Reference

1. Pearson F, Johnson MJ, Leaf AA. Milk osmolality: does it matter? *Arch Dis Child Fetal Neonatal Ed.* 2013;98:F166-F169.

Variability in human milk composition: benefit of individualized fortification in very-low-birth-weight infants

de Halleux V, Rigo J (Univ of Liege, Belgium)

Am J Clin Nutr 98:529S-535S, 2013

Background.—Preterm infants fed fortified human milk (HM) grow more slowly than those fed preterm formulas. These differences could be related to the variability in the macronutrient composition of expressed HM, resulting in inadequate nutrient intake in relation to the estimated needs of the preterm infants.

Objectives.—The aim of this article was to show the variability in HM composition from an infant's own mother's milk (OMM) or pooled HM from the milk bank. The second objective was to evaluate the advantages of individual fortification on nutritional intakes over standard fortification.

Design.—The macronutrient composition of 428 OMM, 138 HM pools from single donors, 224 pools from multiple donors, and 14 pools from colostral milk was determined by using a mid-infrared analyzer. Individualized fortification was performed after analysis of the milk samples in 2 steps: adjustment of fat content up to 4 g/dL, followed by the addition of an HM fortifier to provide 4.3 $g \cdot kg^{-1} \cdot d^{-1}$ according to the daily prescribed volume of feeding. Nutritional intakes resulting from the individualized fortification were compared with calculated intakes resulting from standard fortification (HM fortifier: 4 packets/dL).

Results.—The variability in contents of fat, protein, and energy was high for all types of HM samples. Compared with standard fortification, individual fortification significantly reduced the variability in nutritional intakes, allowing the maintenance of protein intake and the protein:energy ratio in the range of the nutritional recommendations.

Conclusions.—The variability in expressed HM with respect to its protein and energy content is high. This variability persists after standard fortification, possibly resulting in under- or overnutrition. Because both over- and undernutrition confer risks in later development, individualized fortification optimizes protein and energy intake.

▶ The de Halleux and Rigo studies, using a mid-infrared analyzer on 428 samples from own mother's milk for very low-birth-weight (VLBW) infants (138 single human milk [HM] pools, 224 multiple donor HM pools, and 14 colostral milks), showed a widely variable macronutrient content especially for protein, fat, and energy. For example, the range of protein (including all 804 samples) was from 0.8 to 2.4 g/dL, fat from 1.8 to 6.6 g/dL, and energy from 47 to 85 kcal/dL. Protein, the most growth-limiting macronutrient, was less than 1.5 g/dL in 56% of the samples, and 67% had energy values less than 67 cal/dL (values considered as reference values for preterm milk composition). After standard fortification versus HM analyses and individual fortification, there was 21% less variability in protein intake versus standard fortification.

Standard fortification, as recommended by the manufacturer, does not meet the nutritional requirements of immature infants, thereby creating conditions for under- or overnutritional risks. Another method of fortification is based on using the blood urea nitrogen (BUN) to avoid excessive protein intake.[1] However, it has been found that BUN is not correlated to protein intakes during the first weeks of life but reflects the renal immaturity of VLBW infants.[2,3] We have not found the BUN to be useful even beyond the first few weeks in these infants, as similar infants with very modest BUN values (6–10 mg/dL) were growing more than 15 g/k/d.[4]

We recently published our experience with another midinfrared analyzer on 83 samples of HM from mothers delivering VLBW infants and confirmed similar observations as Halleux and Rigo. Over the first 6 weeks of life, we found the expected decline in protein and that a mother's own milk always had a higher protein value than that of the donor milk pool.[5] We also showed not only that nutritional inadequacy was common with standard fortification, but some women with higher protein content of their milks could actually reach a protein level above the nutrient recommendation.[5]

Using the same analyzer, we compared milk samples analyzed with the mid-infrared analyzer versus the same samples spun on a creamatocrit.[6] The creamatocrit appeared to overestimate fat and consequently energy. The mid-infrared-analyzed samples were within 1% of values obtained on a sample group sent out to a reference laboratory.

On-site, real-time analysis of HM with these new spectrometric devices is easy, can be very informative, and can allow individualized fortification to tailor nutritional management to the individual patient. Whether these analyses need to be daily or only triggered by poor growth and low BUN needs more study.

D. H. Adamkin, MD

References

1. Arslanoglu S, Moro GE, Ziegler EE. Adjustable fortification of human milk fed to preterm infants: does it make a difference? *J Perinatol.* 2006;26:614-621.
2. Ridout E, Melara D, Rottinghaus S, Thureen PJ. Blood urea nitrogen concentration as a marker of amino-acid intolerance in neonates with birthweight less than 1250 g. *J Perinatol.* 2005;25:130-133.
3. Roggero P, Giannì ML, Morlacchi L, et al. Blood Urea Nitrogen Concentrations in low-birth-weight Preterm Infants During Parenteral and Enteral Nutrition. *J Pediatr Gastroenterol Nutr.* 2010;51:213-215.
4. Radmacher PG, Sparks B, Lewis SL, Serke L, Northam AT, Adamkin DH. Real time human milk analysis contributes to more comprehensive nutrional management. *J Investig Med.* 2013;61:208A.
5. Radmacher PG, Lewis SL, Adamkin DH. Individualizing fortification of human milk using real time human milk analysis. *J Neonatal Perinatal Med.* 2013;6: 319-323.
6. O'Neill EF, Radmacher PG, Sparks B, Adamkin DH. Creamatocrit analysis of human milk overestimates fat and energy content when compared to a human milk analyzer using mid-infrared spectroscopy. *J Pediatr Gastroenterol Nutr.* 2013;56:569-572.

A standardized nutrition approach for very low birth weight neonates improves outcomes, reduces cost and is not associated with increased rates of necrotizing enterocolitis, sepsis or mortality

Butler TJ, Szekely LJ, Grow JL (Akron Children's Hosp, OH)
J Perinatol 33:851-857, 2013

Objective.—To assess how a standard practice for nutrition support in very low birth weight (VLBW) neonates would impact on their hospital course.

Study Design.—This was a prospective, single center, before vs after comparison of a non-standardized approach to nutrition in VLBW neonates to a standardized approach. Standardization of feeding initiation, feeding volume and caloric advancement, management of feeding aspirates (residuals), use of starter parenteral nutrition (PN), use of breast milk and donor breast milk, initiation and discontinuation of intravenous (IV) intralipids, documentation of protein use, and utilization of percutaneously inserted central venous catheters were performed. Multiple outcome measures were evaluated. Fisher's exact, Mann–Whitney *U*-tests and χ^2 tests were used for statistical analysis.

Result.—Sixty-nine infants in the pre-standardization (non-standardized) group were compared with 154 infants in the standardized approach group. Analysis was performed for each group as a whole. Statistically significant improvements were seen in multiple areas for the standardized group including the day of life birth weight was regained ($P < 0.0005$), use of breast milk as the initial feeding ($P < 0.0001$), use of starter PN on admission ($P < 0.0001$), earlier time for initiation of PN ($P < 0.0001$), decreased use of PN overall ($P < 0.0001$), enteral protein use ($P < 0.0001$), earlier time for initiation of IV intralipids ($P < 0.002$), day of life for full enteral feeds ($P < 0.0005$) and first day for initiation of enteral feeds ($P < 0.0001$). Fewer infants born microcephalic at birth remained so at discharge in the standardized group as compared with the pre-standardized group ($P < 0.02$). Similarly, less infants born small for gestational age at birth remained so at discharge in the standardized group as compared with the pre-standardized group ($P < 0.05$). Two cases of necrotizing enterocolitis (NEC) occurred in the pre-standardization group and one in the standardized group. No coagulase-negative *Staphlococcal* infections or line infections occurred during the entire study period. Two cases of sepsis occurred in the pre-standardization group, both in infants <750 g. No cases of sepsis occurred in the standardized group. Cost savings were remarkable from decreased PN usage in the standard group.

Conclusion.—Implementation of a standardized approach to nutrition in VLBW infants reduces the use of PN thereby reducing cost, causes a more rapid regain of birth weight, decreases the number of babies that are small for gestational age and microcephalic at discharge, and decreases the time to full enteral feeds. No adverse increases in mortality, sepsis, NEC, coagulase-negative *Staphlococcal* infections or line infections occurred.

▶ In 1978, Brown and Sweet reported experience at Mount Sinai Medical Center (New York) with a standardized protocol for initiation and slow advancement of feedings in infants at risk for necrotizing enterocolitis (NEC).[1] In the 4 years after its adoption, they observed only one case of NEC among 932 low birth weight (LBW) infants, compared with 14 cases among 1745 infants in the preceding 3.5 years ($P < .05$ by χ^2). Over the ensuing 3.5 decades, several other observational studies have described benefits accruing after standardization of approaches to feeding advancement in very LBW infants. This study adds another report to that collection, documenting that those observations remain consistent despite evolution in the characteristics of the LBW population in our intensive care nurseries and differences among the regimens used. In this study, feedings for infants ≤1500 g at birth were initiated with colostrum at 10 to 20 mL/kg/d and advanced by 10 to 20 mL/kg/d daily, beginning on the second or third day (see report for a more complete description). A detailed, if complicated, protocol for assessment and management of gastric residuals, emphasizing strategies for continuation rather than interruption of feedings, is also provided. Adoption was associated with a number of process improvements, as listed in the abstract. Most notably, the age at initiation of feedings was reduced by more than 2 days (4.6 to 2 days), the number of days of parenteral nutrition by 5 days (13 to 8 days), and the age at removal of the percutaneously inserted central venous catheter (PICC) line by 7 days (15 to 8 days). The proportion of infants who weighed less than the tenth percentile at discharge decreased from 100% to 67%—still high, but a substantial improvement. Although the sample size was far from sufficient to detect even a doubling of the NEC rate, the NEC rate was low both before and after the change (2.9% and 0.6%, respectively). The cumulative message of these studies is that predefined strategies are better than ad hoc decisions about feeding adjustments. It is time to move beyond arguments about the utility of standardized feeding protocols (just do it!) and turn attention to systematic optimization of the elements of those regimens.

W. E. Benitz, MD

Reference

1. Brown EG, Sweet AY. Preventing necrotizing enterocolitis in neonates. *JAMA*. 1978;240:2452-2454.

Cohort Study of Probiotics in a North American Neonatal Intensive Care Unit

Janvier A, Malo J, Barrington KJ (Centre Hospitalier Universitaire Sainte Justine, Montréal, Quebec, Canada)
J Pediatr 164:980-985, 2014

Objective.—To determine whether routine probiotic administration to very preterm infants would reduce the incidence of necrotizing enterocolitis (NEC) without adverse consequences.

Study Design.—Since the end of July 2011, we have administered a probiotic mixture to all admitted infants of <32 weeks' gestation. We give 0.5 g of a mixture of 4 bifidobacteria (*Bifidobacterium breve, bifidum, infantis, and longum*) and *Lactobacillus rhamnosus* GG (2×10^9 colony-forming units) per day, starting with the first feed, until the infant reaches 34 weeks. We compared complications among infants admitted during the first 17 months of routine use with those admitted during the previous 17 months.

Results.—Two hundred ninety-four infants received probiotics, and 317 infants formed the comparison group. Introduction of probiotics was associated with a reduction in NEC (from 9.8% to 5.4%, $P < .02$), a nonsignificant decrease in death (9.8% to 6.8%), and a significant reduction in the combined outcome of death or NEC (from 17% to 10.5%, $P < .05$). After adjustment for gestational age, intrauterine growth restriction, and sex, the improvements remained significant (OR for NEC, 0.51; 95% CI, 0.26-0.98; OR for death or NEC, 0.56; 95% CI, 0.33-0.93). There was no effect of probiotics on health care–associated infection.

Discussion.—A product that is readily available in North America, that has excellent quality control, and that contains strains similar to those that have been shown effective in randomized controlled trials substantially reduced the frequency of NEC in our neonatal intensive care unit.

▶ Probiotics seem like an inherently good idea, and our window to do proper randomized, controlled trials is rapidly closing because of a lack of equipoise. This study by Janvier et al suggests the safety of administering a bifidobacteria mix, but because it was historically controlled, conclusions about the efficacy of probiotics to reduce death or necrotizing enterocolitis (NEC) remain unconvincing, given the variability of the prevalence of NEC in any neonatal intensive care unit. The good news is that this is another positive trial—and bad news, another shift in equipoise without a definitive trial.

Acceptance of probiotics into routine practice has been hampered by many factors. Regulatory agencies have viewed probiotics as a nutritional supplement, not a drug. The number of formulations, dosages, and regimens tested has been countless, and NEC as the outcome measure remains an elusive and shifting endpoint.

Although it may seem trite, it's high time we did the definitive trial and settled this issue once and for all.

S. M. Donn, MD

Randomized controlled trial of prophylactic rectal stimulation and enemas on stooling patterns in extremely low birth weight infants

Sáenz de Pipaón Marcos M, Teresa Montes Bueno M, Sanjosé B, et al (La Paz Univ Hosp, Madrid, Spain)

J Perinatol 33:858-860, 2013

Objective.—We hypothesized that rectal stimulation and small volume enemas would accelerate normalization of stooling patterns in extremely low birth weight infants.

Study Design.—In a randomized controlled trial, infants with a gestational age ≤28 weeks received one of the following: twice daily rectal stimulation and/or enemas until two stools were passed daily, without enemas or stimulation, for three consecutive days. Intervention only occurred when symptoms, abdominal distension and no defecation, occurred in the previous 24 h. Enema administration occurred if abdominal distension persisted without defecation occurring after rectal stimulation. Multivariable linear regression was used to determine the contribution of a patent ductus arteriosus (PDA) on normalization of stooling patterns and feeding tolerance.

Result.—Rectal stimulation and/or small volume enemas did not accelerate the median (quartile range) time normalization of stooling patterns, 13 (11–20) days in control group and 16 (12–25.5) days in intervention group. A higher frequency of PDA occurred in the intervention than the non-intervention group. Infants with a persistent PDA had a longer duration of parenteral nutrition, worse feeding tolerance and more days to achieve normal stooling patterns. In multivariable regression analysis, a PDA, not repeated rectal stimulation and/or enemas, was significantly related to stooling and feeding tolerance.

Conclusion.—Twice daily administration of rectal stimulation and/or enemas did not normalize stooling patterns (fecal frequency). A PDA is

an important determinant of acquisition of normal stooling patterns and feeding tolerance of very immature newborns.

▶ The notion that preterm infants need to stool at least once a day in the neonatal intensive care unit is quite pervasive. Because of this, many neonatal intensive care units routinely incorporate the use of the enemas or glycerin chip suppositories to induce defecation. It is thought that this practice may actually improve feeding tolerance and, in some cases, may decrease the incidence of necrotizing enterocolitis, even though the studies on which this is based are nonexistent. This study evaluated the effects of rectal stimulation and small-volume enemas versus nonintervention to determine whether they would accelerate normalization of defecation in these infants. The intervention group was stimulated by twice-daily enemas until the complete evacuation of meconium and with rectal stimulation every 12 hours thereafter. If the infant did not pass stools during 8 hours after the stimulation, an enema was administered. The control group was provided intervention only when symptoms, abdominal distention, and no defecation occurred in the previous 24 hours. The primary study outcome was interestingly defined as the time when normal defecation patterns occurred. They defined the normal defecation pattern established when stools were passed each day without enemas or stimulation for 3 consecutive days.

After randomization, the birth weight of the intervention group was approximately 90 g less than that of the control group, but this was not statistically significant. There were several outcomes that differed between the 2 groups. The days to reach full enteral feedings were approximately 11 days longer in the intervention group; the days on parenteral nutrition were approximately 9 days longer in the intervention group, which appears to be contrary to common opinions about stimulation of defecation increasing the tolerance to feedings and improving the babies' ability to feed. Also of interest was the fact that there was only one baby in the control group that developed necrotizing enterocolitis and 7 in the intervention group that developed necrotizing enterocolitis or intestinal perforation, which approaches a statistical significance. The rate of retinopathy of prematurity greater than the grade one was also higher in the intervention group. The authors claim that this may be because the incidence of ductus arteriosus was higher in the intervention group. However, the intervention group did trend toward being lower in birth weight by approximately 90 g, as previously mentioned, and this may actually have contributed to some of these differences.

Neither this study, in which enemas were used, nor a previous study by Khadr et al,[1] in which glycerin suppositories were administered, showed a reduced time to full enteral feedings nor were there any other benefits shown by these interventions. In fact, this study suggests an association with increased necrotizing enterocolitis, increased retinopathy of prematurity, and a longer time to reach full enteral feedings and days on parenteral nutrition. Whether this was actually due to the smaller birth weight in this group or an association with a patent ductus arteriosus as claimed by the authors remains in question. Nevertheless, these articles do not support the need for routine stimulation of defecation in preterm babies.

J. Neu, MD

Reference

1. Khadr SN, Ibhanesebhor SE, Rennix C, et al. Randomized controlled trial: impact of glycerin suppositories on time to full feeds in preterm infants. *Neonatology.* 2011;100:169-176.

Epidemiology and Trends of Necrotizing Enterocolitis in Sweden: 1987–2009

Ahle M, Drott P, Andersson RE (Univ Hosp, Linköping, Sweden)

Pediatrics 132:e443-e451, 2013

Objective.—To investigate temporal, seasonal, and geographic variations in the incidence of necrotizing enterocolitis (NEC) and its relation to early infant survival in the Swedish population and in subgroups based on gestational age, birth weight, and gender.

Methods.—In the Swedish birth cohort of 1987 through 2009 all children with a diagnosis of NEC were identified in the National Patient Register, the Swedish Medical Birth Register, and the National Cause of Death Register. NEC incidence, early mortality, and seasonality were analyzed with descriptive statistics, Poisson regression, and auto regression.

Results.—The overall incidence of NEC was 3.4 in 10 000 live births, higher in boys than in girls (incidence rate ratio 1.22, 95% confidence interval 1.06–1.40, $P = .005$), with a peak in November and a trough in May, and increased with an average of ~5% a year during the study period. In most subgroups, except the most immature, an initial decrease was followed by a steady increase. Seven-day mortality decreased strongly in all subgroups over the entire study period (annual incidence rate ratio 0.96, 95% confidence interval 0.95–0.96, $P < .001$). This was especially marked in the most premature and low birth weight infants.

Conclusions.—After an initial decrease, the incidence of NEC has increased in Sweden during the last decades. An association with the concurrent dramatically improved early survival seems likely.

▶ The fact that necrotizing enterocolitis (NEC) rates differ from country to country has been known for a long time. However, the reasons behind this have been largely speculative. Good epidemiologic studies to evaluate this have been largely hampered by lack of good nationwide data sets from various countries. One of the countries known to have a relatively low NEC rate is Sweden. However, in this study of neonates that involved more than 2 000 000 newborns from 1987 through 2009 showed an initial decrease in NEC during the early years with a subsequent increase in more recent years. The periods analyzed spanned back to the times before the institution of some of our modern therapies such as surfactant. Of major interest in the study is the marked increase in the survival of the preterm infants during these years with 7-day mortality in babies less than 31 weeks of gestational age decreasing by more than half. Thus, a larger number of very small and highly susceptible infants survived to be exposed to the factors that cause NEC. Also of major interest is that the incidence of NEC, which was initially lower in Sweden than in the United Kingdom and Ireland, became similar to those of the United Kingdom and Ireland during the latter years of this study. In fact, the overall incidence among infants that developed NEC in Sweden became similar to that of the white population in the United States.

Even though factors such as breast feeding are highly prevalent in certain countries such as Sweden, the incidence of NEC has still continued to increase. It would be a major interest to see similar data from other countries in which the incidence of NEC has been reported to be very low, such as from Japan, especially because of the reports of the a large number of babies down to 22 weeks of gestation surviving in Japan.

J. Neu, MD

Abnormal heart rate characteristics before clinical diagnosis of necrotizing enterocolitis

Stone ML, Tatum PM, Weitkamp J-H, et al (Univ of Virginia, Charlottesville; Wake Forest Univ, Winston-Salem, NC; Vanderbilt Univ, Nashville, TN; et al)
J Perinatol 33:847-850, 2013

Objective.—Earlier diagnosis and treatment of necrotizing enterocolitis (NEC) in preterm infants, before clinical deterioration, might improve outcomes. A monitor that measures abnormal heart rate characteristics (HRC) of decreased variability and transient decelerations was developed as an early warning system for sepsis. As NEC shares pathophysiologic features with sepsis, we tested the hypothesis that abnormal HRC occur before clinical diagnosis of NEC.

Study Design.—Retrospective review of Bells stage II to III NEC cases among infants <34 weeks gestation enrolled in a prospective randomized clinical trial of HRC monitoring at three neonatal intensive care units.

Result.—Of 97 infants with NEC and HRC data, 33 underwent surgical intervention within 1 week of diagnosis. The baseline HRC index from 1 to 3 days before diagnosis was higher in patients who developed surgical vs medical NEC (2.06 ± 1.98 vs 1.22 ± 1.10, $P = 0.009$). The HRC index increased significantly 16 h before the clinical diagnosis of surgical NEC and 6 h before medical NEC. At the time of clinical diagnosis, the HRC index was higher in patients with surgical vs medical NEC (3.3 ± 2.2 vs 1.9 ± 1.7, $P < 0.001$).

Conclusion.—Abnormal HRC occur before clinical diagnosis of NEC, suggesting that continuous HRC monitoring may facilitate earlier detection and treatment.

▶ The need to find better diagnostic biomarkers for necrotizing enterocolitis (NEC) is a major challenge in neonatal intensive care. The authors of this article have previously developed a technique that evaluates termed heart rate characteristic (HRC) evaluation to detect sepsis in premature neonates. This study is a retrospective evaluation of the babies who had surgical or medical NEC and an evaluation of the HRC before diagnosis of either medical or surgical NEC. One limiting factor in this study is that the time of diagnosis of NEC was when the diagnosis was first definitively made by radiographic evaluation showing signs such as pneumatosis intestinalis. The evaluators did not compare the time of first suspicion on the clinical symptomatology such as distended abdomen, bloody stools, or other indicators that suggested NEC with HRC measurements. Thus, a major benefit to the use of clinical signs is not shown. Furthermore, this study did not specifically evaluate differences between sepsis and NEC HRC scores and, thus, may be highly nonspecific. Nevertheless, it is of interest that electrocardiographic signals become abnormal early in the development of NEC. Further evaluation may evolve into a very useful test and, therefore, is necessary. However, it will be necessary to differentiate NEC from sepsis because the treatment, such as continuing or discontinuing enteral feeding, currently is very different for those infants.

J. Neu, MD

Association of cord blood digitalis-like factor and necrotizing enterocolitis

Graves SW, for the *Eunice Kennedy* Shriver National Institute of Child Health and Human Development Maternal-Fetal Medicine Units Network (Brigham Young Univ, Provo, UT; et al)

Am J Obstet Gynecol 210:328.e1-328.e5, 2014

Objective.—Endogenous digoxin-like factor (EDLF) has been linked to vasoconstriction, altered membrane transport, and apoptosis. Our objective was to determine whether increased EDLF in the cord sera of preterm infants was associated with an increased incidence of necrotizing enterocolitis (NEC).

Study Design.—Cord sera from pregnant women enrolled in a randomized trial of $MgSO_4$ for fetal neuroprotection were analyzed for EDLF using a red cell Rb^+ uptake assay in which the inhibition of sodium pump-mediated Rb^+ transport was used as a functional assay of EDLF. Specimens were assayed blinded to neonatal outcome. Cases (NEC, $n = 25$) and controls (neonates not developing stage 2 or 3 NEC, $n = 24$) were matched by study center and gestational age. None of the women had preeclampsia. Cases and controls were compared using the Wilcoxon test for continuous and the Fisher exact test for categorical variables. A conditional logistic regression analysis was used to assess the odds of case vs control by EDLF level.

TABLE 4.—EDLF Levels as a Function of NEC Severity

Variable	Mean EDLF (%) ± SD	Cases or Controls
No NEC	15.7 ± 17.5	22 controls, no cases
NEC level 1	20.9 ± 29.6	2 controls, no cases
NEC level 2	20.1 ± 22.0	12 cases
NEC level 3	40.5 ± 26.9	13 cases

Trend $P = .008$.
EDLF, endogenous digoxin-like factor; *NEC*, necrotizing enterocolitis.

Results.—Cases and controls were not significantly different for gestational age, race, maternal steroid use, premature rupture of membranes, or $MgSO_4$ treatment. In logistic models adjusted for treatment group, race, premature rupture of membranes, and gestational age, cord sera EDLF was significantly associated with development of NEC ($P = .023$).

Conclusion.—These data demonstrated an association between cord sera EDLF and NEC (Table 4).

▶ There is a need to find predictive biomarkers for necrotizing enterocolitis (NEC). Endogenous digoxin-like factor (EDLF) is a Na-K-ATPase inhibitor that resembles digoxin in many of its actions. As part of a randomized controlled trial of $MgSO_4$ for neuroprotection, cord sera were collected and analyzed for EDLF. According to the authors, some data suggest that antibody treatment to EDLF may reduce some of the complications of prematurity. The authors hypothesized that there may be an association between the level of EDLF in the cord blood and the subsequent development of NEC. In a case-control analysis, they found an almost 2-fold increase in EDLF in patients who developed NEC, with higher levels in those patients with worse disease (Table 4). This relationship held true after controlling for several variables including gestational age. Although this association is of interest, a strong biological mechanistic link is not present, and thus this may simply be part of an epiphenomenon related to prematurity and susceptibility to several diseases related to prematurity. For example, late-onset sepsis was not evaluated, and it is possible that this could also be related to increased cord sera levels of EDLD. Thus, despite skepticism, this is a lead that should not be ignored.

J. Neu, MD

Brain Magnetic Resonance Imaging in Infants with Surgical Necrotizing Enterocolitis or Spontaneous Intestinal Perforation versus Medical Necrotizing Enterocolitis

Merhar SL, Ramos Y, Meinzen-Derr J, et al (Cincinnati Children's Hosp Med Ctr, OH)
J Pediatr 164:410-412.e1, 2014

Magnetic resonance imaging of the brain was performed in 26 preterm infants with necrotizing enterocolitis (NEC) or spontaneous intestinal

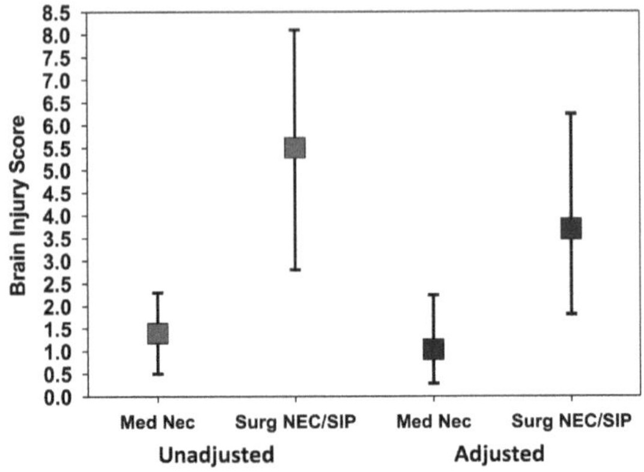

FIGURE 2.—Brain injury scores in infants with medical NEC vs those with surgical NEC/SIP, unadjusted analysis and after adjustment for possible confounding variables. (Reprinted from Journal Pediatrics. Merhar SL, Ramos Y, Meinzen-Derr J, et al. Brain magnetic resonance imaging in infants with surgical necrotizing enterocolitis or spontaneous intestinal perforation versus medical necrotizing enterocolitis. *J Pediatr.* 2014;164:410-412.e1, Copyright 2014, with permission from Elsevier.)

perforation at term equivalent age. Infants with surgical NEC or spontaneous intestinal perforation had significantly more brain injury on magnetic resonance imaging compared with infants with medical NEC, even after adjustment for confounders (Fig 2).

▶ As stated by the authors, "preterm infants with necrotizing enterocolitis are known to have worse neurodevelopmental outcomes than the gestational age matched controls." It is also known that infants with surgical necrotizing enterocolitis have worse outcomes than those with the medical necrotizing enterocolitis. In this study, the authors used their opportunity of doing routine magnetic resonance imaging before discharge in all of their preterm infants to evaluate differences in brain injury scores in babies with medical necrotizing enterocolitis versus surgical necrotizing enterocolitis versus spontaneous intestinal perforations. As seen in Fig 2, surgical necrotizing enterocolitis and spontaneous intestinal perforations had higher brain injury scores at the time of discharge from the hospital than medical necrotizing enterocolitis. However, there was still a very significant overlap, and it is not clear whether spontaneous intestinal perforations actually resulted in a different injury score then medical necrotizing enterocolitis or surgical necrotizing enterocolitis. A couple of questions arise from this study. First, were there predisposing factors that resulted in both brain injury as well as intestinal injury where the necrotizing enterocolitis itself did not actually cause the brain injury seen on the MRI? Second, because the spontaneous intestinal perforations were not separated from the surgical necrotizing enterocolitis results, were there actually differences between these 2 entities in terms of radiologic imaging studies? The extent of intestinal necrosis and inflammation with the necrotizing enterocolitis would likely be greater than that seen with spontaneous intestinal perforation unless the spontaneous intestinal perforation resulted in a spillage of intestinal contents with peritonitis and systemic inflammation. Nevertheless, these results are of interest and show that use of magnetic resonance imaging at the time of discharge from the hospital may be helpful in providing some clues about subsequent neurodevelopmental problems. A clinical correlation study with additional follow-up would be of interest.

J. Neu, MD

Intestinal location of necrotizing enterocolitis among infants with congenital heart disease

Cozzi C, Aldrink J, Nicol K, et al (The Ohio State Univ of College and Medicine, Columbus)

J Perinatol 33:783-785, 2013

Objective.—To determine whether differences exist in the location of necrotizing enterocolitis (NEC) in infants with congenital heart disease (CHD) versus those without CHD.

Study Design.—Retrospective cohort study utilizing 11 years of patient data. Inclusion criterion was surgical exploration for NEC. Presence or absence of CHD was determined. Surgical and/or pathology reports were reviewed to identify the location of NEC. Data were analyzed by *t*-tests and χ^2 analyses.

Result.—One hundred and sixty-seven patients met the inclusion criteria. CHD infants had a higher percentage of mortality. There was no difference in the location of NEC between non-CHD and CHD patients, with the predominant location being the small intestine in both. In addition, there was no difference in the location of NEC between preterm non-CHD patients and full-term CHD patients with the small intestine again being the primary site.

Conclusion.—Despite differences in gestational age between non-CHD and CHD patients, the location of NEC in these infants did not differ.

▶ As stated in this article, previous reports of necrotizing enterocolitis in non-congenital heart disease patients have documented principally small intestinal involvement in preterm infants. In full-term infants, these reports documented primarily colonic involvement. This study was a retrospective review designed to determine if differences exist in the location of necrotizing enterocolitis in infants with congenital heart disease versus those without congenital heart disease.

Evaluation of records from patients less than 6 months of age who underwent exploratory laparotomy over an 11-year period at a large Children's Hospital was done. Infants with necrotizing enterocolitis and congenital heart disease were compared with those infants with necrotizing enterocolitis but no congenital heart disease. The types of cardiac disease in the congenital heart included coarctation of the aorta, tetralogy of fallot, atrial ventricular septal defects, bicuspid aortic valves with severe aortic regurgitation, or hypoplastic left heart syndrome. When comparing infants without congenital heart disease with those with congenital heart disease, the location of necrotizing enterocolitis did not differ between the groups. Furthermore evaluation of the location of necrotizing enterocolitis in infants greater than 37 weeks of gestation compared with the preterm infants less than 37 weeks of gestation without congenital heart disease also showed no differences in intestinal location of the intestinal necrosis.

The major take-away message from this study is that the location of necrotizing enterocolitis in infants with congenital heart disease does not differ from that in preterm infants. Despite previous studies suggesting that the term infants have a greater incidence of colonic necrotizing enterocolitis, one can suggest that many of these cases may actually be secondary to causes other than ischemia to the intestine, such as might be seen in infants with Hirschsprung disease or viral enteropathy, that may mimic necrotizing enterocolitis. Nevertheless, the types of lesions seen in the term infants in this study certainly do not rule out an ischemic etiology. The likelihood of an ischemic etiology being a primary pathophysiologic event in the preterm infant is highly unlikely given the fact that most of these infants get the disease well beyond the time of birth when these ischemic events primarily occur.

J. Neu, MD

Cronobacter: an emerging opportunistic pathogen associated with neonatal meningitis, sepsis and necrotizing enterocolitis

Hunter CJ, Bean JF (Ann and Robert H. Lurie Children's Hosp of Chicago, IL)
J Perinatol 33:581-585, 2013

Members of the genus *Cronobacter* are an emerging group of opportunist Gram-negative pathogens. This genus was previously thought to be a single species, called *Enterobacter sakazakii*. *Cronobacter spp.* typically affect low-birth-weight neonates, causing life-threatening meningitis, sepsis and necrotizing enterocolitis. Outbreaks of disease have been associated with contaminated infant formula, although the primary environmental source remains elusive. Advanced understanding of these bacteria and better classification has been obtained by improved detection techniques and genomic analysis. Research has begun to characterize the virulence factors and pathogenic potential of Cronobacter. Investigations into sterilization techniques and protocols for minimizing the risk of contamination have been reviewed at national and international forums. In this review, we explore the clinical impact of Cronobacter neonatal and pediatric infections, discuss virulence and pathogenesis, and review prevention and treatment strategies (Fig 2).

▶ *Cronobacter* is the name of a genus of gram-negative microorganisms known to be pathogenic that cause meningitis and necrotizing enterocolitis in premature babies. This microorganism may be better known to some of us as *Enterobacter sakazakii*, but the name was changed in 2007 because of refinements in taxonomic identification technologies. This microbe became notorious after babies developed severe infection after exposure to powdered milk formulas, but this was not always a consistent predisposing factor.

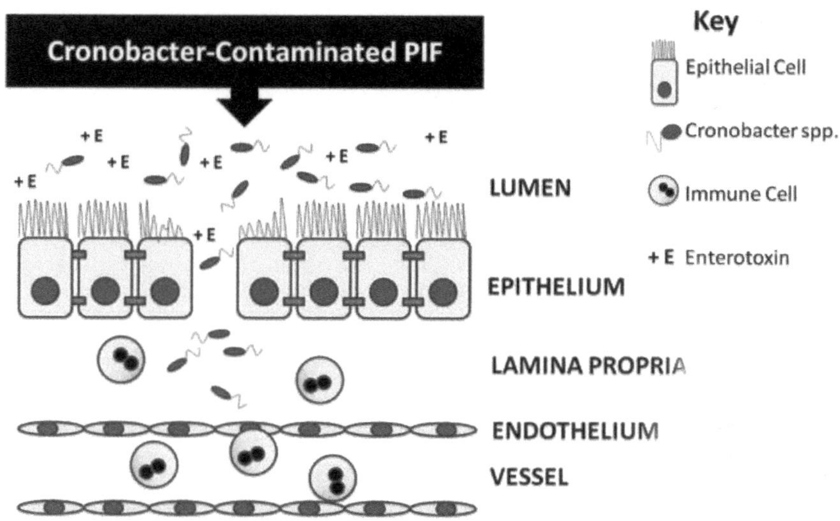

FIGURE 2.—Model of *Cronobacter* infection following ingestion of contaminated PIF. Oral inoculation of *Cronobacter* into an infant after ingestion of contaminated PIF. The bacteria release enterotoxin (+E), which may increase bacterial virulence and disrupt the intestinal barrier causing necrotizing enterocolitis. *Cronobacter* adheres to the intestinal layer. In the setting of a disrupted epithelial barrier, microbes traverse the mucosal layers, gaining access to lower immune and nonimmune cell populations. Mucosal microvascular endothelial cells, which represent the final anatomic border before the host's microcirculation, sense microbial antigens and respond rapidly by mounting an immune response. Cronobacter may enter to vasculature thereby gaining access to the blood–brain barrier resulting in bacteremia and meningitis. (Reprinted from Hunter CJ, Bean JF. Cronobacter: an emerging opportunistic pathogen associated with neonatal meningitis, sepsis and necrotizing enterocolitis. *J Perinatol.* 2013;33:581-585, with permission from Nature America, Inc.)

This article reviews some of the history of *Cronobacter* and its pathogenicity. It proposes a mechanism of how *Cronobacter* in contaminated premature infant formula powder may cause necrotizing enterocolitis (Fig 1 in the original article). The mechanism includes a breakdown of the intercellular junctional barrier with subsequent translocation into the highly immunoreactive subepithelium, where an inflammatory response can be initiated.

The article also discusses some strategies for prevention of *Cronobacter* infection, which include encouraging the use of breast milk or liquid milk formula rather than powdered formulations, reconstitution with water at greater than 70°C with the rapid cooling before feeding to 37°C, and, in general, avoidance of powdered infant formulas whenever possible. The latter may be difficult in some settings, especially because powdered formulas tend to be less expensive than the liquid ready-to-feed formulas.

Also of major interest is the fact that this microorganism appears to cause necrotizing enterocolitis fairly consistently, and if one is able to isolate a specific virulence factor from this microorganism, it may hold a very important clue for the pathogenesis of necrotizing enterocolitis. More research in this area is certainly indicated.

J. Neu, MD

Usefulness of abdominal ultrasound in diagnosing necrotising enterocolitis

Bohnhorst B (Hannover Med School, Germany)

Arch Dis Child Fetal Neonatal Ed 98:F445-F450, 2013

Necrotising enterocolitis is a serious disorder in preterm infants with a mortality of up to 60%. Therefore, early and precise diagnosis and rapid initiation of proper treatment are essential. Clinically suspected diagnosis is usually confirmed by typical findings on plain abdominal radiograph, for example, pneumatosis intestinalis, portal venous gas and, in case of intestinal perforation, pneumoperitoneum. Recently, there has been growing evidence that with real-time ultrasound, intramural air and portal gas can be better detected than with x-ray. Furthermore, ultrasound is able to assess the bowel wall directly and detect bowel wall thickening or thinning, reduced peristalsis or disturbed bowel wall perfusion. Intra-abdominal fluid, both intraluminal or extraluminal is also visible. However, data regarding the diagnostic validity and prognostic value of abdominal ultrasound are limited and often focused on a single finding rather than a combination of them. Additionally, until now, ultrasound findings seem to have little influence on therapeutic decisions. Therefore, the value of abdominal ultrasound in the diagnosis of necrotising enterocolitis has to be determined by further studies until its use can be generally recommended.

▶ The definitive diagnosis of necrotizing enterocolitis (NEC) is one of the most vexing problems in neonatal intensive care. There has been considerable interest over the past decade in the use of abdominal ultrasound scan in the diagnosis of NEC. Currently, the standard is the use of clinical examination and abdominal radiography. The diagnosis of NEC has classically been categorized into 3 stages, with stage I primarily indicating a suspicion of the disease. Stage I can be diagnosed if the infants have the abdominal distention, increased gastric residuals, changes in apnea and bradycardia, and other nonspecific signs. Thus, this is a classification that probably should not even be used because most very preterm babies exhibit these signs during their hospital course. Stage II is usually defined as clinical symptoms plus abdominal radiographic findings that consist of pneumatosis intestinalis and/or portal venous gas. Thickening of the bowel wall, persistent bowel loops, and bowel distention have been considered as suspicious indicators for NEC but are not considered to be definitive. Stage III is usually a surgical disease that is defined at the time of surgery, but the increasing use of peritoneal drainage systems has very likely confounded some of the definitive cases of NEC when they were actually spontaneous intestinal perforations.

This article on the use of ultrasound scan is interesting from the perspective that there are several factors that may make this a useful adjunct in the diagnosis of NEC but at the same time may actually lead us astray. It is obvious from this article that this is not something that should be done by either neonatologists or radiologists who are not highly trained in its use. Some of the ultrasound examinations that the author considers reasonable for evaluation of NEC include bowel wall thickness, peristalsis, and bowel wall perfusion. However, standards for bowel wall thickness have not been established, and thinness of the bowel wall less than 1.0 mm indicates an abnormal thinning that may result from ischemia or necrosis. Thus, this may not be a useful modality. Intramural gas or pneumatosis intestinalis can be detected readily using this technique. However, it appears that it can be so sensitive that it can detect many patients with Stage I disease. In other words, it is so highly sensitive that it may not be able to discern individuals with any kind of intestinal disease at all. On the other hand, portal venous gas appears to be a more reliable indicator, but, unfortunately, the gold standard for the diagnosis of NEC without surgery and direct visualization of a necrotic bowel is still missing, making studies of sensitivity and specificity a challenge.

There are often infants with a distended abdomen in whom there is a high suspicion for NEC where there is no definitive pneumatosis intestinalis or portal venous gas by abdominal radiography. A decision needs to be made whether these infants need surgical exploration. In these cases, evaluation for free abdominal fluid could be highly suspicious of bowel perforation when done by ultrasound scan. In addition, absent bowel wall perfusion can also be highly sensitive and specific compared with abdominal radiography in the detection of severe NEC when a decision needs to be made on whether the infant should go to surgery.

Overall, it appears that if used by experienced individuals, abdominal ultrasound scan may be a useful adjunct in the diagnosis of NEC. However, as stated by the author, additional studies will need to be done before this can be generally recommended. Perhaps a combination of physical examination abdominal radiography, ultrasound scan, and the use of biochemical diagnostic biomarkers will be combined in the future to aid in the early and accurate diagnosis of NEC.

J. Neu, MD

A prospective comparison of intestinal sonography and abdominal radiographs in a neonatal intensive care unit

Silva CT, Daneman A, Navarro OM, et al (The Univ of Toronto, Canada)

Pediatr Radiol 43:1453-1463, 2013

Background.—No study reported in the literature comprehensively compares findings on neonatal abdominal radiographs with sonography.

Objective.—To compare the findings on abdominal radiographs and sonograms in infants in intensive care, to better understand how the various intestinal gas patterns on radiographs relate to the spectrum of appearances on sonography and, second, to evaluate the ability of sonography to differentiate necrotizing enterocolitis from other intestinal pathology.

Materials and Methods.—We prospectively evaluated sonograms and radiographs, blinded to the other modality and to clinical information. Patients' charts were reviewed by a third blinded reader and used as a reference standard for diagnosis. We made associations between sonographic findings, radiographic intestinal gas patterns and clinical diagnoses.

Results.—We included 75 infants with gestational ages between 23 weeks and 41 weeks. Sonographic abnormalities were present in infants with all radiographic intestinal gas patterns, including normal patterns. We only saw absent intestinal perfusion and fluid collections on sonography (suggesting intestinal necrosis and sealed perforation) in infants with intestinal dilatation with elongation on radiographs. Separation of intestinal loops on radiographs was most commonly caused by reasons other than intestinal wall thickening. Increased intestinal echogenicity or free fluid with echoes on sonography correlated with a diagnosis of necrotizing enterocolitis, whereas anechoic free fluid correlated with absence of necrotizing enterocolitis.

Conclusion.—Sonography is complementary to radiographs in infants with suspected intestinal pathology, with a spectrum of appearances seen on each modality. Some sonographic findings either strongly suggest necrotizing enterocolitis or supply evidence against this diagnosis.

▶ Abdominal sonography is a long-established modality for diagnostic imaging of solid and fluid-filled organs. Application to evaluation of bowel structure and integrity has been much slower to develop, despite accumulation of cases showing informative findings over more than 30 years. Although conventional radiography has the advantage of better spatial resolution and a large body of prior experience, sonography allows visualization of the bowel wall, assessment of peristalsis, dynamic imaging of gas in the portal circulation, and Doppler measurements of bowel perfusion. This report attempts to synthesize those earlier reports through systematic comparison of contemporaneous sonographic and radiographic images in 75 neonates with suspected or proven bowel pathology. In this experience, these imaging modalities were found to be complementary, revealing limitations to the sensitivity and specificity for both. Sonographic abnormalities were evident in 75% of infants with normal radiographs and 75% of those with a clinical diagnosis of no bowel disease, suggesting that such findings should be approached with some circumspection regarding their clinical importance. However, 90% of infants with necrotizing enterocolitis (NEC) had at least one sonographic abnormality, including bowel wall echogenicity in two-thirds and echogenic free peritoneal fluid in half. Anechoic free fluid was most often associated with conditions other than NEC. Sonography appears to be more sensitive than radiography for detection of free peritoneal air, but the management implications of that incremental sensitivity is not clear. This collection of case data provides a foundation for accrual of additional clinical experience to guide integration of bowel sonography into our everyday practices. Until that experience is sufficient to inform correlation of imaging findings, management choices, and ultimate outcomes, it behooves us to remember that our knowledge base for this technology is still under development.

W. E. Benitz, MD

Interleukin-8 predicts 60-day mortality in premature infants with necrotizing enterocolitis

Benkoe T, Reck C, Pones M, et al (Med Univ of Vienna, Austria)
J Pediatr Surg 49:385-389, 2014

Objective.—The purpose of this study was to evaluate the predictiveness of circulating interleukin (IL)-8 for 60-day mortality in premature infants with necrotizing enterocolitis (NEC).

Background.—NEC affects up to 5% of premature infants and remains a leading cause of mortality among neonates.

Methods.—A total of 113 infants with surgically ($n = 50$) or medically ($n = 63$) treated NEC were retrospectively analyzed. Laboratory parameters including serum IL-8 were assessed at the diagnosis of NEC and during the preoperative workup.

Results.—The 60-day mortality was 19% (22/113), 10% (6/63) in medical and 33% (16/50) in surgical NEC. IL-8 levels significantly correlated with 60-day mortality (odds ratio: 1.38; CI 1.14—1.67; $p = 0.001$). Median IL-8 levels at diagnosis were significantly higher in neonates who were later treated surgically (median = 2625 pg/ml; range: 27—7500) compared with those treated medically (median = 156 pg/ml; range: 5-7500; $p < 0.001$). The AUC to discriminate between medical and surgical NEC was 0.82 (CI, 0.74—0.90), and an exploratory IL-8 cutoff point could be established at 1783 pg/ml (sensitivity of 90.5%; specificity of 59.2%).

Conclusions.—Our findings that serum IL-8 (i) correlates directly with 60-day mortality and (ii) differs significantly between medically and surgically treated infants may change the process of therapeutic decision making in NEC (Fig 2).

► This retrospective analysis of the relationship of interleukin-8 (IL-8) to necrotizing enterocolitis (NEC) starts with a very interesting introduction on the difficulties in the diagnosis of NEC. The diagnosis of this disease is complicated by the limited diagnostic accuracy of radiographs and other imaging techniques. The early radiologic features, such as dilated bowel loops, positive intestinal gas, and even pneumatosis intestinalis is distinctly hampered by interobserver variability. The presence of pneumoperitoneum is commonly considered a definite sign for surgical intervention. However, as stated in this article, pneumoperitoneum is absent on plain radiographs in 50% to 60% of the cases. Thus, there is a tremendous need for sensitive and specific diagnostic biomarkers of this disease.

There is a considerable excitement about the use of intestinal fatty acid-binding proteins, claudin and calprotectin, as indicators for the diagnosis of NEC.[1,2] However, IL-8, an inflammatory chemokine with potent neutrophil chemotactic capability, was studied in this article using blood samples of patients suspicious of having had NEC. The results showed that there was a considerable concordance of high levels of IL-8 and NEC, especially surgical NEC, where the levels of this marker were several-fold higher than in NEC, requiring only medical management. This finding suggests that levels of the IL-8 in the serum could potentially be used for discrimination between cases

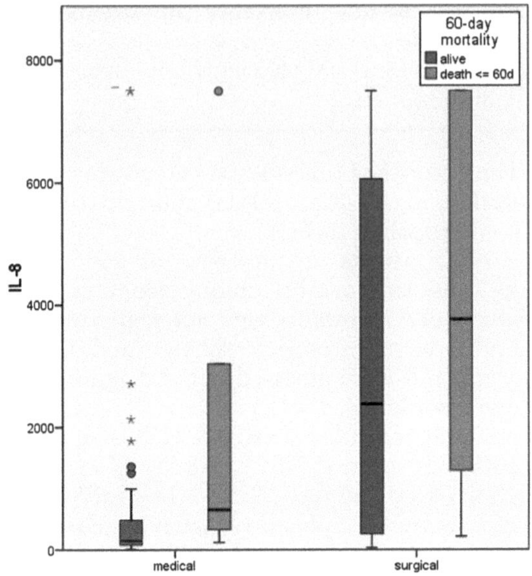

FIGURE 2.—Box-whiskers plots. Distribution of IL-8 values by 60-day mortality of surgically versus medically treated infants with NEC. (Reprinted from Benkoe T, Reck C, Pones M, et al. Interleukin-8 predicts 60-day mortality in premature infants with necrotizing enterocolitis. *J Pediatr Surg.* 2014;49:385-389, Copyright 2014, with permission from Elsevier.)

in which surgery is required rather than just medical therapy. In addition to the potential discrimination between surgical and medical NEC, the high levels of IL-8 also corresponded strongly with mortality at 60 days (Fig 2). Thus, these high levels could be used as the potential indicators of prognosis.

Difficulties in making a definitive diagnosis of this disease using clinical and radiographic techniques necessitates better diagnostic biomarkers, especially when attempting to discriminate the need for surgical intervention versus medical intervention. This article suggests that IL-8 may actually be useful for this. A caveat is that the retrospective nature of this study diminishes its strength but at the same time strongly supports the need for additional more prospective studies of IL-8 and other biomarkers of NEC.

J. Neu, MD

References

1. Gregory KE, Winston AB, Yamamoto HS, et al. Urinary Intestinal Fatty Acid Binding Protein Predicts Necrotizing Enterocolitis. *J Pediatr.* 2014 Mar 14 [Epub ahead of print].
2. Thuijls G, Derikx JP, van Wijck K, et al. Non-invasive markers for early diagnosis and determination of the severity of necrotizing enterocolitis. *Ann Surg.* 2010;251: 1174-1180.

Cytokine Levels in the Preterm Infant with Neonatal Intestinal Injury

Bhatia AM, Stoll BJ, Cismowski MJ, et al (Emory Univ School of Medicine, Atlanta, GA; Nationwide Children's Hosp, Columbus, OH; et al)

Am J Perinatol 31:489-496, 2014

Objectives.—The purpose of this study is to characterize the cytokine response of preterm newborns with surgical necrotizing enterocolitis (NEC) or spontaneous intestinal perforation (SIP) before surgical treatment and to relate these finding to intestinal disease (NEC vs. SIP).

Study Design.—The study was a 14-month prospective, cohort study of neonates undergoing surgery or drainage for NEC or SIP or surgical ligation of patent ductus arteriosus (PDA). Multiplex cytokine detection technology was used to analyze six inflammatory markers: interleukin-2, interleukin-6 (IL-6), interleukin-8 (IL-8), interleukin-1 β (IL-1β), interferon-gamma, and tumor necrosis factor-α (TNF-α).

Results.—Patients with NEC had much higher median preoperative levels of IL-6 (NEC: 8,381 pg/mL; SIP: 36 pg/mL; PDA: 25 pg/mL, $p < 0.001$), IL-8 (NEC: 18,438 pg/mL; SIP: 2,473 pg/mL; PDA: 1, 110 pg/mL, $p = 0.001$), TNF-α (NEC: 161 pg/mL; SIP: 77 pg/mL; PDA: 71 pg/mL, $p < 0.001$), and IL-1β (NEC: 85 pg/mL; SIP: 31 pg/mL; PDA: 24 pg/mL, $p = 0.001$). Patients with NEC totalis (NEC-totalis had the highest levels of IL-8 and were significantly different from infants with limited NEC (28,141 vs. 11,429 pg/mL, $p = 0.03$).

Conclusion.—Surgical NEC is a profoundly more proinflammatory disease than SIP. The cytokine profiles of patients with SIP are closer to those of a nonseptic surgical neonate.

▶ In this interesting article, Bhatia et al compared the proinflammatory cytokine response in 3 neonatal surgical conditions—necrotizing enterocolitis (NEC), spontaneous intestinal perforation (SIP), and ligation of the patent ductus arteriosus (PDA)—and concluded that NEC necessitating surgical intervention was a profoundly more proinflammatory condition compared with SIP or the nonseptic surgical procedure of PDA ligation.

These results correspond closely with our own findings of cytokine profiles, in both blood[1] and tissue[2] samples during our search for novel biomarkers and investigation into the pathophysiology of NEC. In addition to upregulation of the circulating proinflammatory cytokines, we also performed differential whole genome microarray on human intestinal tissues from NEC, SIP, and surgical control infants with noninflammatory intestinal conditions.[2] Extensive changes of gene expression involving multiple inflammatory pathways were observed in NEC compared with SIP or surgical control infants. This finding further reinforces the concept that surgical NEC is a highly proinflammatory disease. It has important clinical implications. Not only could the upregulation of proinflammatory cytokines explain the association between NEC and neurodevelopmental impairment, it also provides insights into why various inflammatory biomarkers fail to identify SIP with minimal intraabdominal contamination at an early stage.[3] The markedly elevated proinflammatory cytokine levels in surgical NEC totalis is likely attributed to the intense inflammation of the disease process together with the extent (or length) of bowel involvement, rather than a unique phenomenon specific to this disease entity. Another potential confounding factor might be systemic or intraabdominal sepsis (ie, Gram-negative septicemia or peritonitis), which frequently coexists with NEC, and could trigger a profound proinflammatory host response. Nonspecific mediators of the inflammatory cascade, such as cytokines and chemokines, are unlikely useful biomarkers for differentiating NEC from septicemia or accurately separating different degrees of severity of NEC because of overlapping mediator levels. However, recent studies indicate that gut-associated biomarkers such as intestinal-fatty acid binding protein and trefoil factor-3 are more specific biomarkers for identifying surgical or severe cases of NEC.[4,5]

In summary, both clinical and molecular evidence suggest that NEC is a substantially more proinflammatory disease than SIP, and NEC and SIP are likely 2 different disease entities associated with different etiologies. Understanding the basic pathophysiologic mechanisms of NEC would enable the discovery of novel disease-specific or organ-specific biomarkers for early diagnosis and new therapeutic strategies for revolutionizing its treatment.

P. C. Ng, MD

References

1. Chan KY, Leung FW, Lam HS, et al. Immunoregulatory protein profiles of necrotizing enterocolitis versus spontaneous intestinal perforation in preterm infants. *PLoS ONE*. 2012;7:e36977.
2. Chan KY, Leung KT, Tam YH, et al. Genome-wide expression profiles of necrotizing enterocolitis versus spontaneous intestinal perforation in human intestinal tissues: dysregulation of functional pathways. *Ann Surg*. 2013 [Epub ahead of print].
3. Lam HS, Wong SP, Cheung HM, et al. Early diagnosis of intra-abdominal inflammation and sepsis by neutrophil CD64 expression in newborns. *Neonatology*. 2011;99:118-124.
4. Thuijls G, Derikx JP, van Wijck K, et al. Non-invasive markers for early diagnosis and determination of the severity of necrotizing enterocolitis. *Ann Surg*. 2010;251:1174-1180.
5. Ng EW, Poon TC, Lam HS, et al. Gut-associated biomarkers L-FABP, I-FABP, and TFF3 and LIT score for diagnosis of surgical necrotizing enterocolitis in preterm infants. *Ann Surg*. 2013;258:1111-1118.

Randomized Controlled Trial of Slow vs Rapid Enteral Feeding Advancements on the Clinical Outcomes of Preterm Infants With Birth Weight 750–1250 g

Karagol BS, Zenciroglu A, Okumus N, et al (Children's Education and Res Hosp, Ankara, Turkey; et al)

JPEN J Parenter Enteral Nutr 37:223-228, 2013

Objective.—To evaluate the effect of slow vs rapid rates of advancement of enteral feed volumes on the clinical outcomes in preterm infants with 750–1250 g birth weight.

Study Design.—A total of 92 stable neonates 750–1250 g and gestational age <32 weeks were randomly allocated to enteral feeding advancement of 20 mL/kg/d (n = 46) or 30 mL/kg/d (n = 46). The primary outcome was days to reach full enteral feeding, defined as 180 mL/kg/d. Secondary outcomes included rates of necrotizing enterocolitis (NEC) and culture-proven sepsis, days of parenteral nutrition (PN), length of hospital stay, and growth end points.

Results.—Neonates in the rapid-feeding advancement group achieved full enteral volume of feedings earlier than the slower advancement group. They received significantly fewer days of PN, exhibited a shorter time to regain birth weight, and had a shorter duration of hospital stay. The incidence of NEC and the number of episodes of feeding intolerance were not significantly different between the groups, whereas the incidence of culture-proven late-onset sepsis was significantly less in infants receiving a rapid feeding advancement. Excluding infants who were small for gestational age at birth, the incidence of extrauterine growth restriction was significantly reduced in the rapid-advancement group at 28 days and at hospital discharge.

Conclusion.—Rapid enteral feeding advancements in 750–1250 g birth weight infants reduce the time to reach full enteral feeding and the use of PN administration. Rapid-advancement enteral feed also decreases extrauterine growth restriction with improved short-term outcomes for these high-risk infants.

▶ Extrauterine growth failure continues to be a major clinical problem for premature neonates. In many institutions, fear of necrotizing enterocolitis (NEC) limits the rate and management of feeding advancements in these infants. In this randomized comparison of advancement of feedings by either 20 or 30 mL/kg/d, the authors concluded that more rapid advancement of enteral feeding volumes in preterm infants weighing 750 to 1250 g was associated with significantly earlier achievement of full enteral feedings, reduced use of parenteral nutrition, and reduced duration of central line placement. They did not observe an increased risk of NEC or mortality. The incidence of NEC in this study was 10%, which is high compared with rates reported from the California Perinatal Quality Care Collaborative for similar infants during the same period (approximately 4%), potentially obscuring effects that might be apparent at lower background attack rates. Additionally, the sample size was not sufficient to reliably evaluate effects of the rate of feeding advancement on the incidence of NEC. There are several ambiguities about implementation of the standard feeding protocol in this study. The authors do not report the number of infants who received maternal breast milk vs formula or outcomes for those groups. It is unclear which fortifier(s) were used and if the same was used in all infants. Lastly, the authors do not define "temporary" cessation of feedings or report how many infants in each group (breast milk vs formula, or rapid vs slow advancement) required such feeding cessation. These limitations may limit general application of the conclusions drawn from this study, particularly with respect to relative safety of different strategies. Nevertheless, this study does provide further evidence for feasibility of and short-term benefits from adoption of scheduled feeding advancement protocols for very low-birth-weight infants.

N. K. Yamada, MD

Enteral L-Arginine Supplementation for Prevention of Necrotizing Enterocolitis in Very Low Birth Weight Neonates: A Double-Blind Randomized Pilot Study of Efficacy and Safety

Polycarpou E, Zachaki S, Tsolia M, et al (General District Hosp Athens "Alexandra," Greece; Athens Univ, Greece; et al)

JPEN J Parenter Enteral Nutr 37:617-622, 2013

Background.—Necrotizing enterocolitis (NEC) is the most common acquired gastrointestinal disease in premature infants and has high mortality and morbidity. Endothelial nitric oxide is an important regulator of vascular perfusion and is synthetized from the amino acid L-arginine. Hypoargininemia is frequently observed in preterm neonates and may predispose them to NEC. Our objective was to determine the effect of enteral L-arginine supplementation on the incidence and severity of NEC in very low birth weight (VLBW) neonates.

Materials and Methods.—We conducted a parallel blind randomized pilot study, comprising VLBW neonates with birth weight ≤1500 g and gestational age ≤34 weeks. VLBW neonates were randomly assigned to receive enteral L-arginine supplementation (1.5 mmol/kg/d bid) between the 3rd and 28th day of life or placebo. Diagnosis and classification of NEC were done according to modified Bell's criteria.

Results.—Eighty-three neonates were randomized to the arginine (n = 40) or placebo (n = 43) group. No adverse effects were observed in neonates receiving L-arginine supplementation. The incidence of NEC stage III was significantly lower in the arginine-supplemented group (2.5% vs 18.6%, $P = .030$).

Conclusions.—Enteral L-arginine supplementation of 1.5 mmol/kg/d bid can be safely administered in VLBW neonates from the 3rd to the 28th day of life. Enteral L-arginine supplementation appears to reduce the incidence of stage III NEC in VLBW infants. Larger studies are needed to further evaluate the effect of L-arginine supplementation in preventing NEC in VLBW infants (Table 2).

▶ The pathogenesis of necrotizing enterocolitis (NEC) has not been fully elucidated, but diverse observations implicate vascular compromise as a very important, if not critical, initiating factor. The authors hypothesized that provision of arginine, the precursor molecule for production of nitric oxide, which is often in short supply in preterm infants, may ameliorate the risk of NEC, reducing the incidence or severity of this disease. This small, randomized, controlled trial provides some evidence in support of that hypothesis, but these promising and intriguing results must be interpreted with caution. Of 7 outcomes examined, only the rate of stage III NEC differed between treatment and placebo

TABLE 2.—Incidence of Necrotizing Enterocolitis (NEC), Morbidity, and Mortality Due to NEC in the Arginine and Control Groups

	Neonates Receiving Arginine (n = 40)	Neonates Not Receiving Arginine (n = 43)	*P* Value
Incidence of NEC (all stages)	9 (22.5)	16 (37.2)	NS
Incidence of NEC (stages II and III)	4 (10.0)	10 (23.3)	NS
Incidence of NEC (stage II)	3 (7.5)	2 (4.7)	NS
Incidence of NEC (stage III)	1 (2.5)	8 (18.6)	.030
Age of NEC diagnosis, d, median	17	15	NS
Incidence of death due to NEC	0	4 (9.3)	.045
Incidence of death due to other causes	8 (20.0)	8 (18.6)	NS

Values are presented as No. (%) unless otherwise indicated. NS, not statistically significant.

groups (as tested by Fisher Exact test without correction for multiple comparisons; $P = .03$; see abstract). Rates of all NEC (stage I–III), stage II–III NEC, stage II NEC alone, death caused by NEC, or mortality from other causes were not significantly different, however (see Table 2; note that the recalculated *P* value for death from NEC is .12, not .045). It may be argued that the study is simply underpowered to show statistical significance of the lower rate of stage II–III NEC (10 vs 23%) and shift to less severe disease (75% vs 20% stage II), but those results do need confirmation in a larger trial. In addition, the high rate of NEC in this population (17% overall, 23% in the placebo group, and 10% even in the arginine-supplemented group) compared with benchmark rates of 5% to 7% in recent North American cohorts, raises the concern that the putative benefit, even if validated, may not be achievable in settings in which the baseline attack rate is lower. If these preliminary observations can be confirmed in a population with a background rate more representative of current benchmarks, they may add a significant new tool to the limited collection currently available for prevention of this often devastating disorder. For the moment, however, it is not yet time to adopt enteral arginine supplementation into routine practice.

W. E. Benitz, MD

Growth and Fatty Acid Profiles of VLBW Infants Receiving a Multicomponent Lipid Emulsion From Birth

Vlaardingerbroek H, Vermeulen MJ, Carnielli VP, et al (Sophia Children's Hosp, Rotterdam, The Netherlands, Salesi Children's Hosp, Ancona, Italy, Emma Children's Hosp, Amsterdam, The Netherlands)
J Pediatr Gastroenterol Nutr 58:417-427, 2014

Objectives.—Very-low-birth-weight (VLBW) infants are dependent on parenteral nutrition after birth. A parenteral lipid emulsion with a multicomponent composition may improve growth and neurodevelopment and may prevent liver injury, which is often observed in association with long-term parenteral nutrition with pure soybean oil. Our aim was to evaluate the safety and efficacy of a multicomponent lipid emulsion containing 30% soybean oil, 30% medium-chain triacylglycerol, 25% olive oil, and 15% fish oil compared with a conventional pure soybean oil emulsion in VLBW infants.

Methods.—We conducted a double-blind randomized controlled trial in VLBW infants randomized to parenteral nutrition with the multicomponent (study group) or pure soybean oil emulsion (control group) from birth at a dose of 2 to 3 g · kg^{-1} · day^{-1} until the infants were receiving full enteral nutrition. We assessed efficacy by growth rates and measuring plasma fatty acid profiles (representative subset). Safety was evaluated by assessing hematologic and biochemical parameters, potentially harmful phytosterol concentrations (same subset), and clinical neonatal outcome parameters.

Results.—Ninety-six infants were included (subsets n = 21). The multicomponent emulsion was associated with higher weight and head circumference z scores during admission. Plasma eicosapentaenoic acid and docosahexaenoic acid concentrations were higher in the study group. The hematological, biochemical, and neonatal outcomes were not different between groups, whereas the plasma concentrations of phytosterols were higher in the control group.

Conclusions.—The multicomponent lipid emulsion was well tolerated and associated with improved growth and higher plasma fatty acid profiles in VLBW infants in comparison with the pure soybean oil emulsion (Fig 3, Table 6).

▶ The use of soybean oil emulsions has been the mainstay of intravenous lipid nutrition for premature infants for more than 30 years. During this time, it has been well understood that lipid needs are different for preterm infants compared with adults and that this is not the optimal lipid composition for these infants. Complications such as cholestatic liver disease, chronic lung disease, and systemic inflammatory processes have been attributed to use of these soybean oil emulsions. The relatively high levels of phytosterols as well as the balance of omega 3 to 6 fatty acids being suboptimal are considered the major reasons for these complications. Neonatologists have been concerned about the use of these soybean-based emulsions and have used a traditional approach of slowly advancing them over the first week after birth—a practice that results in suboptimal calorie intake. The concern is that an early overload of lipid may cause some of these previously mentioned complications. Over the past decade, several new lipid emulsions have been formulated and tested in newborn infants. One of these, a fish oil-based emulsion (Omegaven), has been evaluated, and it has been suggested that this may be preventative against cholestatic liver disease, especially in infants who have undergone surgery and require long-term parenteral nutrition. However, this is not a balanced emulsion, and there is concern that it does not supply adequate quantities of omega 6 fatty acids, which are required for growth.

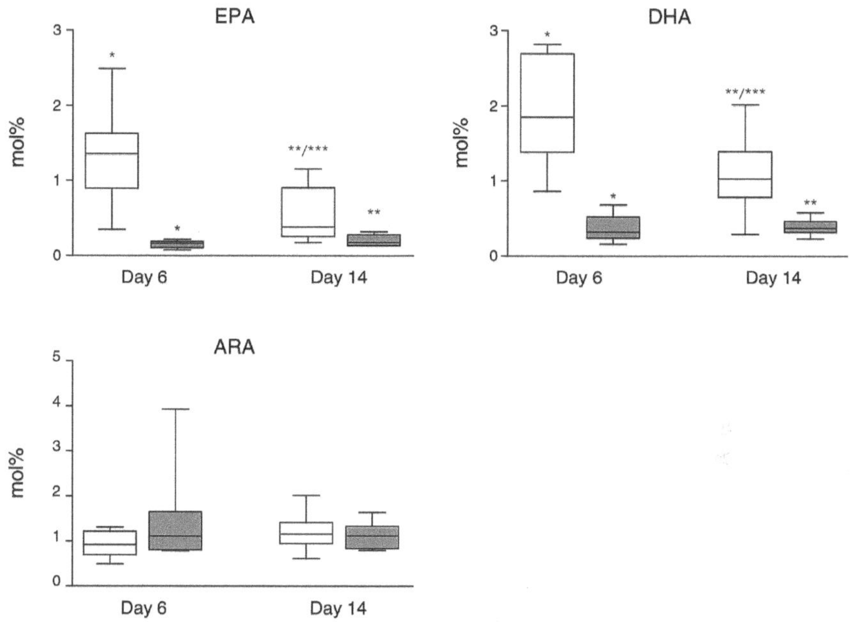

FIGURE 3.—Plasma triacylglycerol content of eicosapentaenoic acid (EPA), docosahexaenoic acid (DHA), and arachidonic acid (ARA) (in mol%) in the study group (white bars, n = 10) and the control group (gray bars, n = 11). Box-and-whiskers plots indicate the medians, interquartile ranges, and the 2.5th and 97.5th percentiles. *There was a significant difference (Mann-Whitney *U* test, $P < 0.05$) between the study group and the control group on day 6. **There was a significant difference (Mann-Whitney *U* test, $P < 0.05$) between the study group and the control group on day 14. ***There was a significant change from day 6 to 14 (Wilcoxon signed-rank test, $P < 0.05$). (*Reprinted from*Vlaardingerbroek H, Vermeulen MJ, Carnielli VP, et al. Growth and fatty acid profiles of VLBW infants receiving a multicomponent lipid emulsion from birth. *J Pediatr Gastroenterol Nutr.* 2014;58:417-427, Copyright 2014, with permission by the AAP.)

TABLE 6.—Growth During the Hospital Stay

	Study Group, $N = 48$		Control Group, $N = 48$	
	First 28 days	Discharge*	First 28 days	Discharge
No. days until discharge		87 (66–110)		95 (72–114)
Weight gain, g · kg^{-1} · day^{-1}	13.8 ± 5.6	27.6 ± 6.5†	11.9 ± 4.9	24.5 ± 6.0
Change in weight *z* score from birth	−1.2 ± 1.1	0.2 ± 1.1†	−1.6 ± 1.0	−0.5 ± 1.3
Head circumference gain, mm/wk	5.8 ± 2.7	8.5 ± 1.4	5.8 ± 2.6	8.0 ± 1.4
Change in head circumference *z* score from birth	−0.9 ± 0.9	0.7 ± 0.9†	−0.9 ± 0.9	0.1 ± 1.1
Lower leg length gain, mm/day	0.26 ± 0.14		0.28 ± 0.14	

The data are presented as the median (IQR) or mean ± standard deviation.
*The growth data were measured until discharge home or postmenstrual age of 40 weeks, whichever event came first.
†Significantly different from the control group ($P < 0.05$). The weight z scores from birth to the time of discharge increased in the study group, whereas the *z* scores for the control infants decreased.

In this study, another lipid emulsion, which consists of a combination of soybean oil, medium chain lipids, olive oil, and fish oil (SMOF), was compared with a standard soybean oil emulsion. The primary outcome was the balance of lipid composition between the 2 groups. Secondary outcomes included growth, complications such as cholestasis, liver enzymes, and length of stay in the hospital. The SMOF lipid emulsion resulted in significant differences in eicosapentaenoic acid and docosahexanoic acid on days 6 and 14 after instituting the lipid infusion (Fig 3), with a lower concentration of phytosterols in the SMOF group. Of interest is that in this study, 2 to 3 grams per kilo per day of intravenous lipid was instituted in these infants shortly after birth, a practice that many neonatologists in the United States are still afraid to institute, based more on tradition than science. Secondary outcomes also showed some interesting differences in improved growth and increased head circumference with the SMOF lipid at the time of discharge (Table 6). No complications were seen with the SMOF lipid.

This study is promising. It is the first randomized trial of these lipids evaluating the stated outcomes and could potentially result in a paradigm shift in care of preterm infants. Further studies will be helpful in terms of safety and efficacy. The question is raised whether an enteral preparation similar to the SMOF lipid composition could actually be provided in lieu of a parenteral preparation.

J. Neu, MD

Safety and Efficacy of Early Parenteral Lipid and High-Dose Amino Acid Administration to Very Low Birth Weight Infants

Vlaardingerbroek H, Vermeulen MJ, Rook D, et al (Erasmus MC-Sophia Children's Hosp, Rotterdam, The Netherlands; et al)

J Pediatr 163:638-644.e5, 2013

Objective.—To assess the efficacy and safety of early parenteral lipid and high-dose amino acid (AA) administration from birth onwards in very low birth weight (VLBW, birth weight <1500 g) infants.

Study Design.—VLBW infants (n = 144; birth weight 862 ± 218 g; gestational age 27.4 ± 2.2 weeks) were randomized to receive 2.4 g of AA $kg^{-1} \cdot d^{-1}$ (control group), or 2.4 g AA $kg^{-1} \cdot d^{-1}$ plus 2-3 g lipids $kg^{-1} \cdot d^{-1}$ (AA + lipid group), or 3.6 g AA $kg^{-1} \cdot d^{-1}$ plus 2-3 g lipids $kg^{-1} \cdot d^{-1}$ (high AA + lipid group) from birth onwards. The primary outcome was nitrogen balance. The secondary outcomes were biochemical variables, urea rate of appearance, growth rates, and clinical outcome.

Results.—The nitrogen balance on day 2 was significantly greater in both intervention groups compared with the control group. Greater amounts of AA administration did not further improve nitrogen balance compared with standard AA dose plus lipids and was associated with high plasma urea concentrations and high rates of urea appearance. No differences in other biochemical variables, growth, or clinical outcomes were observed.

Conclusions.—In VLBW infants, the administration of parenteral AA combined with lipids from birth onwards improved conditions for anabolism and growth, as shown by improved nitrogen balance. Greater levels of AA administration did not further improve the nitrogen balance but led to increased AA oxidation. Early lipid initiation and high-dose AA were well tolerated.

► Before about 15 years ago, the common practice in neonatal intensive care units was to use the traditional approach of intravenous nutrition that included a glucose infusion to maintain glucose blood concentrations within normal limits. Concurrently, introduction of amino acids and lipids was slow, sometimes taking more than a week to attain levels of 3 g/kg/d of either amino acids or intravenous lipids. Several studies in the last 10 to 15 years have discussed the safety aspects of providing amino acids at levels that more closely approach the amounts that the premature infant would be receiving had that infant remained in utero, that is, approximately 3 to 4 g/kg/d. Not only was the safety of starting these amino acids very early, even on the first day after birth, shown to be safe and beneficial in terms of protein balance using several different techniques, the fear that previously existed that these infants would have high blood urea nitrogen concentrations and acidosis was not shown to be true.

Lipids, when provided intravenously, are a rich source of energy and, because of this, should be protein sparing. Despite this fact, the tradition of maintaining low lipid infusions over the first several days and slowly increasing them persists in many neonatal intensive care units.

This study evaluated 3 groups of infants who were provided different quantities of intravenous amino acid and lipid intakes. The data clearly showed that provision of early lipids, on the first day after birth, was not only safe as shown in previous metaanalyses, but also resulted in improved conditions for anabolism, through increased nitrogen balance. The group receiving the highest quantity of amino acids, 3.6 g/kg/d, did not show increased nitrogen balance over the group receiving 2.6 g/kg/d and the same amount of lipid, but did show increased amino acid oxidation. The higher nutritional intakes did not result in an improvement in growth over the first 8 days, but this was not surprising because of the high variability of water fluxes during this period and the fact that little lean body mass is actually added during this first week after birth, as very aptly described by the authors.

The authors also describe the phenomena of hypokalemia and hypophosphatemia that can occur in those babies receiving higher quantities of amino acid intake, but this can be readily ameliorated by adjustments in the intravenous infusion of these agents.

This study aptly shows that it is safe and efficacious to not only initiate amino acid infusions in very low birth weight babies right after birth but also lipids at approximately 3 g/kg/d.

J. Neu, MD

Vitamin D status of early preterm infants and the effects of vitamin D intake during hospital stay

Monangi N, Slaughter JL, Dawodu A, et al (Cincinnati Children's Hosp Med Ctr/Univ of Cincinnati, OH; Nationwide Children's Hosp, Columbus, OH; et al)

Arch Dis Child Fetal Neonatal Ed 2013 [Epub ahead of print]

Objectives.—To evaluate vitamin D (vitD) status in early preterm infants (EPTIs) at birth and during birth hospitalisation on current vitD intake.

Design/Methods.—Serum 25-hydroxyvitamin-D [25(OH)D] concentrations, vitD intake and risk factors for low vitD status were assessed in 120 infants born at ≤32 weeks gestation.

Results.—Mean (SD) serum 25(OH)D at birth was 46.2 (14.0) nmol/L with lower concentrations in infants born <28 weeks than at 28-32 weeks gestation, p=0.02. Serum 25(OH)D was <50 nmol/L in 63% of mothers, 64% of infants at birth and 35% of infants at discharge. Mean daily vitD intake was 289 ± 96 IU at 4 weeks of age and 60% achieved 400 IU/day intake at discharge.

Conclusions.—Serum 25(OH)D <50 nmol/L was widespread in parturient women and in EPTIs at birth and at discharge. Optimising maternal vitD status during pregnancy and improving postnatal vitD intake may enhance infant vitD status during hospitalisation.

▶ Vitamin D deficiency and preterm birth share antecedent risk factors. Investigators in Cincinnati evaluated serum 25-hydroxyvitamin-D (25[OH]D) concentrations from 120 mother/preterm (< 32 weeks' gestation) infant pairs. They analyzed maternal blood at delivery and infant dried blood spots using liquid chromatography/tandem mass spectrometry (ZRT Laboratories). Infant blood spots were obtained at 48 hours, 4 weeks, and 36 weeks or discharge. Sixty-three percent of mothers and 64% of infants had low 25(OH)D levels at birth (< 50 nmol/L). Maternal and infant levels were highly correlated ($r = 0.77$, $P = .001$). Despite supplementation starting at 2 weeks of age, of 200 IU daily in the neonatal intensive care unit above feedings, more than 30% of infants at 36 weeks or discharge had levels less than 50 nmol/L. The authors, however, do not discuss the limitations of the methods of 25(OH)D measurement using blood spots, nor do they correlate these findings with clinical outcomes of interest. Nonetheless, this study highlights the need to study the implications (or lack thereof) of low 25(OH)D levels in preterm infants.

H. H. Burris, MD

10 Hematology and Bilirubin

A Randomized, Masked, Placebo-Controlled Study of Darbepoetin Alfa in Preterm Infants

Ohls RK, Christensen RD, Kamath-Rayne BD, et al (Univ of New Mexico, Albuquerque; Intermountain Health Care, Salt Lake City, UT; Cincinnati Children's Hosp, OH; et al)

Pediatrics 132:e119-e127, 2013

Background.—A novel erythropoiesis stimulating agent (ESA), darbepoetin alfa (Darbe), increases hematocrit in anemic adults when administered every 1 to 3 weeks. Weekly Darbe dosing has not been evaluated in preterm infants. We hypothesized that infants would respond to Darbe by decreasing transfusion needs compared with placebo, with less-frequent dosing than erythropoietin (Epo).

Methods.—Preterm infants 500 to 1250 g birth weight and ≤48 hours of age were randomized to Darbe (10 μg/kg, 1 time per week subcutaneously), Epo (400 U/kg, 3 times per week subcutaneously) or placebo (sham dosing) through 35 weeks' gestation. All received supplemental iron, folate, and vitamin E, and were transfused according to protocol. Transfusions (primary outcome), complete blood counts, absolute reticulocyte counts (ARCs), phlebotomy losses, and adverse events were recorded.

Results.—A total of 102 infants (946 ± 196 g, 27.7 ± 1.8 weeks' gestation, 51 ± 25 hours of age at first dose) were enrolled. Infants in the Darbe and Epo groups received significantly fewer transfusions ($P = .015$) and were exposed to fewer donors ($P = .044$) than the placebo group (Darbe: 1.2 ± 2.4 transfusions and 0.7 ± 1.2 donors per infant; Epo: 1.2 ± 1.6 transfusions and 0.8 ± 1.0 donors per infant; placebo: 2.4 ± 2.9 transfusions and 1.2 ± 1.3 donors per infant). Hematocrit and ARC were higher in the Darbe and Epo groups compared with placebo ($P = .001$, Darbe and Epo versus placebo for both hematocrit and ARCs). Morbidities were similar among groups, including the incidence of retinopathy of prematurity.

Conclusions.—Infants receiving Darbe or Epo received fewer transfusions and fewer donor exposures, and fewer injections were given to

Darbe recipients. Darbepoetin and Epo successfully serve as adjuncts to transfusions in maintaining red cell mass in preterm infants.

▶ Darbepoetin alfa (Darbe) is a novel long-acting erythropoiesis-stimulating agent. The increased half-life of Darbe allows for dosing every 1 to 4 weeks in adults with anemia secondary to renal disease or cancer, and prior single-dose pharmacokinetic studies have found a similarly prolonged half-life in preterm infants. In this study, Ohls and collaborators randomly assigned 102 preterm infants 500 to 1250 g birth weight and less than 48 hours old to receive either Darbe once weekly as a subcutaneous (SQ) injection, erythropoietin (Epo) 3 times weekly SQ injection, or placebo (sham injections 3 times weekly). Dosing continued until 35 weeks postconceptional age, discharge, transfer to another unit, or death. Enrolled infants received iron supplementation over the duration of the study, and the dose was adjusted based on ferritin levels. Red cell transfusions were given following standardized restrictive transfusion guidelines. Overall, infants in the Darbe and Epo groups had significantly higher hematocrit levels and required significantly fewer transfusions (1.2 ± 2.4 vs 2.4 ± 2.9 in Darbe and placebo groups, respectively) and donor exposures during the study. Importantly, 59% of Darbe-, 52% of Epo-, and 38% of placebo-treated infants did not receive any transfusions during their hospitalization. To some extent, this low rate of transfusion was attributable to the use of very restrictive transfusion guidelines and carefully monitored iron supplementation in all infants. Mortality and all preterm morbidities evaluated (including retinopathy of prematurity (ROP)) were similar among groups, and no adverse effects directly attributed to Darbe were noted. With increasing awareness of the adverse effects of transfusions (ie, necrotizing enterocolitis) and growing concerns about old blood, the potential use of erythropoiesis-stimulating agents to help avoid transfusions in this population might become a clinically appealing option. The very restrictive transfusion guidelines applied in this study were well tolerated in the short term, although their impact on neurodevelopmental outcome remains controversial.

M. Sola-Visner, MD

Cognitive Outcomes of Preterm Infants Randomized to Darbepoetin, Erythropoietin, or Placebo

Ohls RK, Kamath-Rayne BD, Christensen RD, et al (Univ of New Mexico, Albuquerque; Cincinnati Children's Hosp, OH; Intermountain Health Care, Salt Lake City, UT; et al)

Pediatrics 133:1023-1030, 2014

Background.—We previously reported decreased transfusions and donor exposures in preterm infants randomized to Darbepoetin (Darbe) or erythropoietin (Epo) compared with placebo. As these erythropoiesis-stimulating agents (ESAs) have shown promise as neuroprotective agents, we hypothesized improved neurodevelopmental outcomes at 18 to 22 months among infants randomized to receive ESAs.

Methods.—We performed a randomized, masked, multicenter study comparing Darbe (10 μg/kg, 1×/week subcutaneously), Epo (400 U/kg, 3×/week subcutaneously), and placebo (sham dosing 3×/week) given through 35 weeks' postconceptual age, with transfusions administered according to a standardized protocol. Surviving infants were evaluated at 18 to 22 months' corrected age using the Bayley Scales of Infant Development III. The primary outcome was composite cognitive score. Assessments of object permanence, anthropometrics, cerebral palsy, vision, and hearing were performed.

Results.—Of the original 102 infants (946 ± 196 g, 27.7 ± 1.8 weeks' gestation), 80 (29 Epo, 27 Darbe, 24 placebo) returned for follow-up. The 3 groups were comparable for age at testing, birth weight, and gestational age. After adjustment for gender, analysis of covariance revealed significantly higher cognitive scores among Darbe (96.2 ± 7.3; mean ± SD) and Epo recipients (97.9 ± 14.3) compared with placebo recipients (88.7 ± 13.5; $P = .01$ vs ESA recipients) as was object permanence ($P = .05$). No ESA recipients had cerebral palsy, compared with 5 in the placebo group ($P < .001$). No differences among groups were found in visual or hearing impairment.

Conclusions.—Infants randomized to receive ESAs had better cognitive outcomes, compared with placebo recipients, at 18 to 22 months. Darbe and Epo may prove beneficial in improving long-term cognitive outcomes of preterm infants.

▶ The primary outcome of this small, randomized trial, as stated in the body of the article, was to compare the cognitive outcome in early childhood of preterm infants randomized to Darbepoetin (Darbe) therapy to that of infants randomized to placebo. Yet the study design included a third cohort that was randomized to erythropoietin (Epo) therapy, and nowhere in the article do the authors give a rationale for including the Epo cohort. Based on the results of an earlier pilot study, each group required 22 infants to identify a difference of 15 in the Bayley Scales of Infant and Toddler Development III composite cognitive score between the Darbe and placebo group, using an α of 0.05 and 80% power. In fact, the mean difference in the cognitive composite score between the Darbe and placebo groups was 7.7, and the median scores were 95 and 90, respectively. The rate of cerebral palsy in the placebo group was 21%, an unexpectedly high rate compared with the unexpectedly low rate of 0% in either the Epo or Darbe group. These unusual rates most likely reflect the small sample sizes.

The jury is still out concerning the role of erythropoiesis stimulating agents as a potential neuroprotective strategy for newborn infants. The results of this study, although promising, are insufficient to provide an answer.

L. A. Papile, MD

Association, among very-low-birthweight neonates, between red blood cell transfusions in the week after birth and severe intraventricular hemorrhage

Christensen RD, Baer VL, Lambert DK, et al (Inst for Healthcare Delivery Res, Salt Lake City, UT)

Transfusion 54:104-108, 2014

Background.—Previous reports describe a statistical association, among very-low-birthweight (VLBW, <1500 g) neonates, between red blood cell (RBC) transfusion in the first days after birth and development of severe intraventricular (brain) hemorrhage (IVH).

Study Design and Methods.—We hypothesized that after we established a neonatal intensive care unit (NICU) transfusion management program in 2009, a decrease in early (first week after birth) RBC transfusion rate and a decrease in the incidence of severe IVH occurred concomitantly.

Results.—During a 9-year period 2716 VLBW neonates were admitted to our NICUs. In 2004, 58% of VLBW neonates received one or more RBC transfusions during the first week. After a transfusion compliance program was established in 2009, this rate declined, reaching 25% by 2012. In parallel, the severe IVH rate also declined, from 17% in 2004 to 8% in 2012 ($R^2 = 0.73$). IVH occurred in 27% of those who received a RBC transfusion during the first week versus less than 2% of those with no early transfusion ($p < 0.001$). The decrease in IVH rate occurred exclusively among neonates born in an Intermountain Healthcare perinatal center and not among those initially cared for in an "outside" hospital and subsequently transported to an Intermountain NICU.

Conclusions.—It remains unclear whether transfusing VLBW neonates during the first days after birth is a proximate cause of IVH. However, the present report is consistent with previous studies showing that successful efforts to reduce early RBC transfusions is associated with a decrease in the incidence of severe IVH (Fig 1).

▶ Once again, Christensen and colleagues at Intermountain Healthcare in Utah describe a striking association between transfusion practices and an important complication of prematurity, severe intraventricular hemorrhage (IVH) in this instance. These same authors have previously reported a statistical association between red blood cell (RBC) transfusion and development of or progression to severe IVH. In this report, they describe reduction in the rate of severe IVH closely paralleling reduction in early RBC transfusion rates (Fig 1). By logistic regression, the odds ratio for severe IVH associated with transfusion in the first postnatal week was an impressive 21.4 (95% confidence interval, 13.2–32.2). In their Discussion (which is highly recommended reading), the authors are careful not to assert that this strong association is causal in nature. In particular, they postulate that milking or delayed clamping of the umbilical cord and reduction of early phlebotomy losses may reduce both the need for transfusion and the risk of

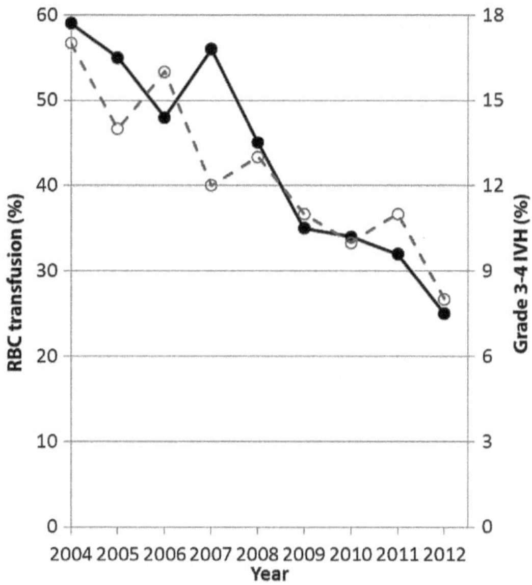

FIGURE 1.—RBC transfusion and severe IVH among VLBW neonates in the Intermountain Healthcare NICUs. The figure shows the annual percentage, from 2004 to 2012, of VLBW (<1500 g) neonates that received a RBC transfusion during their first week after birth (●). Also shown is the annual percentage of VLBW neonates that developed a severe (Grade 3 or 4) IVH (○). Both are shown as "percentage" (number of VLBW neonates with these variables divided by births < 1500 g). (Reprinted from Christensen RD, Baer VL, Lambert DK, et al. Association, among very-low-birthweight neonates, between red blood cell transfusions in the week after birth and severe intraventricular hemorrhage. *Transfusion.* 2014;54:104-108, with permission from Transfusion and John Wiley and Sons, www.interscience.wiley.com.)

severe IVH. Neither the mechanisms by which those measures might reduce IVH nor those by which transfusion might lead to IVH have been elucidated. However, the absence of an increased risk of severe IVH in the liberal transfusion arms of randomized trials of restricted vs liberal transfusion criteria (including the PINT trial,[1] which was adequately powered to detect a difference of the magnitude reported in this study) suggests that the explanation is most likely confounding by indication, so our attention should be directed toward adoption of practices that avoid or prevent anemia or hypovolemia, rather than a more tolerant attitude toward those findings.

W. E. Benitz, MD

Reference

1. Kirpalani H, Whyte RK, Andersen C, et al. The Premature Infants in Need of Transfusion (PINT) study: a randomized, controlled trial of a restrictive (low) versus liberal (high) transfusion threshold for extremely low birth weight infants. *J Pediatr.* 2006;149:301-307.

The effect of hematocrit on the efficacy of phototherapy for neonatal jaundice

Lamola AA, Bhutani VK, Wong RJ, et al (Stanford Univ School of Medicine, CA)

Pediatr Res 74:54-60, 2013

Background.—The therapeutic phototherapy action spectrum ranges from 420 to 500 nm. However, a recent report of improved efficacy of fluorescent "turquoise" light (~490 nm) as compared with blue light (~450 nm) underscores the need to define an optimal action spectrum for precision-targeted phototherapy using very narrow wavelength ranges.

Methods.—We used a current semi-empirical model of the optical properties of skin for robust calculations of the fraction of light absorbed by bilirubin at various wavelengths that could be confounded by hemoglobin (Hb), melanin, and skin thickness. Applying assumptions regarding the wavelength dependence of bilirubin photochemistry, "action spectra" were assembled from the calculated values.

Results.—All the calculated action spectra displayed a peak between 472 and 480 nm (most at 476 nm), which is a significant shift from the well-reported 460 nm absorption peak of bilirubin. Of note, the relative amplitudes of the action spectra showed an inverse relationship with hematocrit (Hct).

Conclusion.—We speculate that a narrow range of light at 476 nm would be 60% more effective than blue (broadband) fluorescent lamps. Because Hb serves as a major competitor of bilirubin for light absorption, the calculations also predict that the efficacy of phototherapy is dependent on the Hct. A high Hct could reduce therapeutic efficiency.

▶ Phototherapy works because bilirubin in the skin and subcutaneous tissue absorbs the light energy delivered, causing the bilirubin to be converted to molecules that can be excreted even when normal conjugation is deficient. The 2 pigments that compete with bilirubin for light absorption are hemoglobin and melanin. In this elegant analysis, Lamola and colleagues draw our attention to the effect of the hemoglobin concentration on the efficacy of phototherapy. They show that most of the calculated action spectra of bilirubin are at ~476 nm and that the amplitudes of the action spectra are inversely related to the hematocrit. Hemoglobin is the primary competitor with bilirubin for the absorption of light and this competition is most intense in the range of 400 to 460 nm. Thus the ideal "action spectrum" for phototherapy is in the range of 475 to 480 nm. Competition for light absorption from hemoglobin suggests that infants with higher hematocrits might be expected to respond less effectively to phototherapy and Lamola et al calculate that an increase in hematocrit from 50% to 67% would result in a 28% reduction in the rate of bilirubin decrement with phototherapy.

The absorption of light by hemoglobin and bilirubin also generates heat. With broader light spectrums, such as those generated by fluorescent lamps, more heat is generated by the heat load the absorption of less effective light produces, whereas a narrow-band LED light that delivers a narrower spectrum should produce a lower heat load. Vreman et al have shown that broadband light leads to more production of carbon monoxide than light-emitting diode (LED) light, suggesting that broadband light is producing oxidative stress.[1]

We need studies in newborn infants to confirm that these calculations of the effect of the hematocrit on the efficacy of phototherapy have clinical application. We also need clinical studies of narrow-band LED phototherapy systems with peak emission at 476 nm to confirm that such systems are, in fact, more effective than systems with broader-band emission spectra.

M. J. Maisels, MD, DSc

Reference

1. Vreman HJ, Knauer Y, Wong RJ, Chan ML, Stevenson DK. Dermal carbon monoxide excretion in neonatal rats during light exposure. *Pediatr Res.* 2009;66:66-69.

Causes of hemolysis in neonates with extreme hyperbilirubinemia

Christensen RD, Nussenzveig RH, Yaish HM, et al (Intermountain Healthcare, Salt Lake City, UT; Univ of Utah School of Medicine, Salt Lake City, UT)
J Perinatol 2014 [Epub ahead of print]

Objective.—We instituted a quality improvement process to enhance our capacity to diagnose genetic hemolytic conditions in neonates with extremehyperbilirubinemia.

Study Design.—During a 1-year period, whenever the total serum bilirubin (TSB) was >25 mg dl^{-1} a special evaluation was perfomed. If we deemed an erythrocyte membrane defect likely, based on red blood cell morphology, EMA-flow cytometry was performed. Otherwise 'next-generation' sequencing was performed using a panel of genes involved in neonatal hyperbilirubinemia.

Result.—Ten neonates had a TSB ≥25 mg dl^{-1}. Two others were evaluated as part of this process at the request of their attending neonatologists, because each had a TSB >14 mg dl^{-1} in the first hours after birth and required phototherapy for ≥1 week. Explanations for the jaundice were found in all 12 neonates. Five had hereditary spherocytosis, three of which also had ABO hemolytic disease. Two had pyruvate kinase deficiency. One had severe G6PD deficiency. The other four had ABO hemolytic disease.

Conclusion.—On the basis of the present small case series, we suggest that among neonates with extreme hyperbilirubinemia, it can be productive to pursue a genetic basis for hemolytic disease.

▶ It has long been a frustrating aspect of caring for the jaundiced newborn that initiating a "hyperbilirubinemia workup" (total and direct serum bilirubin, blood types on mother and baby, direct antiglobulin test, complete blood count, reticulocyte count) more often than not yields no useful information. In a study of 360 newborns readmitted with hyperbilirubinemia (serum bilirubin 12.7—29.1 mg/dL), we could identify a putative cause other than breast-milk jaundice or "unknown" in only 5% of cases.[1] In the US kernicterus registry, 91% of infants had bilirubin levels > 25 mg/dL, but no cause for the hyperbilirubinemia was identified in 43% of infants.[2] In the study, Christensen and colleagues could not identify a specific diagnosis in 66% of neonates with total serum bilirubin levels > 30 mg/dL in the Intermountain Healthcare system.

To address this problem, these investigators implemented a structured approach in 10 neonates whose total serum bilirubin was ≥25 mg/dL and in 2 neonates with early significant hyperbilirubinemia. As illustrated in their supplementary figure, this approach included attention to the mean corpuscular hemoglobin concentration, careful evaluation of the peripheral smear, flow cytometry if hereditary spherocytosis was suspected, and testing for G6PD and pyruvate kinase deficiency. If all of these tests were unrevealing, DNA sequencing was performed. They were able to identify a hemolytic cause for jaundice in all 12 infants, in 4 of whom the diagnosis was made by DNA sequencing.

The longer I am involved in evaluating jaundiced newborns, the more I am convinced that, absent the diagnosis of Crigler-Najjar syndrome, some degree of hemolysis is involved in any infant with significant hyperbilirubinemia,[3] a view that is now accepted by many bilirubinologists. The hemolysis may not have a specific (or currently known) diagnosis, but there is certainly an increase in red cell turnover and bilirubin production.

The lessons to be learned from this important study are clear: with the appropriate evaluation including genetic diagnosis, we should be able to identify a cause for the elevated bilirubin in the majority of significantly jaundiced newborns, and it is highly likely that the cause will be some form of hemolytic disease.

M. J. Maisels, MD, DSc

References

1. Maisels MJ, Kring E. Risk of sepsis in newborns with severe hyperbilirubinemia. *Pediatrics*. 1992;90:741-743.
2. Bhutani VK, Johnson LH, Jeffrey Maisels M, et al. Kernicterus: epidemiological strategies for its prevention through systems-based approaches. *J Perinatol*. 2004;24:650-662.
3. Maisels MJ, Kring E. The contribution of hemolysis to early jaundice in normal newborns. *Pediatrics*. 2006;118:276-279.

Unbound Free Fatty Acids from Preterm Infants Treated with Intralipid Decouples Unbound from Total Bilirubin Potentially Making Phototherapy Ineffective

Hegyi T, Kathiravan S, Stahl GE, et al (UMDNJ-Robert Wood Johnson Med School, New Brunswick, NJ; Phoenix Children's Hosp, Ariz; Cooper Med School of Rowan Univ, Camden, NJ; et al)

Neonatology 104:184-187, 2013

Extremely low birth weight (ELBW; <1,000 g) infants have poor outcomes, often compromised by bilirubin neurotoxicity. We measured unbound bilirubin (B_f) and unbound free fatty acid (FFA_u) levels in 5 ELBW infants in a trial examining the effects of pharmacologic ductal closure on infants treated with Intralipid infusion (3 g/kg/day). The levels for all infants (mean ± SD) were: total serum bilirubin (TSB) 4.6 ± 1.7 mg/dl, FFA u 376 ± 496 nM , and B f 42 ± 30 nM . Of the 3 infants who died, 2 had TSB <5.9 mg/dl but FFA_u >580 nM and B_f >75 nM . Multiple regression revealed a major effect on B_f levels due to FFA_u, indicating that Intralipid elevated levels of FFA_u and B_f. Indomethacin or ibuprofen reduced B_f levels, most likely by reducing FFA_u levels through lipase inhibition. Because displacement of B f by FFA_u decouples B f from TSB, phototherapy may not reduce the risk of bilirubin or FFA u toxicity in Intralipid-treated ELBW infants.

► Most of the extremely low birth weight (ELBW) infants in our nurseries received Intralipid, and we know that this leads to an increase in plasma free fatty acid (FFA), although FFAs are not measured routinely. We have long known that FFA displaces bilirubin from its binding to albumin. The infusion of 1 g/kg of Intralipid over a 15-hour period in infants of < 30 weeks of gestation produced a fatty acid:albumin (F:A) ratio of less than 3:1 and minimal increases in unbound bilirubin concentrations.[1] In infants of ≤32 weeks' gestation who received 2 to 3 g/kg of intravenous fat given as a continuous infusion of 2 g/kg for 7 days, the resulting F:A ratios were only 0.1 to 0.8.[2]

Now Hegyi and colleagues demonstrate that some ELBW infants receiving 3 g/kg/day of Intralipid will develop markedly elevated unbound FFA levels and that these levels of unbound FFA will displace bilirubin from albumin, producing potentially neurotoxic levels of free bilirubin. The disturbing feature of these observations is that the total bilirubin levels in two-fifths of such infants were only 3.9 and 5.9 mg/dL, yet they had a dramatic elevation of both their FFA levels (1331 and 581 nM) and their unbound bilirubin levels (79.4 and 94.2 nM), respectively. Both of these infants died. In such infants, aggressive phototherapy might have already lowered the total bilirubin level or prevented it from increasing,[3] but clearly, phototherapy did not affect the unbound bilirubin level in the presence of elevated unbound FFA.

In the Neonatal Network phototherapy study,[4] aggressive (prophylactic) phototherapy led to a 5% increase (unexplained to date) in mortality among infants weighing 501 to 750 g, and there was an increase in death or neurodevelopmental impairment with increasing levels of unbound bilirubin.[5] No data were provided regarding the levels of FFA. Is it possible that an increase in these levels contributed to the mortality in some of these infants? The principle of *primum non nocere* is a fundamental component of any intervention, and lipid infusion in ELBW infants is no exception.

M. J. Maisels, MD, DSc

References

1. Spear ML, Stahl GE, Paul MH, Egler JM, Pereira GR, Polin RA. The effect of 15-hour fat infusions of varying dosage on bilirubin binding to albumin. *JPEN J Parenter Enteral Nutr.* 1985;9:144-147.

2. Nizar L, Vyhmeister N, Ross R, et al. A jaundiced look at intravenous fat administration and the risk factor for kernicterus. *Clin Res.* 1990;38:197A.
3. Maisels MJ, Watchko JF, Bhutani VK, Stevenson DK. An approach to the management of hyperbilirubinemia in the preterm infant less than 35 weeks of gestation. *J Perinatol.* 2012;32:660-664.
4. Morris BH, Oh W, Tyson JE, et al. Aggressive vs. conservative phototherapy for infants with extremely low birth weight. *N Engl J Med.* 2008;359:1885-1896.
5. Oh W, Stevenson DK, Tyson JE, et al. Influence of clinical status on the association between plasma total and unbound bilirubin and death or adverse neurodevelopmental outcomes in extremely low birth weight infants. *Acta Paediatr.* 2010;99: 673-678.

Bilistick: A Low-Cost Point-of-Care System to Measure Total Plasma Bilirubin

Coda Zabetta CD, Iskander IF, Greco C, et al (Liver Res Centre, Trieste, Italy; Cairo Univ, Egypt; et al)
Neonatology 103:177-181, 2013

Background.—Severe neonatal hyperbilirubinemia, with consequent encephalopathy, remains a common cause of morbidity and death in many regions of the world. Poor access to clinical laboratory resources and screening programs to measure plasma bilirubin levels is a major contributor to delayed treatment in developing countries, and the cost of existing point-of-care screening instruments precludes their dissemination.

Objectives.—We are evaluating the accuracy of a low-cost, minimally invasive point-of-care system (Bilistick) requiring a 25-μl blood sample that could be used in low-resource environments to evaluate patients with neonatal jaundice.

Methods.—We compared plasma bilirubin levels in divided blood samples by clinical laboratories and by Bilistick at two medical centers serving term and near-term newborns from ethnically different populations.

Results.—118 neonates with bilirubin levels ranging from 24.8 to 501.0 μmol/l were analyzed. The mean bilirubin concentration (±SD) was 215.6 ± 85.5 μmol/l for Bilistick and 226.1 ± 86.4 μmol/l by laboratory determination. Pearson's correlation coefficient between all paired results was 0.961, and the Bland-Altman analysis showed a mean difference of 10.3 μmol/l with a 95% interval of agreement of −38.0 to 58.7 μmol/l.

Conclusion.—Bilistick is a minimally invasive method for measuring total bilirubin concentration over a wide range of values and should provide an affordable and accurate system for pre-discharge and follow-up screening of jaundiced infants, particularly in low-resource environments.

▶ Measuring the plasma bilirubin level in the Western world is a routine procedure readily available in hospital and outpatient laboratories. The same cannot be said for low-resource countries, even when a laboratory is available. Laboratory measurements require a consistent source of electricity, an unpredictable resource in these countries, even in urban areas. No bilirubin quantification of any kind can be done in most remote areas. The development of a low-cost, point-of-care method for measuring plasma bilirubin is a welcome advance that could make an important contribution to the care of newborns in these countries where extreme hyperbilirubinemia and kernicterus are distressingly common.

The Bilistick (Bilimetrix, Trieste, Italy) is a handheld rechargeable battery-operated system that can measure the plasma Bilirubin from a 25-μL sample of whole blood, and the data provided by Zabetta et al suggest that its accuracy is comparable to standard laboratory techniques. The authors estimate that the cost of this instrument is < 150 euros (approximately $200 US), an amount that should make it possible for governments to place this instrument in most rural locations.

We look forward to additional field testing and then implementation of this promising instrument.

M. J. Maisels, MD, DSc

Predischarge Screening for Severe Neonatal Hyperbilirubinemia Identifies Infants Who Need Phototherapy

Bhutani VK, on behalf of the Initial Clinical Testing Evaluation and Risk Assessment for Universal Screening for Hyperbilirubinemia Study Group (Stanford Univ, CA; et al)

J Pediatr 162:477-482, 2013

Objective.—To test whether the combined use of total plasma/serum bilirubin (TSB) levels and clinical risk factors more accurately identifies infants who receive phototherapy than does the use of either method alone.

Study Design.—We recruited healthy infants of ≥35 weeks' gestation at 6 centers that practiced universal predischarge TSB screening. Transcutaneous bilirubin (TcB) was measured at 24 hours, with TSB at 24-60 hours and at 3- to 5- and 7- to 14-day follow-up visits. Clinical risk factors were identified systematically.

Results.—Of 1157 infants, 1060 (92%) completed follow-up, and 982 (85%) had complete datasets for analysis. Infant characteristics included 25% were nonwhite and 55% were Hispanic/Latino; >90% were breastfed. During the first week, jaundice was documented in 84% of subjects. Predischarge TSB identified the 41 (4.2%) and 34 (3.5%) infants who received phototherapy before and after discharge, respectively. Prediction of postdischarge phototherapy was similar for combined clinical risk factors (earlier gestational age [GA], bruising, positive direct antiglobulin test, Asian race, exclusive breastfeeding, blood type incompatibility, jaundice extent) and age-adjusted TSB (area under the curve [AUC] = .86 vs .87), but combined screening was better (AUC = .95). TcB/TSB combined with GA alone was equally predictive (AUC = .95; 95% CI .93-.97).

Conclusions.—Jaundice is present in 4 of 5 (84%) healthy newborns. Predischarge TcB/TSB (adjusted for postnatal age) combined with specific clinical factors (especially GA) best predicts subsequent phototherapy use.

Universal implementation of this strategy in the US should improve outcomes of healthy newborns discharged early.

▶ This prospective multicenter cohort study confirmed what has been observed in 2 single-center studies[1,2]—if you combine the predischarge, hour-specific, measurement of a total serum bilirubin (TSB) or transcutaneous bilirubin (TcB), with the infant's gestational age, you get a better prediction of the likelihood of the need for phototherapy than provided by either the bilirubin level or clinical risk factors alone. Keren et al[1] found that these 2 measurements provide a level of positive and negative prediction that is indistinguishable from models that use additional clinical risk factors. The advantage of using this parsimonious model is obvious, and it deserves to be universally adopted. It is easy to obtain a TSB or TcB before discharge and when the gestational age is usually known. Plugging these 2 factors into a simple algorithm[3] provides immediate information regarding the need (or lack of need) for, and timing of, a repeat TSB level and follow-up.

The data of Bhutani et al also help to delegitimize a myth that has long persisted. Textbook chapters and journal articles, for several decades, have stated that about 60% of all newborns become clinically jaundiced during the first week of life although, until recently, there has never been a careful prospective study of this. Keren et al[4] found that 83% of infants aged 3 to 5 days had some degree of jaundice and, in the current study, Bhutani et al documented jaundice in 84% of infants (90% breastfed) in the first 7 days. We found that 79% of breastfed infants were jaundiced on day 3.[5]

There is only 1 important problem with this article. The authors provide a figure on which the peak bilirubin levels for the study infants are plotted on what is said to be a reproduction of the American Academy of Pediatrics (AAP) Clinical Practice Guideline for the use of phototherapy.[6] I'm not sure where the authors obtained the bilirubin thresholds shown on their figure, but they are not the thresholds provided in the AAP guideline.

M. J. Maisels, MD, DSc

References

1. Keren R, Luan X, Friedman S, Saddlemire S, Cnaan A, Bhutani VK. A comparison of alternative risk-assessment strategies for predicting significant neonatal hyperbilirubinemia in term and near-term infants. *Pediatrics*. 2008;121:e170-e179.
2. Maisels MJ, DeRidder JM, Kring EA, Balasubramaniam M. Routine transcutaneous bilirubin measurements combined with clinical risk factors improve the prediction of subsequent hyperbilirubinemia. *J Perinatol*. 2009;29:612-617.
3. Maisels MJ, Bhutani VK, Bogen D, Newman TB, Stark AR, Watchko JF. Hyperbilirubinemia in the newborn infant > 35 weeks' gestation: an update with clarifications. *Pediatrics*. 2009;124:1193-1198.
4. Keren R, Tremont K, Luan X, Cnaan A. Visual assessment of jaundice in term and late preterm infants. *Arch Dis Child Fetal Neonatal Ed*. 2009;94:F317-F322.
5. Maisels MJ, Clune S, Coleman K, et al. The natural history of jaundice in predominantly breast-fed infants. *Pediatrics*. 2014;134:e340-e345.
6. Maisels MJ, Baltz RD, Bhutani V, et al. Management of hyperbilirubinemia in the newborn infant 35 or more weeks of gestation. *Pediatrics*. 2004;114:297-316.

Severe Neonatal Hyperbilirubinemia in the Netherlands

Gotink MJ, Benders MJ, Lavrijsen SW, et al (Univ Med Ctr Groningen, the Netherlands; Univ Med Ctr Utrecht, the Netherlands)

Neonatology 104:137-142, 2013

Background.—The occurrence of severe neonatal hyperbilirubinemia (SH) is partly attributed to nonhospitalized perinatal care. The Netherlands have a high frequency of home births and nonhospitalized perinatal care, and the incidence of SH is unknown.

Objective.—To assess the effects of home births and early hospital discharge on the incidence of SH in term-born infants in the Netherlands.

Methods.—In this nationwide prospective surveillance study between 2005 and 2009, infants (≥37 weeks GA) were included if total serum bilirubin (TSB) was ≥ 500 μmol/l or if they received an exchange transfusion when TSB was ≥ 340 μmol/l.

Results.—Seventy-one infants had SH (incidence 10.4/100,000); 43 had a TSB ≥ 500 μmol/l (incidence 6.3/100,000) and 45 (63%) underwent an exchange transfusion. 26% of the infants with SH were born at home, which is similar to 22% of all term infants who are born at home in the Netherlands ($p = 0.41$). Maximum TSB levels were similar in infants born at home (523 ± 114 μmol/l) and infants born in hospital (510 ± 123 μmol/l; $p = 0.70$). Of the 51 infants born in hospital, 33 were discharged and readmitted with SH, with maximal TSB levels (567 ± 114 μmol/l), which were higher than in infants who remained hospitalized (406 ± 47 μmol/l; $p = 0.0001$).

Conclusion.—The incidence of severe hyperbilirubinemia in term-born infants in the Netherlands is 10.4 per 100,000, which is similar to other developed countries. Home birth and early hospital discharge do not necessarily lead to a higher incidence of SH, provided that perinatal home care is well organized (Table 5).

▶ The Netherlands is a country with an advanced system of health care available to all citizens. In addition, much of the outpatient perinatal care is provided by midwives and maternity nurses, and 22% of term newborns are born at home. Of those born in hospital, more than 50% are discharged within 24 hours. Thus, Gotink et al wanted to know what effect this system of perinatal, intrapartum, and postpartum care might have on the incidence of severe hyperbilirubinemia. Infants ≥37 weeks' gestation were included in the sample if their total bilirubin (TSB) was ≥500 μmol/L (29.2 mg/dL) or they received an exchange transfusion when the TSB was ≥340 μmol/L (20 mg/dL). This population-based study found no difference in maximum TSB levels between those born at home and those born in the hospital. The incidence of TSB levels ≥510 μmol/L (30 mg/dL) was 5.1/100 000 live births, similar to other European populations (see Table 5)

From their data, it is not possible to conclude how many infants developed kernicterus or chronic bilirubin encephalopathy, but they report that 8 infants had "advanced acute bilirubin encephalopathy," which they defined as acute

TABLE 5.—Epidemiological Data on SH from Several Developed Countries

	United States [2, 4, 17]	Canada [18]	Denmark [19]	UK-Ireland [20]	Switzerland [21]	The Netherlands
Study years	1995–2008	2002–2004	2002–2005	2003–2005	2007–2008	2005–2009
Inclusion criteria	TSB ≥420 μmol/l	TSB ≥425 μmol/l and/or ET	TSB ≥450 μmol/l	TSB ≥500 μmol/l	TSB ≥limit for ET	TSB ≥500 μmol/l or TSB ≥340 μmol/l and ≥limit for ET
Incidence of TSB ≥425 μmol/l	25–36/100,000	40.3/100,000	45/100,000	NA	17/100,000	NA
Incidence of TSB ≥510 μmol/l	3–12/100,000	NA	12/100,000	7.1/100,000	2/100,000	5.1/100,000

NA = Not available.
Editor's Note: Please refer to original journal article for full references.

bilirubin encephalopathy that included retrocollis-opisthotonos and convulsions. Such infants are most likely to develop chronic bilirubin encephalopathy, or kernicterus, in which case their incidence of kernicterus is 1.2/100 000 live births. If a TSB ≥510 umol/L (30 mg/dL) occurs in 5.1 and kernicterus in 1.2/100 000 live births, then, in the Netherlands, the risk of an infant with a bilirubin of ≥30 mg/dL developing kernicterus is about 23.5% (1.2 divided by 5.1).

These calculations pose the question of why some 77% of infants whose TSBs exceed 30 mg/dL do not develop kernicterus and what makes those who do more susceptible to the neurologic consequences of extreme hyperbilirubinemia. In the Egyptian population, Rh hemolytic disease and sepsis were the only comorbidities that contributed to the development of kernicterus.[1] None of the Dutch cases were septic, and only 6% had Rh isoimmunization.

M. J. Maisels, MD, DSc

Reference

1. Gamaleldin R, Iskander I, Seoud I, et al. Risk factors for neurotoxicity in newborns with severe neonatal hyperbilirubinemia. *Pediatrics*. 2011;128:e925-e931.

Iron supplementation in premature infants using the zinc protoporphyrin to heme ratio: short- and long-term outcomes

Miller SM (New York Presbyterian Hosp)

J Perinatol 33:712-716, 2013

Objective.—The objective of this study was to determine the effect of incrementally higher doses of iron on the zinc protoporphyrin to heme ratio (ZnPP/H) and serum ferritin, and developmental outcomes in premature infants at risk for iron deficiency.

Study Design.—Infants eligible for this prospective, randomized blinded trial were between 27 and 30 completed weeks of gestation, older than 1 week of age and tolerating 100 ml kg^{-1} per day of enteral feedings. The control group was treated with 2.2 mg kg^{-1} per day of ferrous sulfate and the treatment group was treated with 3 to 12 mg kg^{-1} per day based on the ZnPP/H. Infants had follow-up with Bayley exams at 6 and 24 months corrected age. Statistical evaluation included Student's t-tests and Fisher's exact test.

Result.—Eighty-one infants were enrolled (40 control, 41 treatment). The average total iron dose for the control group was 2.2 mg kg^{-1} per day and for the treatment group was 10.4 mg kg^{-1} per day ($P < 0.05$). The ZnPP/H was not different between the two groups. The ferritin at the end of the study was decreased in the control group but remained stable in the treatment group (control initial 202 ± 109 ng ml^{-1}, final 168 ± 141 ng ml^{-1} ($P < 0.05$); treatment initial 187 ± 131 ng ml^{-1}, final 176 ± 118 ng ml^{-1}). At 24 months, infants with psychomotor development index <85 occurred in 25% of the subjects in the control group and in 7% of subjects in the treatment group in a post hoc analysis (odds ratio, 4.2; 95% confidence interval, 0.7 to 43, $P = 0.07$).

Conclusion.—The ZnPP/H may not be a reliable marker of iron status when used in a short period of time during iron supplementation. Infants treated with a lower dose of ferrous sulfate had a decreasing serum ferritin and a trend toward increased motor delays at 24 months.

▶ Preterm infants are at high risk of iron deficiency because of a combination of low iron stores, phlebotomy losses, and rapid growth. Iron supplementation is critical in this population, because iron is essential for brain development. Classically, iron deficiency is diagnosed by anemia, low serum ferritin, elevated total iron-binding capacity, and elevated soluble transferrin receptor. In preterm infants, however, some of these measures are unreliable, and anemia is a late finding. The zinc protoporphyrin-to-heme ratio (ZnPP/H) has been proposed as an indicator of pre-anemic iron deficiency in preterm infants. In this study, Miller randomly assigned 81 infants 27 to 30 weeks of gestation and greater than 1 week old to receive iron at either 2 mg/kg/d or 3 to 12 mg/kg/d based on the ZnPP/H level (mean, 10.4 mg/kg/d). Infants were enrolled at mean corrected age of 32 weeks, and were treated for an average of 3 weeks. ZnPP/H levels at study entry and completion were no different between and within groups. Serum ferritin levels decreased in the control group but remained stable in the treatment group. At 24 months of follow-up, there were no significant differences between treatment and control groups in cognitive, motor, and language scores (Bayley Scale of Infant Development), although the mean scores tended to be higher in the treated group. In a post hoc analysis, motor delays (psychomotor development index <85) were identified in 7% of treatment vs 25% of control infants ($P = .07$). Although not significant, this is an intriguing trend. Overall, this study suggested that ferritin might be a better measure of iron status than ZnPP/H in preterm infants and supports the importance of adequate iron supplementation for neurodevelopment. The results need to be interpreted with caution, however, because the study period was very short (3 weeks), and no data are provided regarding iron supplementation before and after study.

M. Sola-Visner, MD

11 Renal, Metabolism, and Endocrine Disorders

Neonatal Thyrotoxicosis

Bisschop PH, van Trotsenburg ASP (Academic Med Ctr Amsterdam, the Netherlands)

N Engl J Med 370:1237, 2014

Background.—Neonatal thyrotoxicosis may develop in the fetuses of mothers with Graves' disease. A case occurring before the mother was diagnosed with Graves' disease was reported.

Case Report.—Male infant born after 36 weeks of gestation was admitted to the intensive care unit to receive empirical treatment for sepsis. His mother, 22, had been assessed for oligohydramnios at 31 weeks of gestation. At that time the fetal heart rate was 158 beats per minute. At 35 weeks of gestation, intrauterine growth retardation was detected on ultrasonography, which had been performed every 2 weeks since the oligohydramnios assessment. The fetal heart rate was 150 beats per minute, but no goiter was found. Birth weight was 1800 g and Apgar scores were normal, although his pulse was 200 beats per minute. Upper eyelids were retracted and subcutaneous fat nearly absent. One day after delivery, the mother was diagnosed with Graves' disease. She reported having lost 28 kg over the past year and 6 kg during pregnancy. The infant was diagnosed with neonatal thyrotoxicosis and had a thyrotropin level under 0.01 μU per liter, free thyroxine level over 70 pmol per liter, and thyrotropin-binding inhibitory immumoglobulin level of 56 U per liter. Treatment consisted of propranolol, methimazole, and potassium iodide, which led to normalized thyrotoxin levels and resolution of tachycardia within 5 days. Levothyroxine was also given at this point.

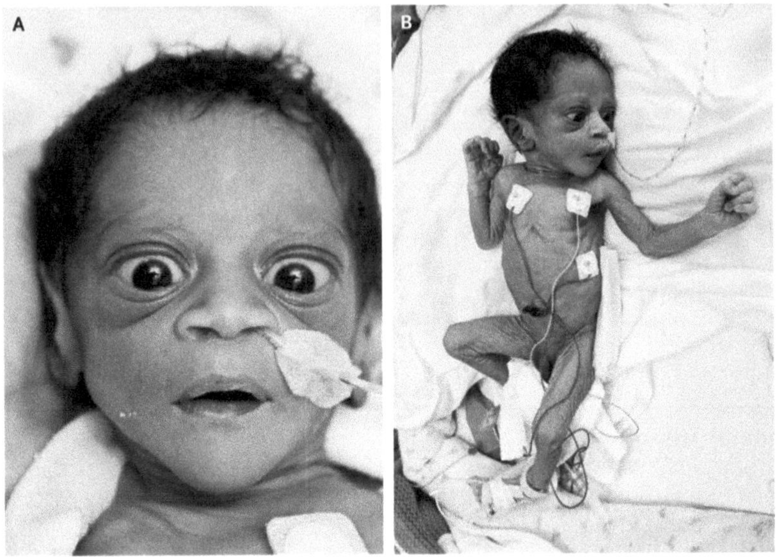

FIGURE 1.—(Reprinted from Bisschop PH, van Trotsenburg ASP. Neonatal thyrotoxicosis. *N Engl J Med.* 2014;370:1237, Copyright 2014, with permission from Massachusetts Medical Society.)

Conclusion.—This infant suffered intrauterine growth retardation related to his mother's undiagnosed Graves' disease (Fig 1).

▶ This is an excellent example of an infant with the thyrotoxicosis. The picture showing severe proptosis and retraction of the upper eyelids with almost absent subcutaneous fat is very typical of this disease in the newborn. The case report describes a baby who also had a rapid heartbeat at 200 bpm, very typical of the infant with the thyrotoxicosis or Graves disease. Of interest, it appears that the thyrotoxicosis was not suspected in the mother initially because she was referred for assessment of oligohydramnios and had an unexplained weight loss. Diagnosis was not made during the pregnancy, and she was treated for Graves disease, which was diagnosed one day after the delivery. This boy had very low levels of thyrotropin and high levels of thyroxine. Treatment with propranolol, methimazole and potassium iodide was provided. Of interest is that it only took 5 days for the thyroxine levels to become normalized and the tachycardia to resolve.

J. Neu, MD

Dextrose gel for neonatal hypoglycaemia (the Sugar Babies Study): a randomised, double-blind, placebo-controlled trial

Harris DL, Weston PJ, Signal M, et al (Waikato District Health Board, Hamilton, New Zealand; Univ of Canterbury, Christchurch, New Zealand; et al)

Lancet 382:2077-2083, 2013

Background.—Neonatal hypoglycaemia is common, and a preventable cause of brain damage. Dextrose gel is used to reverse hypoglycaemia in individuals with diabetes; however, little evidence exists for its use in babies. We aimed to assess whether treatment with dextrose gel was more effective than feeding alone for reversal of neonatal hypoglycaemia in at-risk babies.

Methods.—We undertook a randomised, double-blind, placebo-controlled trial at a tertiary centre in New Zealand between Dec 1, 2008, and Nov 31, 2010. Babies aged 35–42 weeks' gestation, younger than 48-h-old, and at risk of hypoglycaemia were randomly assigned (1:1), via computer-generated blocked randomisation, to 40% dextrose gel 200 mg/kg or placebo gel. Randomisation was stratified by maternal diabetes and birthweight. Group allocation was concealed from clinicians, families, and all study investigators. The primary outcome was treatment failure, defined as a blood glucose concentration of less than 2·6 mmol/L after two treatment attempts. Analysis was by intention to treat. The trial is registered with Australian New Zealand Clinical Trials Registry, number ACTRN12608000623392.

Findings.—Of 514 enrolled babies, 242 (47%) became hypoglycaemic and were randomised. Five babies were randomised in error, leaving 237 for analysis: 118 (50%) in the dextrose group and 119 (50%) in the placebo group. Dextrose gel reduced the frequency of treatment failure compared with placebo (16 [14%] *vs* 29 [24%]; relative risk 0·57, 95% CI 0·33–0·98; $p = 0{\cdot}04$). We noted no serious adverse events. Three (3%) babies in the placebo group each had one blood glucose concentration of 0·9 mmol/L. No other adverse events took place.

Interpretation.—Treatment with dextrose gel is inexpensive and simple to administer. Dextrose gel should be considered for first-line treatment to manage hypoglycaemia in late preterm and term babies in the first 48 h after birth.

▶ Jane Hawdon[1] has written a wonderful, at times almost tongue in check, article on the dilemma of diagnosing hypoglycemia in newborns. In describing some of her early research on the topic, she notes that when she was called in for a baby with the admitting diagnosis of hypoglycemia (<2.6 mmol/L–45 mg/dL), "Many babies on my arrival seemed surprisingly well and were physically resisting all efforts to site nasogastric tubes and intravenous cannulae, and were returning to the sender the volumes of formula milk that were given to them with the best of intentions.

Imagine my dismay, especially on the part of the babies and their mothers, when laboratory measurements demonstrated that for many babies, the admission glucose was not confirmed as being in the hypoglycemic range and that the initial near patient testing strip had proved to be an inaccurate measurement." Later she notes "Further, as the study elapsed and following discussion with experts such as the late Marvin Cornblath, it became evident that many babies did not have a pathological condition, rather they were simply doing what babies do in the process of adaptation after birth, mounting a metabolic response to a physiological fall in blood glucose."

The conundrum of defining hypoglycemia has resulted in many discussions, reports, and conferences, none with truly a true gold standard. Later in the article, Hawdon writes, "Groups of experts have reviewed the evidence base in the light of more recent publications[2-5] and have presented no arguments to move from the pragmatic consensus of 2000." The Committee of the Fetus and Newborn of the American Academy of Pediatrics statement on hypoglycemia, spearheaded by David Adamkin,[6] concluded, "Current evidence does not support a specific concentration of glucose that can discriminate normal from abnormal or can potentially result in acute or chronic irreversible neurologic damage. Early identification of the at-risk infant and institution of prophylactic measures to prevent neonatal hypoglycemia are recommended as a pragmatic approach despite the absence of a consistent definition of hypoglycemia in the literature." Hawdon[1] noted, "The suggested blood glucose thresholds for intervention are:

- any single value < 1.0 mmol/l (17 mg/dl)
- baby with abnormal clinical signs—single value < 2.5 mmol/l (45 mg/dl)
- baby at risk of impaired metabolic adaptation but without physical signs—< 2.0 mmol/l (35 mg/dl) and remaining < 2.0 mmol/l at next measurement."

With this rather lengthy background, we examine the Sugar Babies Study, a well-controlled randomized trial that demonstrated that "Treatment with 40% dextrose gel 200 mg/kg was more effective than feeding alone for reversal of neonatal hypoglycemia in at-risk late preterm and term babies in the first 48 h after birth." The treatment is simple, inexpensive, well tolerated, and effective. It is easy to administer, can be made up in every pharmacy, and supports breastfeeding because there is less of a need for formula supplementation. There was no rebound hypoglycemia and fewer admissions to the intensive care unit of babies who did not need admission for other reasons. The authors request that dextrose gel should be considered for first-line management of late preterm and term hypoglycemic babies in the first 48 hours after birth. This seems like a reasonable request provided we know when we are dealing with hypoglycemia and not a physiologic drop in blood glucose that will return spontaneously and quickly to normal levels.

A. A. Fanaroff, MD, FRCPE

References

1. Hawdon JM. Definition of neonatal hypoglycaemia: time for a rethink? *Arch Dis Child Fetal Neonatal Ed.* 2013;98:F382-F383.
2. Williams AF. Neonatal hypoglycaemia: clinical and legal aspects. *Semin Fetal Neonatal Med.* 2005;10:363-368.

3. Boluyt N, van Kempen A, Offringa M. Neurodevelopment after neonatal hypoglycemia: a systematic review and design of optimal future study. *Pediatrics.* 2006; 117:2231-2243.
4. Rozance PJ, Hay WW. Hypoglycemia in newborn infants: features associated with adverse outcomes. *Biol Neonate.* 2006;90:74-86.
5. Hay WW Jr, Raju TN, Higgins RD, Kalhan SC, Devaskar SU. Knowledge gaps and research needs for understanding and treating neonatal hypoglycemia: workshop report from Eunice Kennedy Shriver National Institute of Child Health and Human Development. *J Pediatr.* 2009;155:612-617.
6. Committee on Fetus and Newborn, Adamkin DH. Postnatal glucose homeostasis in late-preterm and term infants. *Pediatrics.* 2011;127:575-579.

Early Hyperglycemia Is Associated With Poor Gross Motor Outcome in Asphyxiated Term Newborns

Spies EE, Lababidi SL, McBride MC (Akron Children's Hosp, Hudson, OH; Northeast Ohio Med Univ, Rootstown, OH)
Pediatr Neurol 50:586-590, 2014

Background.—Hyperglycemia after ischemic stroke in adults and after near-drowning in children is associated with a poor neurological outcome. Anaerobic metabolism of glucose leads to buildup of lactic acid, free radical production, mitochondrial failure, and ultimately an increase in neurological injury. In asphyxiated infants, high lactate peaks are seen in the basal ganglia with magnetic resonance spectroscopy. Because motor disability in asphyxiated full-term newborns often relates to injury in the basal ganglia, we hypothesized that hyperglycemia and associated buildup of lactic acid may lead to worse gross motor outcome.

Methods.—Glucose, blood gas values, and demographic data were abstracted from the medical records of 41 term infants with asphyxia and without confounding diagnoses. Their Gross Motor Function Classification System scores were determined from the medical record or by structured telephone interviews.

Results.—The outcomes of 14 infants were considered poor on the basis of death within the first 6 months or moderate-to-severe cerebral palsy (Gross Motor Function Classification System score 1-5). The other 27 infants had no gross motor disability (Gross Motor Function Classification System score 0). The highest recorded blood glucose correlated with poor outcome ($P = 0.046$ by logistic regression). Infants with hyperglycemia (blood glucose > 150 mg/dL) were more likely to have poor outcome ($P = 0.017$; odds ratio: 5.9; 95% confidence interval: 1.4-24.7).

Conclusions.—High blood glucose in the first 12 hours is associated with poor gross motor outcome in this cohort of asphyxiated term infants. Clinicians should avoid hyperglycemia in managing term infants with asphyxia.

► In this retrospective observation, a correlation between hyperglycemia and poor outcome was established in a population of full-term infants with birth asphyxia. Poorest outcomes were found in babies with the highest blood glucose concentrations. Although this forms an interesting hypothesis, it is difficult to determine whether the hyperglycemia represents pancreatic dysfunction, an exaggerated endogenous stress response, or an iatrogenic complication. Providing specific glucose infusion rates might have helped discern this.

The inclusion criteria selected are somewhat soft. I would have used the same criteria used in the hypothermia trials; a pH of 7.20 seems too high. No information is provided about either oxygenation or ventilation. Are we dealing with asphyxia or merely acidosis?

Younger investigators should also be reminded that Apgar scores are discontinuous and cannot be averaged. Levels of pH, which are logarithmic, can only be expressed as an average if they are first converted to hydrogen ion concentration, averaged, then reconverted by taking the antilog. Shame on the reviewers for missing this.

In view of these findings, it might be interesting to see if the same observation can be made from examination of the datasets of the 3 major cooling trials.

S. M. Donn, MD

ACTH and cortisol cord plasma concentrations in preterm and term infants

Bagnoli F, Mori A, Fommei C, et al (Univ Hosp of Siena, Italy)

J Perinatol 33:520-524, 2013

Objective.—To measure the adrenocorticotropic hormone (ACTH) and cortisol (F) cord plasma levels in preterm and term infants in relation to their mode of delivery.

Study Design.—We studied 180 newborns appropriate for gestational age (GA) with birth weights between 365 and 4380 g and GAs between 21 and 41 weeks divided into three groups: born by vaginal delivery (VD), elective cesarean section (ECS) and emergency cesarean section (EMCS). ACTH and F levels were valued with enzyme-linked immunosorbent assay testing. Median concentrations were compared between groups by Student's *T*-test for independent and paired data. Multiple regression analysis was used to investigate the effect of GA on F and ACTH concentrations.

Result.—A significant positive correlation between GA and plasma concentrations of ACTH ($P < 0.05$) was found in the whole population, but not between GA and F ($P = \text{NS}$). A significant positive correlation was found between GA and plasma concentrations of both ACTH ($P = 0.01$) and F ($P = 0.03$) in VD. In those born by ECS, we demonstrated a positive correlation not only between plasma concentrations of ACTH ($P = 0.0000$) and F ($P = 0.00002$), respectively, with GA, but also a correlation between ACTH and F ($P = 0.0004$). No significant correlations were found in the EMCS group ($P = \text{NS}$).

Conclusion.—Our results suggest simultaneous pituitary-adrenal maturation, which is complete only at term. The responsiveness of preterm babies to different stressful stimulations is similar to the terms' but quantitatively lower, and the secretion of ACTH and F may not suffice in severe pathological circumstances (Fig 1).

▶ Recognition of the critical role of cortisol in supporting function of virtually every organ system led to awarding of the Nobel Prize to Kendall, Reichstein, and Hench in 1950. By the 1970s, it had become apparent that corticosteroids

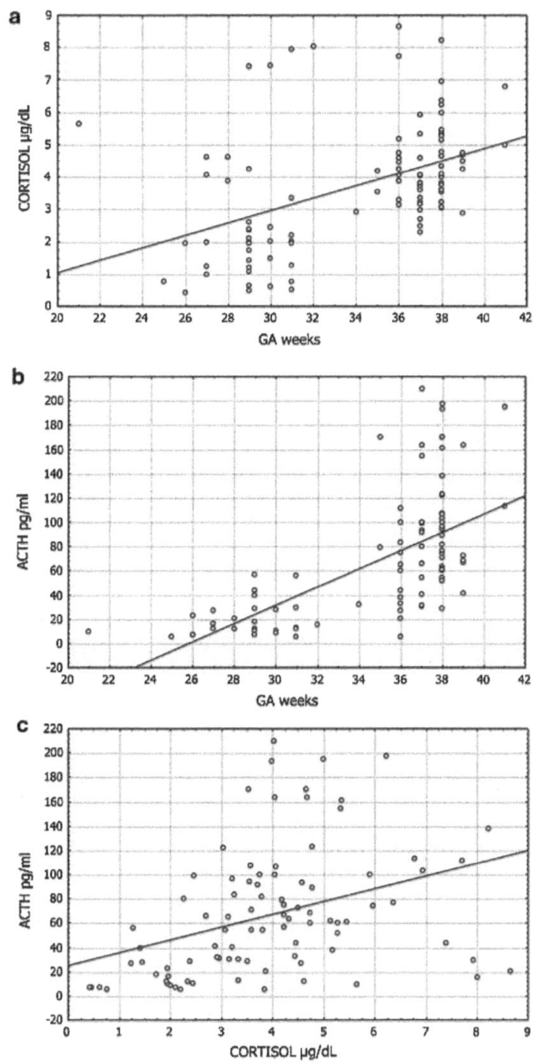

FIGURE 1.—Correlation between (**a**) cortisol and gestational age (GA), (**b**) adrenocorticotropic hormone (ACTH) and GA, (**c**) cortisol and ACTH in elective cesarean section (ECS) population. (Reprinted from Bagnoli F, Mori A, Fommei C, et al. ACTH and cortisol cord plasma concentrations in preterm and term infants. *J Perinatol.* 2013;33:520-524, with permission from Nature America, Inc.)

had substantial effects on pulmonary physiology in preterm infants with severe respiratory failure. However, strategies for optimal application of that knowledge to care of such infants in our nurseries remain elusive, in part because of incomplete understanding of normal fetal and neonatal homeostasis of the pituitary-adrenal axis. This carefully constructed observational study provides important insights into that biology. These authors measured cord blood levels of adrenocorticotropic hormone (ACTH) and cortisol in a convenience sample of 180 infants. Segregation of those who had not experienced labor but were delivered by elective cesarean delivery, allowed demonstration of increasing levels of ACTH and cortisol with advancing gestation (Fig 1). In addition, both ACTH and cortisol levels were significantly higher in preterm (≤32 weeks) but not in term (≥38 weeks) infants who had been exposed to the stress of labor, demonstrating the ability of preterm fetuses to respond to stress with ACTH and cortisol release. This contrasts the postnatal clinical observation that extremely preterm infants release cortisol in response to exogenous ACTH but choose not to release ACTH or cortisol in response to stress. This may be related to a unique aspect of gestational biology in primates. Unlike other mammals, the placenta is the primary source of corticotropin-releasing hormone (CRH) in primates. Plasma levels of CRH of placental origin steadily increase in late gestation, driving the increase in ACTH and cortisol in unstressed fetuses described in this article. Thus, it appears that the hypothalamus of the preterm human neonate may be developmentally unprepared to assume responsibility for control of the pituitary-adrenal access, resulting in the signs of adrenal insufficiency prevalent in this population. Investigation of this hypothesis may lead to a much deeper understanding of the nature and time course of maturation of this facet of hypothalamic function, which is necessary to guide development of optimal strategies for replacement of cortisol while awaiting developmental maturation, much as we provide surfactant replacement pending maturation of pulmonary type II cells.

W. E. Benitz, MD

12 Miscellaneous

Randomized controlled trial of Family Nurture Intervention in the NICU: assessments of length of stay, feasibility and safety

Welch MG, the FNI Trial Group (Columbia Univ College of Physicians & Surgeons, NY)

BMC Pediatr 13:148, 2013

Background.—While survival rates for preterm infants have increased, the risk for adverse long-term neurodevelopmental and behavioral outcomes remains very high. In response to the need for novel, evidence-based interventions that prevent such outcomes, we have assessed Family Nurture Intervention (FNI), a novel dual mother-infant intervention implemented while the infant is in the Neonatal Intensive Care Unit (NICU). Here, we report the first trial results, including the primary outcome measure, length of stay in the NICU and, the feasibility and safety of its implementation in a high acuity level IV NICU.

Methods.—The FNI trial is a single center, parallel-group, randomized controlled trial at Morgan Stanley Children's Hospital for mothers and their singleton or twin infants of 26–34 weeks gestation. Families were randomized to standard care (SC) or (FNI). FNI was implemented by nurture specialists trained to facilitate affective communication between mother and infant during specified calming interactions. These interactions included scent cloth exchange, sustained touch, vocal soothing and eye contact, wrapped or skin-to-skin holding, plus family-based support interactions.

Results.—A total of 826 infants born between 26 and 34 weeks during the 3.5 year study period were admitted to the NICU. After infant and mother screening plus exclusion due to circumstances that prevented the family from participating, 373 infants were eligible for the study. Of these, we were unable to schedule a consent meeting with 56, and consent was withheld by 165. Consent was obtained for 150 infants from 115 families. The infants were block randomized to groups of N = 78, FNI and N = 72, SC. Sixteen (9.6%) of the randomized infants did not complete the study to home discharge, 7% of those randomized to SC and 12% of FNI infants. Mothers in the intervention group engaged in 3 to 4 facilitated one- to two-hour sessions/week. Intent to treat analyses revealed no significant difference between groups in medical complications. The mean length of stay was not significantly affected by the intervention.

Conclusion.—There was no significant effect demonstrated with this intervention amount on the primary short-term outcome, length of stay. FNI can be safely and feasibly implemented within a level IV NICU.

Trial Registration.—Clinicaltrials.gov: NCT01439269.

▶ The aim of the Family Nurture Intervention protocol is to mitigate the adverse consequences of prolonged separation of mother and baby after preterm birth.[1] Specifically, the intervention promotes dyadic interaction between mother and infant using repeated experience with calming sessions, including scent cloth exchange, firm sustained touch and holding. The sessions are facilitated by Nurture Specialists, former neonatal intensive care unit nurses trained in implementing the protocol.

It is not surprising that the length of stay did not differ between the intervention and control groups. As noted by the authors, a large number of families declined to participate because of the considerable study burden imposed by the trial. Thus, those most likely to participate were families who had better support systems, more time, and fewer responsibilities. This is supported by the demographic characteristics of the participating families; mothers were on average 32 to 34 years of age; approximately 70% were married; 62% to 65% had a graduate or higher education; and the majority had a family income greater than $70 000. The fact that there was little if any difference in the amount of specified nurture activities may imply that mothers in both groups were more likely to give lots of attention to the baby, regardless of group assignment. In addition, study contamination due to communication between subjects in the 2 groups was inevitable.

L. A. Papile, MD

Reference

1. Welch MG, Hofer MA, Brunelli SA, et al. Family nurture intervention (FNI): methods and treatment protocol of a randomized controlled trial in the NICU. *BMC Pediatr.* 2012;12:14.

Online support for parents of preterm infants: a qualitative and content analysis of Facebook 'preemie' groups

Thoren EM, Metze B, Bührer C, et al (Charité Univ Med Ctr, Berlin, Germany)
Arch Dis Child Fetal Neonatal Ed 98:F534-F538, 2013

Objective.—To qualitatively evaluate the content of communication in Facebook communities dedicated to preterm infants.

Design.—The 25 largest public English-language Facebook groups focusing on preterm infants were identified. For each group, the 20 most recent wallposts and a maximum of the 15 first comments to these wallposts, and the 15 most recent discussion topics were analysed according to a thematic coding scheme. The purpose of each group was determined and personal characteristics of administrators and active posters were analysed.

Results.—1497 individual Facebook groups focusing on preterm infants were found, wherein the 25 largest had between 391 and 14 986 members. Non-profit fundraising groups comprised 48% of analysed groups and had the greatest number of members (median 1450, IQR 548–5435), followed by general awareness (24% of all groups, members: median 1183, IQR 658–2116) and interpersonal support groups (28% of all groups, members: median 823, IQR 484–1022). 85.0% of administrators and 91.5% of posters were women, and two-thirds of posts had been written by mothers of preterm infants. The analysis of posts, comments and discussion topics (n = 1054) showed that 'information sharing' (31%) and 'interpersonal support' (53%) were the most common purposes.

Conclusions.—Facebook groups related to preterm birth have become a popular tool for fundraising and awareness-raising. However, most group members use these forums for information sharing and interpersonal support. Given their popularity and reach, further research is warranted to understand the motivations, implications and risks of dynamic online communication among parents of preterm infants.

► It is estimated that there are more than 600 million registered users of Facebook. Included are many sites devoted to disease-specific groups that emphasize disease awareness, support for patients and families (sharing personal clinical information, requesting disease-specific guidance, and receiving emotional support), and/or fundraising. In this report, the authors investigated what is available on Facebook that addresses preterm infants, identifying are the individuals actively participating, and what are the official purposes of the Facebook groups.

The search was restricted to Facebook groups; sites for companies or individuals were excluded. To be included in the study, the groups had to address "preterm infants," operate in English, and be public for anyone with a Facebook account to view and join. The 25 largest groups were identified, and their purpose was classified into 1 of the following categories: (1) nonprofit fundraising group, (2) preterm infants general awareness group, or (3) interpersonal support group. Posters were categorized as (1) private person, (2) parent of a premature infant, (3) adult that was born prematurely, (4) medical personnel, (5) person representing an organization, or (6) person representing a company.

In contrast to other disease-related groups on Facebook, the majority of the "premie" groups were officially created for nonprofit fundraising, or general awareness rather than supportive care. Despite this, the analysis of downloaded posts, comments, and discussion topics showed that personal information sharing and interpersonal emotional support were the most common purposes. The fact that medical personnel comprised less than 2% of the posters most likely reflects their reluctance to participate because of the Health Insurance Portability and Accountability Act's Privacy Rule.

L. A. Papile, MD

Neonatal intensive care unit handoffs: a pilot study on core elements and epidemiology of errors

DeRienzo C, Lenfestey R, Horvath M, et al (Duke Univ Hosp, Durham, NC; Duke Univ Health System, Durham, NC)

J Perinatol 34:149-152, 2014

Objective.—To define the core data elements of a neonatal intensive care unit (NICU) handoff compare NICU residents' written and verbal handoff data with real-time, auto-populated data and identify the epidemiology of handoff errors.

Study Design.—We defined nine core data elements for a NICU patient handoff. We then compared residents' written and verbal handoffs against real-time, auto-populated data for each core element.

Result.—A total of 101 NICU patient handoffs (31 unique patients) were analyzed. Per patient, residents made more written errors for infants in critical-care beds than for infants in step-down beds (2.33 vs 1.67, $P = 0.04$). Replacing residents' written handoffs with the gold-standard, auto-populated data would have prevented 92% of written errors.

Conclusion.—NICU infants are subjected to many handoff errors. Sicker infants are at higher risk for error. Auto-population can reduce written handoff errors and allow residents more time for training and educational opportunities.

▶ It would be hard to argue that resident handoffs in the neonatal intensive care unit (NICU) have become more problematic and error-prone as the complexity of care increases and the resident exposure and experience decreases. In this study, the group from Duke compared written and verbal handoffs against a computer-generated data for parameters selected a priori. Not surprisingly, the autopopulated format performed better.

The authors acknowledge that the results were affected by resident competence and experience, as well as the selected cases. It is as yet unclear whether better sign-outs will lead to fewer errors or improved care, but at least there appears to be a mechanism now in place to do an appropriate randomized and controlled trial, although doing it right will be challenging.

Many centers, including my own, are struggling with the evolving electronic medical record. I applaud the efforts of DeRienzo and colleagues for using the technology to assess and improve an age-old problem in the NICU.

S. M. Donn, MD

Examining the effects of a targeted noise reduction program in a neonatal intensive care unit

Wang D, Aubertin C, Barrowman N, et al (Children's Hosp of Eastern Ontario, Ottawa, Ontario, Canada; Children's Hosp of Eastern Ontario Res Inst, Ottawa, Ontario, Canada)

Arch Dis Child Fetal Neonatal Ed 99:F203-F208, 2014

Objectives.—To determine whether implementation of a noise reduction policy followed by the addition of direct audit and feedback reduces noise levels in a tertiary-level neonatal intensive care unit (NICU).

Study Design.—Noise level data was collected in three phases: (1) baseline (preintervention), (2) immediately postimplementation of our noise reduction policy, (3) postunveiling of direct audit and feedback mechanism.

Setting.—A level 3 NICU in Ontario, Canada.

Interventions.—Noise reduction policy and a direct audit and feedback mechanism.

Main Outcome Measures.—Average noise level.

Results.—The baseline level of noise in our unit consistently exceeds guidelines with an average baseline noise of 49 dB (±1.4). Our intervention resulted in a significant reduction in noise levels for one of the four areas in our NICU [−1.06 dB (−1.52, −0.6)], with a trend towards reduction in a second area (−0.21 dB (−0.6, 0.18)). Unexpectedly, two other areas experienced a significant increase in noise (2.05 dB (1.18, 2.94); 0.85 dB (0.11, 1.59)).

Conclusions.—The baseline noise in the NICU consistently exceeds guidelines, but reductions in noise levels are achievable. Nonetheless, more work is needed to find the optimal NICU design and noise reduction strategy.

▶ I found this to be an interesting article describing an educational intervention aimed at noise reduction in the neonatal intensive care unit environment. The investigators validated something many have observed: people make noise. Although we certainly use numerous devices that contribute to the cacophony of the intensive care unit, including high-frequency devices; blaring alarms from ventilators, monitors, and infusion pumps; pagers and telephones (that we could put on vibrate but don't); and public address systems, the reality is that with proper intervention and behavior modification, we can make a significant contribution to noise reduction.

A little over 2 years ago, we moved into a new children's hospital with a single-room care model. I was immediately impressed by the reduction in ambient noise, despite using the same ventilators, monitors, pumps, and so on. The logical conclusion was the segregation of not only babies but of care providers and the compartmentalization of care. Time will tell if there is developmental value for this to the babies, but with a lot less neurosensory overload, I am not quite as fatigued when I leave in the evening.

The other adage this study supports is how hard it is to change human behavior.

S. M. Donn, MD

Breastfeeding Keratosis: This Frictional Keratosis of Newborns May Mimic Thrush

Kiat-Amnuay S, Bouquot J (Univ of Texas School of Dentistry at Houston)
Pediatrics 132:e775-e778, 2013

We report the first example, to our knowledge, of a frictional keratosis from exuberant sucking in a breastfeeding infant. A 2-month-old girl was referred for evaluation of a well-demarcated, nonsloughing white keratotic plaque of the lower lip mucosa, just inside the vermilion border. The plaque had a slightly irregular surface, had no surrounding erythema, and was the only such plaque in the mouth. It had been present for at least 3 weeks and had been unsuccessfully treated by her pediatrician via oral Mycostatin (nystatin). Her parents sought a second opinion when the infant was prescribed a full course of oral Diflucan (fluconazole). A cytopathology smear (Papanicolaou test) revealed abundant mature keratinocytes with no evidence of *Candida*. The mother admitted that the infant "worked hard" at sucking during breastfeeding and continued sucking long after feeding. The parents were unaware of any other habit or potential irritation of the lips. After 3 months of age the infant's sucking pattern became more "normal" and the keratosis disappeared; it did not recur during 3 years of follow-up. We propose the term "breastfeeding keratosis" for this entity (Fig 1).

▶ The authors state "we report the first example, to our knowledge, of the frictional keratosis from exuberant sucking in a breastfeeding infant." They

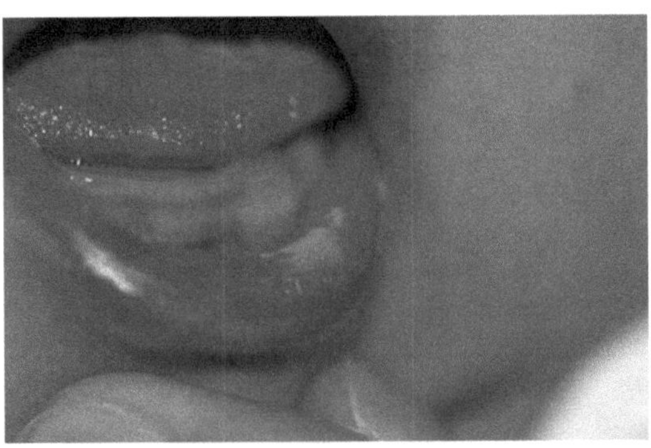

FIGURE 1.—White, moderately well demarcated keratotic plaque of the lower left lip mucosa had a roughened surface and could not be scraped off. (Reprinted from Kiat-Amnuay S, Bouquot J. Breastfeeding keratosis: this frictional keratosis of newborns may mimic thrush. *Pediatrics*. 2013;132:e775-e778, Copyright 2013, with permission from the American Academy of Pediatrics.)

report on a 2-month-old girl who was referred for evaluation of the white keratotic plaque of the lower lip mucosa just inside the vermillion border. The patient had been unsuccessfully treated with oral Mycostatin and also had a course of oral Diflucan, to no avail (Fig 1).

I have seen plaques similar to this on numerous occasions in neonates and have been asked by residents and trainees what they signify. If it could not be removed with gauze or a tongue depressor, the diagnosis often made was a "sucking callus." Thus, this did not appear to be such an unusual case; however, these discrete plaques on the lip at the vermillion border in a vigorously breastfeeding baby are likely to represent something other than oral candidiasis. In this case, cytopathology was done and was positive for clusters of keratinocytes but no mycotic structures.

An eLetter in *Pediatrics* published September 19, 2013, by James W. Antoon and Wallace D. Brown raises the question that the "frictional keratosis" described in this case report actually represents what in the past has been called a *sucking callus*.

Nevertheless, it is important for the clinician to recognize that a plaque on the lip of the vermillion border in a vigorously sucking breastfed baby may not represent a fungal lesion (thrush), and simple diagnostic procedures such as removal with a gauze swab and simple observation may be adequate treatment without exposure to drugs.

J. Neu, MD

Prediction of Neonatal Outcomes in Extremely Preterm Neonates

Ge WJ, on behalf of the Canadian Neonatal Network (Mount Sinai Hosp, Toronto, Ontario, Canada)

Pediatrics 132:e876-e885, 2013

Objective.—To develop and validate a statistical prediction model spanning the severity range of neonatal outcomes in infants born at ≤30 weeks' gestation.

Methods.—A national cohort of infants, born at 23 to 30 weeks' gestation and admitted to level III NICUs in Canada in 2010-2011, was identified from the Canadian Neonatal Network database. A multinomial logistic regression model was developed to predict survival without morbidities, mild morbidities, severe morbidities, or mortality, using maternal, obstetric, and infant characteristics available within the first day of NICU admission. Discrimination and calibration were assessed using a concordance *C*-statistic and the C_g goodness of-fit test, respectively. Internal validation was performed using a bootstrap approach.

Results.—Of 6106 eligible infants, 2280 (37%) survived without morbidities, 1964 (32%) and 1251 (21%) survived with mild and severe morbidities, respectively, and 611 (10%) died. Predictors in the model were gestational age, small (<10th percentile) for gestational age, gender, Score for Neonatal Acute Physiology version II > 20, outborn status, use of antenatal corticosteroids, and receipt of surfactant and mechanical ventilation on the first day of admission. High model discrimination was confirmed by internal bootstrap validation (bias-corrected C-statistic = 0.899, 95% confidence interval = 0.894–0.903). Predicted probabilities were consistent with the observed outcomes (C_g *P* value = .96).

Conclusions.—Neonatal outcomes ranging from mortality to survival without morbidity in extremely preterm infants can be predicted on their first day in the NICU by using a multinomial model with good discrimination and calibration. The prediction model requires additional external validation (Fig, Table 5).

▶ This report from the Canadian Neonatal Network represents another advance in pursuit of the Holy Grail of predicting outcomes for preterm infants born before 30 weeks of gestational age. This work is important in at least 3 respects. First, it provides an update on outcomes for the least mature babies in our units, based on samples collected in 2010 and 2011. Although overall outcomes have not changed dramatically, correlates and predictors of outcomes from this sample are more likely to be generalizable to current practice than those derived from data collected a decade or more earlier (1998–2003 for the National Institute of Child Health and Human Development Neonatal Research Network Outcomes Calculator, for example[1]). Second, the raw data provide a stark reminder that outcomes for the least mature babies are still far from acceptable, as fewer than 20% of babies born before 27 weeks of gestation survive without morbidity and fewer than 25% of those born before 25 weeks survive without severe morbidity (Fig). As has been the case with prior reports, these observations may be skewed by a self-fulfilling expectation of poor outcomes, leading to nonintervention or other care limitations, but these results should give pause

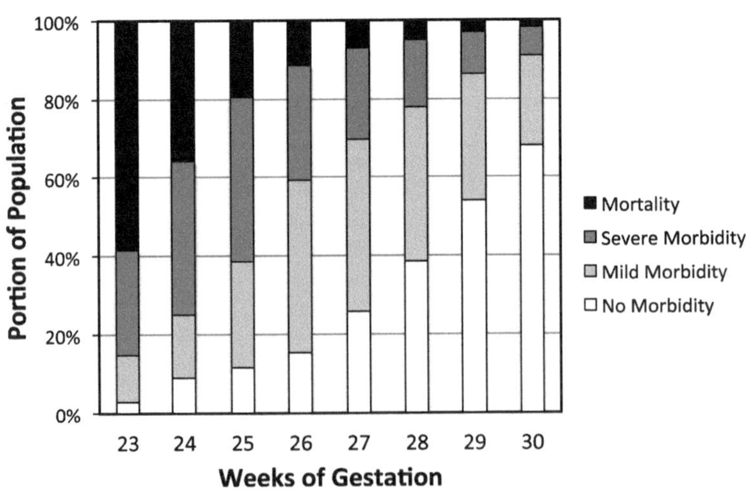

FIGURE.—Observed outcomes for 6106 infants born at 23-30 weeks gestation in the Canadian Neonatal Network in 2010-2011. (Data obtained from Table 2 of Ge WJ, Mirea L, Yang J, et al. Prediction of neonatal outcomes in extremely preterm neonates. *Pediatrics*. 2013;132:e876-e885, Copyright 2013, by the American Academy of Pediatrics.)

TABLE 5.—Change in the Predicted Probability of Each Outcome Level Corresponding to Changes From Baseline for Each Factor Included in the Multivariable Prediction Model Developed Using 6106 Infants Born at ≤30 Weeks' Gestation

Factor	No Morbidity	Mild Morbidity	Severe Morbidity	Mortality	Updated C-Statistic
Baseline infant[a] probability	.76	.20	.04	.004	.75
GA (wk)					.881
23–24	−.58	.11	.31	.16	
25	−.56	.21	.28	.07	
26	−.50	.32	.14	.03	
27	−.36	.25	.10	.02	
28	−.25	.18	.06	.01	
29	−.11	.09	.02	.003	
SGA	−.15	.08	.05	.01	.884
Male	−.01	.01	.003	.002	.885
SNAPII >20	−.11	.04	.05	.02	.896
Outborn	.02	−.02	.01	.001	.897
No antenatal corticosteroids	−.04	.01	.02	.01	.899
Surfactant on day 1	−.04	.02	.02	.001	.901
IPPV or HFV on day 1	−.08	.06	.02	.002	.902

[a]Baseline infant: Female, born 30 at wk GA, SNAPII ≤20, not SGA, inborn, mother received antenatal corticosteroids, infant did not received surfactant or IPPV/HFV on day 1 after admission to NICU. Predicted probabilities for any infant can be computed by starting with the baseline probability and adding or subtracting the values corresponding to the presence of each factor listed in the table.

to providers and be available to inform parents as they make choices about care for their babies in these situations. Third, these authors provide a novel model for prediction across the full range of categorical outcomes (Table 5). Not surprisingly, gestational age provides a very large proportion of the predictive power of the model, but consideration of other factors permits substantial refinement of outcome estimates. Using this model, the probability of each outcome is calculated simply by adding up the coefficients associated with each risk predictor, as listed in the Table 5. Thus, an appropriate-for-age male infant born at 24 weeks estimated gestational age at an outside hospital without antenatal steroids, who received surfactant, remains on intermittent positive pressure ventilation, and has a Score for Neonatal Acute Physiology (SNAPII) of 10 would have a mortality risk of 0.18 (=0.004 + 0.16 + 0.002 + 0.001 + 0.01 + 0.001 + 0.002) and a probability of survival without morbidity of 0.03 (=0.76 − 0.58 − 0.01 + 0.02 − 0.04 − 0.04 − 0.08); probabilities of survival with moderate or severe morbidity are similarly calculated. The components of this model (including the elements of SNAPII) should be readily available in electronic medical records so it is easily adaptable to automatic calculation. Provision of probabilities across the full range of potential outcomes, rather than a single estimate of the probability of one extreme (death or survival without morbidity), should better inform parents and care providers about the prospects for an individual baby. This new model should supplant older tools in counseling parents in these often difficult conversations.

W. E. Benitz, MD

Reference

1. Tyson JE, Parikh NA, Langer J, Green C, Higgins RD. Intensive care for extreme prematurity—moving beyond gestational age. *N Engl J Med.* 2008;358: 1672-1681.

Utility of delayed surgical repair of neonatal brachial plexus palsy

Ali ZS, Bakar D, Li YR, et al (Univ of Pennsylvania, Philadelphia)
J Neursurg Pediatr 13:462-470, 2014

Object.—Neonatal brachial plexus palsy (NBPP) represents a significant health problem with potentially devastating consequences. The most common form of NBPP involves the upper trunk roots. Currently, primary surgical repair is performed if clinical improvement is lacking. There has been increasing interest in "early" surgical repair of NBPPs, occurring within 3-6 months of life. However, early treatment recommendations ignore spontaneous recovery in cases of Erb's palsy. This study was undertaken to evaluate the optimal timing of surgical repair in this group with respect to quality of life.

Methods.—The authors formulated a decision analytical model to compare 4 treatment strategies (no repair or repair at 3, 6, or 12 months of life) for infants with persistent NBPPs. The model derives data from a critical review of published studies and projects health-related quality of life and quality-adjusted life years over a lifetime.

Results.—When evaluating the quality of life of infants with NBPP, improved outcomes are seen with delayed surgical repair at 12 months, compared with no repair or repair at early and intermediate time points, at 3 and 6 months, respectively. ANOVA showed that the differences among the 4 groups are highly significant ($F = 8369$; $p < 0.0001$). Pairwise post hoc comparisons revealed that there are highly significant differences between each pair of strategies ($p < 0.0001$). Meta-regression showed no evidence of improved outcomes with more recent treatment dates, compared with older ones, for either nonsurgical or for surgical treatment ($p = 0.767$ and $p = 0.865$, respectively).

Conclusions.—These data support a delayed approach of primary surgical reconstruction to optimize quality of life. Early surgery for NBPPs may be an overly aggressive strategy for infants who would otherwise demonstrate spontaneous recovery of function by 12 months. A randomized, controlled trial would be necessary to fully elucidate the natural history of NBPP and determine the optimal time point for surgical intervention.

▶ Neonatal brachial plexus palsy (NBPP) has an incidence ranging between 0.5 to 2.6 per 1000 livebirths in the United States. Erb's palsy, affecting C5 and C6, is the most common form of NBPP. Erb's palsy clinically results in loss of function of the supraspinatus, infraspinatus, deltoid, biceps brachii, brachialis, coracobrachialis, and supinator muscles, resulting in loss of shoulder abduction, external rotation, elbow flexion, and forearm supination with the arm in the "waiters tip" position.

The severity of the injury range includes neurapraxic injury, seen in two-thirds of the cases and characterized by spontaneous resolution, usually within 3 months. The other end of the spectrum is a complete avulsion injury, which has no potential for spontaneous recovery. The debate resolves around the optimal time to intervene surgically when there is no spontaneous recovery, and there is neither a consensus nor a series of randomized trials to provide guidance.

Aly et al have shed some light on the topic by scouring the literature and developing "a decision analytical model that allows one to draw conclusions based on the available evidence with a focus on quality of life (QOL) as a surrogate for functional outcome. Our comparative-effectiveness study suggests that when evaluating the QOL of infants with Erb's and extended Erb's palsy, improved outcomes are seen when surgical repair is delayed until 12 months of age, compared with early and intermediate time points, at 3 and 6 months, respectively (see Table 5 in the original article). These results are contrary to the deeply held notion that good outcomes are only associated with early repair."

I especially appreciated one of their subsequent comments: "While our study provides a decision framework for the clinician to consider the treatment option that would yield the best QOL, it should not substitute for the individualized clinical decision making required to manage these patients effectively. This may, in fact, require a 'decision analysis' at each follow-up time point when a change in clinical status occurs."

This study has several limitations and makes many assumptions, yet it reflects much thoughtful analysis of an extensive literature and an attempt to simplify a complex problem.

Chang et al[1] also reviewed the topic. Of 2836 articles initially identified, 307 were included in the analysis, with 198 articles (9646 patients) reporting results after surgical treatment, 70 articles (4434 patients) reporting results after medical treatment, and 39 articles (4247 patients) reporting results after combined surgical and medical treatment. There were many inconsistencies in the published reports including equivalence in usage of classification, diagnostic, and physical assessment tools as well as functional outcome measures. The authors thus concluded:

"In this review, the authors demonstrate disparities in the use of Neonatal Brachial Plexus Palsy (NBPP) evaluation instruments in the current literature. Additionally, valid and reliable evaluation instruments specifically for the NBPP population are significantly lacking, manifesting in difficulties with evaluating the overall impact and effectiveness of clinical treatments in a consistent and comparative manner, extending across the various subspecialties that are involved in the treatment of patients with NBPP." They plea for better reporting of the use of the affected arm in activities of daily living with attention to the psychosocial impact of the disablement.

A. A. Fanaroff, MD, FRCPE

Reference

1. Chang KW, Justice D, Chung KC, Yanng LJ. A systematic review of evaluation methods for neonatal brachial plexus palsy. *J Neurosurg Pediatr.* 2013;12: 395-405.

A comparison of the infant car seat challenge and the polysomnogram at the time of hospital discharge

Schutzman DL, Salvador A, Janeczko M, et al (Albert Einstein Med Ctr, Philadelphia, PA)

Arch Dis Child Fetal Neonatal Ed 98:F411-F415, 2013

Objective.—The American Academy of Pediatrics recommends all infants born at <37 weeks gestation spend a period of observation in a car seat prior to hospital discharge to assess for apnoea, bradycardia or oxygen desaturation. The most recent Cochrane review suggested further studies to determine if the infant car seat challenge (ICSC) accurately predicts the risk of clinically adverse events. We reviewed our experience with the ICSC and the polysomnogram (PSG) to determine if the ICSC accurately predicts the risk of adverse events when compared with the PSG.

Study Design.—Retrospective chart review of all infants in our institution who had an ICSC and a PSG between January 2005 and December 2008.

Result.—785 infants had ICSCs. In addition, 313 infants (56.6%) had an abnormal PSG, even though the vast majority, 158 (88.3%), passed their ICSC. There were no significant differences in gestational age at birth, birth weight, chronological age at study or postmenstrual age at study between infants who either passed or failed the ICSC with those who passed or failed the PSG. The sensitivity of the ICSC was 0.11 and specificity was 0.96. The positive predictive value of the ICSC was 0.77 and the negative predictive value was 0.45.

Conclusions.—The ICSC has a low negative predictive value (0.45) when compared with the PSG as a reference standard for identifying adverse cardiorespiratory events. Although less time consuming and cumbersome than extended polysomnography, the ICSC is not a reliable substitute.

▶ The American Academy of Pediatrics (AAP) recommends that all infants born at less than 37 weeks' gestation have a period of observation in a car safety seat to monitor for apnea, bradycardia, or oxygen desaturation before discharge to home.[1] A minimum duration of the test should be 90 to 120 minutes or the duration of travel to home, whichever is longer. In most hospital facilities, an infant car seat challenge (ICSC) is performed shortly before hospital discharge. In this retrospective chart review, the authors compared the results of ICSC to that of polysomnogram (PSG) done within 24 hours of ICSC.

Per hospital protocol all infants less than 35 weeks' gestation had a 12- to 24-hour PSG performed within 48 hours of hospital discharge and ICSC of 60 minutes' duration within 24 hours of hospital discharge. Criteria for failing the ICSC included apnea greater than 20 seconds, bradycardia less that 80 beats per minute, or oxygen saturation to less that 85%. Criteria for failing the PSG were the same as those for the ICSC with the addition of esophageal pH <4 for more than 4% of the study. Approximately 55% of the infants who passed the ICSC failed the PSG. Because the period of monitoring with PSG was 12 to 24 times as long as the ICSC, this outcome is not surprising. Based on these data, the authors suggest that the length of time for ICSC testing should be significantly increased beyond the recommended 90 to 120 minutes. This recommendation is unwarranted, because the study infants only underwent a 60-minute ICSC, a duration much shorter than that recommended by AAP. Despite this, the study does call into question the purpose of ICSC. As noted in a recent Cochrane review, there are no data from randomized controlled trials that indicate whether ICSC, as recommended, accurately predicts the risk of clinically significant adverse events in preterm infants.[2]

L. A. Papile, MD

References

1. Bull MJ, Engle WA, Committee on Injury, Violence, and Poison Prevention and Committee on Fetus and Newborn. Safe transportation of preterm and low birth weight infants at hospital discharge. *Pediatrics*. 2009;123:1424-1429.
2. Pilley E, McGuire W. Pre 'car seat challenge' for preventing morbidity and mortality in preterm infants. *Cochrane Database Syst Rev*. 2006;(1):CD005386.

Increased Enamel Hypoplasia and Very Low Birthweight Infants

Nelson S, Albert JM, Geng C, et al (Case Western Reserve Univ, Cleveland, OH; et al)
J Dent Res 92:788-794, 2013

Birth cohort studies of developmental defects of enamel (DDE) and early childhood caries (ECC) in very low birthweight (VLBW) and normal birthweight (NBW) infants are rare. In this birth cohort of 234 VLBW and 234 NBW infants, we report the incidence of ECC and DDE at 8 and 18-20 mos of corrected age. Infant medical and maternal socio-demographic data were abstracted from medical records at birth. Dental assessments for ECC and DDE (enamel hypoplasia, demarcated and diffuse opacities) were completed at 8 and 18-20 mos. The incidence of hypoplasia was significantly higher in VLBW compared with NBW infants (8 mos, 19% *vs.* 2%; 18 mos, 31% *vs.* 8%). The incidence of ECC (International Caries Detection and Assessment System: ICDAS ≥ 2) was 1.4% (8 mos) and 12% (18-20 mos) and was similar between the VLBW and NBW groups. At both ages, using a beta-binomial regression model to control for potential confounders (maternal and infant characteristics), we found increased risk for enamel hypoplasia among the VLBW infants compared with the NBW infants. African Americans had a lower risk for enamel hypoplasia at 18-20 mos. The VLBW infants should be monitored for ECC due to the presence of enamel hypoplasia.

▶ I dare say most clinicians are not aware that preterm birth can lead to defects in tooth enamel and a subsequent increased susceptibility for early childhood caries. Apparently the pediatric dental community is aware of this, given that the first published report was in 1984 and there have been numerous publications since then. This observational study differs from previous ones in that it takes into account numerous potentially confounding maternal, infant, and socioeconomic factors. The only significant factor for enamel hypoplasia was very low birth weight with an adjusted relative risk of 4.77 (95% confidence interval 2.82–9.95). The authors postulate that the enamel hypoplasia is the result of altered calcium homeostasis from systemic causes during the pre- and postnatal period, and/or through local causes because of endotracheal intubation and mechanical ventilation during the postnatal period. The very low birth weight cohort had, on average, fewer erupted teeth at the 18-month visit, which may explain why they were not at greater risk for early childhood cavities despite the greater prevalence of enamel hypoplasia. The association of dental hypoplasia and early childhood cavities will be reexamined at 36 months of age when entire primary dentition is present.

L. A. Papile, MD

Compliance with the Baby-Friendly Hospital Initiative and impact on breastfeeding rates

Hawkins SS, Stern AD, Baum CF, et al (Boston College, Chestnut Hill, MA; Harvard Kennedy School of Government, Cambridge, MA; et al)
Arch Dis Child Fetal Neonatal Ed 99:F138-F143, 2014

Objectives.—To examine compliance with the Baby-Friendly Hospital Initiative (BFHI) as well as evaluate the BFHI and its components on breastfeeding initiation and duration overall and according to maternal education level.

Design.—Quasi-experimental study using data from the Pregnancy Risk Assessment Monitoring System (PRAMS) from 2004 to 2008.

Setting.—Birth facilities in Maine.

Participants.—915 mothers who gave birth in four hospitals that were BFHI-accredited or became accredited and 1099 mothers from six matched non-BFHI facilities. Mothers reported on seven (of 10) BFHI practices (breastfeeding practice score 0–7) and receipt of a gift pack with formula (yes/no).

Main Outcome Measures.—Self-report of breastfeeding initiation, any breast feeding for ≥4 weeks, exclusive breast feeding for ≥4 weeks.

Results.—34.6% of mothers from BFHI-accredited facilities reported experiencing all seven BFHI breastfeeding practices, while 28.4% reported being given a gift pack with formula. Among mothers with lower education, the BFHI increased breastfeeding initiation by 8.6 percentage points (adjusted coefficient, 0.086 [95% CI, 0.01 to 0.16]) and, independently, each additional breastfeeding practice was associated with an average increase in breastfeeding initiation of 16.2 percentage points (adjusted coefficient, 0.162 [95% CI, 0.15 to 0.18]). Among all mothers and mothers with higher education, there was no effect of the BFHI on breastfeeding rates.

Conclusions.—Compliance with BFHI practices among BFHI-accredited facilities is not optimal and needs to be monitored, as greater compliance may have an even larger impact on breastfeeding rates and potentially reduce socio-economic disparities in breast feeding.

▶ The World Health Organization and UNICEF established the Baby-Friendly Hospital Initiative (BFHI) in 1991 to emphasize the importance of promoting and supporting breastfeeding.[1] In the United States, this initiative has led to the formal designation of birthing facilities as Baby-Friendly. The fee schedule for becoming a Baby-Friendly designated facility in 2014–2015 ranges from $9000 for a free-standing birth center to $11 700 for a hospital.[2] Additional costs include the 20 hours of BFHI training that must be completed by staff who care for mothers and their babies.

In this study, data related to 7 of the 10 BFHI breastfeeding practices were abstracted from the Maine Pregnancy Risk Assessment Monitoring System questionnaires sent to women 2 to 6 months after delivery. Adherence to BFHI breastfeeding practices was essentially the same in BFHI-designated and nondesignated hospitals, the largest difference being that BFHI-designated hospitals did not give gift packs with formula to mothers. More than 50% of the women in the study experienced 6 or 7 of the 7 breastfeeding practices consistent with BFHI, regardless of the birth facility's BFHI status. In addition, there was no difference in the overall rate of breastfeeding initiation or duration between designated and nondesignated hospitals. The results of this study call into question the need for Baby-Friendly designation in the United States. It seems that the culture of supporting breastfeeding is already prevalent in hospitals that have maternity services.

L. A. Papile, MD

References

1. World Health Organization, United Nations Children's Fund. *Promoting and Supporting Breastfeeding: the Special Role of Maternity Services.* Geneva, Switzerland: World Health Organization; 1989.
2. Baby-Friendly USA. http://www.babyfriendlyusa.org. Accessed May 20, 2014.

Deaths and near deaths of healthy newborn infants while bed sharing on maternity wards

Thach BT (Washington Univ School of Medicine, Kirkwood, MO)
J Perinatol 34:275-279, 2014

Objective.—Our aim was to evaluate programs promoting bed sharing on maternity wards and determining ways to reduce these risks.

Study Design.—Members of the National Association of Medical Examiners were contacted requesting information on deaths of healthy infants while bed sharing on maternity wards.

Result.—Fifteen deaths and three near deaths are reported. One or more factors that increase the risk of bed sharing were present in all cases. Accidental suffocation was deemed the most likely cause of these incidents.

Conclusion.—Cases of infant deaths and near deaths while bed sharing on maternity wards are under reported. The 'Baby Friendly' (BF) initiative in maternity hospitals to promote breastfeeding is endorsed by the American Academy of Pediatrics and the US Center for Disease Control and Prevention. The BF initiative encourages prolonged skin-to-skin contact and bed sharing. Education of mothers and more efficient monitoring should significantly reduce the risk of maternity ward bed sharing.

▶ To promote breastfeeding, direct skin-to-skin contact of newborn infants with their mother immediately after delivery and as much as possible throughout the postpartum period is recommended.[1] This report is a reminder that applying this practice indiscriminately can result in unintended consequences. The reported incidents occurred between 1999 and 2013. In 12 of the 18 cases illustrated, the mother fell asleep either while breastfeeding or shortly thereafter, and in 5 cases another family member was present in the room when the event occurred. Only 6 of the 12 deaths occurred during the first 24 hours after birth, and 2 occurred at 3 days of age. Risk factors included maternal sedating drugs, excessive maternal fatigue, pillows and/or soft bedding present, infant swaddling, and maternal obesity.

The information presented indicates that suffocation resulting from airway occlusion when the infant's face is in contact with the mother's breast or body as the most likely cause of death. Hopefully the report will heighten awareness among maternity hospital personnel of the risk of suffocation during close maternal contact in the postpartum period. Given the manner in which the information was obtained, the incidents reported are probably a substantial underestimation of the true number of events in the United States. The author suggests that these episodes be included in the mandatory reporting of adverse in-hospital events to public health agencies to ascertain the extent of the problem.

L. A. Papile, MD

Reference

1. Section on Breastfeeding. Breastfeeding and the use of human milk. *Pediatrics.* 2012;129:e827-e841.

13 Pharmacology

Effect of Fluconazole Prophylaxis on Candidiasis and Mortality in Premature Infants: A Randomized Clinical Trial

Benjamin DK Jr, for the Fluconazole Prophylaxis Study Team (Duke Clinical Res Inst, Durham, NC; et al)

JAMA 311:1742-1749, 2014

Importance.—Invasive candidiasis in premature infants causes death and neurodevelopmental impairment. Fluconazole prophylaxis reduces candidiasis, but its effect on mortality and the safety of fluconazole are unknown.

Objective.—To evaluate the efficacy and safety of fluconazole in preventing death or invasive candidiasis in extremely low-birth-weight infants.

Design, Setting, and Patients.—This study was a randomized, blinded, placebo-controlled trial of fluconazole in premature infants. Infants weighing less than 750 g at birth (N = 361) from 32 neonatal intensive care units (NICUs) in the United States were randomly assigned to receive either fluconazole or placebo twice weekly for 42 days. Surviving infants were evaluated at 18 to 22 months corrected age for neurodevelopmental outcomes. The study was conducted between November 2008 and February 2013.

Interventions.—Fluconazole (6 mg/kg of body weight) or placebo.

Main Outcomes and Measures.—The primary end pointwas a composite of death or definite or probable invasive candidiasis prior to study day 49 (1 week after completion of study drug). Secondary and safety outcomes included invasive candidiasis, liver function, bacterial infection, length of stay, intracranial hemorrhage, periventricular leukomalacia, chronic lung disease, patent ductus arteriosus requiring surgery, retinopathy of prematurity requiring surgery, necrotizing enterocolitis, spontaneous intestinal perforation, and neurodevelopmental outcomes - defined as a Bayley-III cognition composite score of less than 70, blindness, deafness, or cerebral palsy at 18 to 22 months corrected age.

Results.—Among infants receiving fluconazole, the composite primary end point of death or invasive candidiasis was 16% (95% CI, 11%-22%) vs 21% in the placebo group (95% CI, 15%-28%; odds ratio, 0.73 [95% CI, 0.43-1.23]; $P = .24$; treatment difference, −5% [95% CI, −13% to 3%]). Invasive candidiasis occurred less frequently in the fluconazole group (3% [95% CI, 1%-6%]) vs the placebo group (9% [95% CI, 5%-14%]; $P = .02$; treatment difference, −6% [95% CI, −11% to −1%]). The cumulative incidences of other secondary outcomes were not statistically different between groups. Neurodevelopmental impairment did not differ between the groups (fluconazole, 31% [95% CI, 21%-41%] vs placebo, 27% [95% CI, 18%-37%]; $P = .60$; treatment difference, 4% [95% CI, −10% to 17%]).

Conclusions and Relevance.—Among infants with a birth weight of less than 750 g, 42 days of fluconazole prophylaxis compared with placebo did not result in a lower incidence of the composite of death or invasive candidiasis. These findings do not support the universal use of prophylactic fluconazole in extremely low-birth-weight infants.

Trial Registration.—clinicaltrials.gov Identifier: NCT00734539.

▶ The history of neonatology prominently features disastrous consequences of prophylactic antibiotic therapy, notably, kernicterus and death with the use of prophylactic sulfonamides, and gray baby syndrome and death with the use of chloramphenicol. Such is not the case with prophylactic fluconazole, for which despite no harm, and reducing the rates of invasive *Candida* infection, it did not reduce the composite of death or invasive candidiasis, hence the conclusion that the findings do not support the universal use of prophylactic fluconazole in extremely low birth weight infants. This was a well-designed study with some unanticipated differences between the treatment and control group. More babies in the control group were the beneficiaries of antenatal corticosteroids and were delivered by caesarean delivery. Both these events would increase survival and would influence one of the primary outcome variables. Indeed, mortality overall was lower than anticipated—a good outcome. Also infection rates were lower, a reflection of increased attention to hand hygiene and improved efforts to prevent central-line blood-stream infections.

Of interest is the report from Aliaga et al,[1] who examined data from 709 325 infants at 322 neonatal intensive care units managed by the Pediatrix Medical Group from 1997 to 2010. Over the study period, the annual incidence of invasive candidiasis decreased from 3.6 episodes per 1000 patients to 1.4 episodes per 1000 patients among all infants, from 24.2 to 11.6 episodes per 1000 patients among infants with a birth weight of 750 to 999 g, and from 82.7 to 23.8 episodes per 1000 patients among infants with a birth weight < 750 g. Fluconazole prophylaxis use increased and the use of broad-spectrum antibacterial antibiotics decreased among all infants during this time period, which may have contributed to these findings.

A report from Adams-Chapman[2] on the follow-up of the National Institute of Child Health and Human Development Neonatal Network *Candida* study confirmed that invasive *Candida* infection and/or meningitis were associated with more significant rates of neurodevelopmental impairment than non-*Candida* sepsis and much higher rates than noninfected babies.

Candida remains a significant contributor to mortality and morbidity in extremely low birth weight infants. Unfortunately, despite some early promise, fluconazole prophylaxis is not the answer to preventing these outcomes.

A. A. Fanaroff, MD, FRCPE

References

1. Aliaga S, Clark RH, Laughon M, et al. Changes in the incidence of candidiasis in neonatal intensive care units. *Pediatrics.* 2014;133:236-242.
2. Adams-Chapman I, Bann CM, Das A, et al. Neurodevelopmental outcome of extremely low birth weight infants with *Candida* infection. *J Pediatr.* 2013;163: 961-967.e3.

Prophylactic Indomethacin Worsens Short-Term Respiratory Outcomes in Extremely Low-Birth-Weight Infants

Mondal T, Chaudhuri D, Li B, et al (McMaster Univ and Hamilton Health Sciences, Ontario, Canada)

Am J Perinatol 31:61-68, 2014

Objective.—To compare the effects of prophylactic indomethacin versus expectant management on short-term respiratory outcomes in extremely low-birth-weight (ELBW) infants.

Methods.—This was a retrospective cohort study of ELBW infants with gestational age less than 28 weeks, born at a level III neonatal intensive care unit from 2004 to 2009. Patients were grouped based on whether they received prophylactic indomethacin or expectant treatment. The key outcome was the cumulative number of days of mechanical ventilation. Other outcomes were cumulative number of days supplemental oxygen and continuous positive airway pressure (CPAP) were required; duration of hospital stay; mortality; and other morbidities such as necrotizing enterocolitis and intraventricular hemorrhage. Multivariable linear regression was performed with treatment group and seven covariates, defined a priori, as predictor variables and cumulative number of days of mechanical ventilation as the outcome.

Results.—There were 144 infants in the prophylaxis group and 221 infants in the expectant treatment group. At baseline, the Score for Neonatal Acute Physiology-Perinatal Extension, incidence of respiratory distress syndrome, and usage of antenatal corticosteroids were significantly higher in the prophylaxis group. The cumulative number of days of mechanical ventilation, supplemental oxygen, and CPAP were significantly higher in the prophylaxis group. On multivariable linear regression, after adjusting for confounders, use of prophylactic indomethacin (unstandardized β coefficient = 12.4; 95% confidence interval [CI]: 6.6, 18.1; $p < 0.001$), birth weight ($\beta = -0.025$; 95% CI: −0.05, −0.001; $p = 0.043$), and gestation ($\beta = -4.5$; 95% CI: −7.24, −1.8; $p = 0.001$) were the independent predictors of cumulative number of days of mechanical ventilation.

Conclusion.—ELBW infants who received prophylactic indomethacin had significantly longer cumulative number of days of mechanical ventilation, supplemental oxygen, and CPAP. Prophylactic indomethacin is an independent predictor of cumulative number of days of mechanical ventilation.

▶ The observation that pretreatment with indomethacin reduced the risk of intraventricular hemorrhage in beagle puppies subjected to hemorrhagic shock led to the proposal that initiation of indomethacin shortly after birth might similarly prevent intraventricular hemorrhage (IVH) in very low-birth-weight infants. Two large randomized, controlled trials confirmed that this prophylactic use of indomethacin does reduce the rate of grade III–IV IVH and, incidentally, the rate of persistent patency of the ductus arteriosus. Follow-up studies of the subjects enrolled in those trials found no improvement in long-term neurodevelopment outcomes, however. Nonetheless, many practitioners have continued to use indomethacin prophylaxis for extremely low birth weight infants, on the assumption that the collateral effect of earlier ductal closure might ameliorate severity of respiratory distress syndrome and reduce subsequent development of chronic lung disease. These benefits have not been borne out by controlled trials, however, and some evidence indicates that early use of indomethacin may actually be associated with more severe lung disease. This retrospective analysis of the experience at a single center between 2004 and 2009 adds to the body of available data related to this question. Despite a substantially lower rate of persistent ductal patency (35% after prophylaxis vs 68% with expectant management; $P < .001$), there were no differences in rates of ductal ligation (18% vs 15%; $P = .52$) or mortality (17% vs 24%, $P = .20$). Contrary to expectation, infants who received prophylaxis required more days of assisted ventilation (median, 37.2 vs 24.3; $P < .001$), more days on continuous positive airway pressure (median, 20.3 vs 16.7; $P = .025$), more days on supplemental oxygen (median, 10.5 vs 7.8; $P = .038$), and longer hospital stays (median, 77.7 vs 58.0 days; $P < .001$). These differences may have resulted from differences in baseline characteristics between groups, but the difference in duration of ventilation persisted even after adjustment for birth weight, gestational age, SNAPPE II score, 10-minute Apgar score, antenatal steroid exposure, respiratory distress syndrome, and chorioamnionitis. (Regression analyses for other outcomes were not reported.) Even more surprisingly, these authors found that indomethacin prophylaxis was associated with an increased, rather than decreased, rate of grade III or IV IVH (42% vs 31%; $P = .033$), drawing attention to previous reports that suggest that IVH reduction with indomethacin prophylaxis may be limited to infants with birth weights greater than 1000 g. The authors conclude that "this study disputes a commonly held perception on the effects of prophylactic indomethacin on PDA and short-term respiratory outcomes ... [providing] yet another reason why health care providers should consider not using prophylactic indomethacin in ELBW infants." These sobering data certainly prove food for thought on this matter.

W. E. Benitz, MD

Characterization of the Population Pharmacokinetics of Ampicillin in Neonates Using an Opportunistic Study Design

Tremoulet A, on behalf of the Administrative Core Committee of the Best Pharmaceuticals for Children Act-Pediatric Trials Network (Univ of California, San Diego; et al)

Antimicrob Agents Chemother 58:3013-3020, 2014

Although ampicillin is the most commonly used drug in neonates, developmental pharmacokinetic (PK) data to guide dosing are lacking. Ampicillin is primarily renally eliminated, and developmental changes are expected to influence PK. We conducted an open-label, multicenter, opportunistic, prospective PK study of ampicillin in neonates stratified by gestational age (GA) (≤34 or >34 weeks) and postnatal age (PNA) (≤7 or >7 days). Drug concentrations were measured by tandem mass spectrometry. PK data were analyzed using population nonlinear mixed-effects modeling in NONMEM 7.2. Monte Carlo simulations were conducted to determine the probability of target attainment for the time in which the total steady-state ampicillin concentrations remained above the MIC (T>MIC) for 50%, 75%, and 100% of the dosing interval. A total of 142 PK samples from 73 neonates were analyzed (median [range] GA, 36 [24 to 41] weeks; PNA, 5 [0 to 25] days). The median ampicillin dose was 200 (100 to 350) mg/kg/day. Postmenstrual age and serum creatinine were covariates for ampicillin clearance (CL). A simplified dosing regimen of 50 mg/kg every 12 h for GA of ≤34 weeks and PNA of ≤7 days, 75 mg/kg every 12 h for GA of ≤34 weeks and PNA of >8 and ≤28 days, and 50 mg/kg every 8 h for GA of >34 weeks and PNA of ≤28 days achieved the prespecified surrogate efficacy target in 90% of simulated subjects. Ampicillin CL was associated with neonatal development. A simplified dosing regimen stratified by GA and PNA achieves the desired surrogate therapeutic target in the vast majority of neonates.

▶ Ampicillin is the most commonly used drug in neonates. However, insufficient developmental pharmacokinetic data contributes to confusion regarding appropriate standard dosing in both preterm and term neonates. This trial was an open-label, prospective pharmacokinetic study collecting opportunistic drug concentrations evaluated by tandem mass spectrometry. A total of 142 samples from 73 neonates were analyzed using population nonlinear mixed-effect modeling, and Monte Carlo simulations were conducted to determine the probability of pharmacodynamic target attainment. Inclusion of neonates across a broad age spectrum enabled construction of a robust population pharmacokinetic model considering developmental changes that affect drug distribution and elimination in the first month of life. To achieve 90% target attainment in simulated subjects, the authors propose a simplified dosing regimen of 50 mg/kg every 12 hours for gestational age ≤34 weeks and postnatal age ≤7 days, 75 mg/kg every 12 hours for gestational age ≤34 weeks and postnatal age 8 to 28 days, and 50 mg/kg every 8 hours for gestational age ≥34 weeks and postnatal age ≤28 days. Notably, this recommendation did not account for ampicillin penetration into the cerebrospinal fluid, and further studies are necessary to define optimal regimens for the treatment of meningitis. This trial is the most recent example of outstanding work by experts in infectious diseases and developmental pharmacokinetics capitalizing on the potential of opportunistic sampling. This sampling method allows determination of serum drug concentrations without increasing invasive sampling in this vulnerable population. Advanced pharmacokinetic modeling allows interpretation of this data and simulation of a diverse neonatal population. Further research using opportunistic sample collection and advanced pharmacokinetic modeling will provide invaluable data necessary to optimize dosing of common and novel therapies in neonates.

C. C. McPherson, PharmD

Accuracy of the concentration of morphine infusions prepared for patients in a neonatal intensive care unit

Aguado-Lorenzo V, Weeks K, Tunstell P, et al (Guy's and St. Thomas' NHS Foundation Trust, London, UK; et al)
Arch Dis Child 98:975-979, 2013

Objective.—To investigate the accuracy of morphine infusions prepared for neonates in relation to the label strength and to identify the differences in deviation between infusions made in neonatal intensive care unit (NICU) and those dispensed ready-to-use from pharmacy.

Methods.—Unused portions of morphine solution for infusion were collected over a 6-weeks period and used to determine the concentration of the drug by high-performance liquid chromatography (HPLC).

Results.—A total of 19.2% of infusions prepared by nurses in the ward and 7.8% prepared in the pharmacy were outside the limit required by the British Pharmacopoeia (±7.5%). Moreover, a deviation in concentration of more than 20% was found in ward-prepared infusions, although this was caused by volume discrepancies of less than 0.2 mL. The frequency and magnitude of deviations found in infusions prepared in pharmacy was lower than in those prepared by NICU. The latter showed significantly higher number of out-of-specification samples ($p = 0.015$); however, deviations from intended concentration occurred in both settings. Significant differences between pharmacy and NICU for volumes of less than 0.5 mL or for less than 1 mL were not identified probably due to small sample size, but statistical data show a trend for differences.

Conclusions.—Current practice of preparation of infusions from strengths intended for older children and adults involves dilution of small volumes in a syringe and leads to inaccuracy in the final concentration of infusions for neonatal use. We propose the implementation of standard concentrations for this patient group to effectively eliminate these errors.

▶ In this study, the authors investigated the accuracy of morphine infusions prepared for neonates in relation to the label strength and identified the differences in deviation between infusions made in the neonatal intensive care unit

(NICU) and those dispensed ready to use from the pharmacy.[1] A difference in accuracy of syringes in relation to strength in label, outside the British Pharmacopeia limits, was found in syringes prepared in the NICU and the pharmacy. The authors suggested that individualized syringes made by weight—either by nurses or in the pharmacy—cannot reliably deliver the intended prescribed concentrations.

The use of standardized concentrations is recommended by numerous agencies, including the Institute for Safe Medication Practices and the Vermont Oxford Network,[2] as a way to reduce administration errors after some preventable medication administration or compounding errors that led to serious adverse effects.[3,4]

However, to implement this change, careful considerations such as agreement on clinically appropriate concentrations and diluents, introduction of a change in prescribing and administration practice, labeling of different strengths to avoid mis-selection, and safety of storage are required. Standard drug concentrations combined with smart pump technologies and the use of bar coding might help avoid many steps in the preparation and administration of continuous infusions by minimizing the selection of concentrations, reducing calculation errors, and providing safety alerts for out-of-range concentrations.[5-8] Although smart technologies and standardized practices prevail in most large academic and community NICUs, many still rely on after hours ward-prepared infusions. Investing in 24-hour pharmacy services, smart pump technologies, and standardized concentration for continuous infusions have reduced the errors significantly where adopted. This should be a global goal to improve neonatal patient safety.

V. Bhatt-Mehta, PharmD, MS, FCCP

References

1. Aguado-Lorenzo V, Weeks K, Tunstell P, et al. Accuracy of the concentration of morphine infusions prepared for patients in a neonatal intensive care unit. *Arch Dis Child.* 2013;98:975-979.
2. Standard concentrations of neonatal drug infusions. A collaborative effort between the Institute for Safe Medication Practices (ISMP) and the Vermont oxford network (VON). http://www.ismp.org/tools/PediatricConcentrations.pdf. Accessed June 11, 2014.
3. Institute of Safe Medication Practice. Medication Safety Alert. Infant's death reinforces need for medications to be dispensed in ready-to-use form. ISMP, 1998. http://www.ismp.org/newsletters/acutecare/articles/19980909_2.asp. Accessed June 13, 2014.
4. Sentinel Event Alert. Issue 39: Preventing Pediatric Medication Errors. The Joint Commission. http://www.jointcommission.org/sentinel_event_alert_issue_39_preventing_pediatric_medication_errors/. Accessed June 13, 2014.
5. Hilmas E, Sowan A, Gaffoor M, Vaidya V. Implementation and evaluation of a comprehensive system to deliver pediatric continuous infusion medications with standardized concentrations. *Am J Health Syst Pharm.* 2010;67:58-69.
6. Larsen GY, Parker HB, Cash J, O'Connell M, Grant MC. Standard drug concentrations and smart-pump technology reduce continuous-medication-infusion errors in pediatric patients. *Pediatrics.* 2005;116:e21-e25.
7. Standardization drives safety. Pharmacy Purchasing and Product Management. http://www.pppmag.com/article/1411/November 2013. Accessed June 13, 2014.
8. Medication Safety in the Neonatal Intensive care Unit. Position statement. National association of neonatal Nurses. July 2011.

Unlicensed and off-label drug use in an Irish neonatal intensive care unit: a prospective cohort study

Kieran EA, O'Callaghan N, O'Donnell CPF (The Natl Maternity Hosp, Dublin, Ireland)

Acta Paediatr 103:e139-e142, 2014

Aim.—Many drugs are not licensed for use in children and drugs that are licensed may be given to them in an unapproved manner. We wanted to determine the extent of unlicensed and off-label prescribing in our neonatal intensive care unit (NICU).

Methods.—All infants admitted to our tertiary-level NICU over 2 months were prospectively studied. We recorded demographic data, and all the drugs prescribed and compared the use of each drug to the licensed indications in the Summary of Product Characteristics.

Results.—All the 110 infants admitted received a prescribed drug, with 69 different drugs prescribed, a median (IQR) of four (range: 3–11) drugs each. Just less than a fifth (19%) were unlicensed and 39% were off-label, with 45 infants (44%) receiving both an unlicensed and off-label drug, three (3%) receiving an unlicensed drug and 35 (32%) receiving just an off-label drug. Most infants <32 weeks received unlicensed (91%) and off-label (94%) drugs, and all infants <28 weeks received an unlicensed and an off-label drug.

Conclusion.—Most drugs prescribed to newborns are unlicensed or used for off-label reasons. Many infants, and the majority of preterm infants, admitted to our NICU received unlicensed and off-label drugs.

▶ Although this prospective observation was performed in Dublin, Ireland, I suspect the findings can be extrapolated to most neonatal intensive care units (NICUs) in the developed world. I am not shocked by the off-label use of pharmaceuticals in the NICU, but the magnitude is indeed surprising. Particularly worrisome were the high percentages of exposure to unlicensed pharmacologic agents and off-label drugs and the percentage of infants (44%) who received both an unlicensed and off-label agent. There appears to be an inverse relationship with gestational age, with increasing use in the more preterm infants, who are likely more susceptible to adverse events and unknown pharmacokinetics and pharmacodynamics. In the era of evidence-based medicine, it is incumbent on us to safeguard the well-being of our vulnerable patient population. Administering an unlicensed drug or using a drug off label is not in accordance with these principles. Nor is it consistent with "Primum non nocere."

S. M. Donn, MD

Transplacental passage of vancomycin from mother to neonate

Onwuchuruba CN, Towers CV, Howard BC, et al (Univ of Tennessee Med Ctr, Knoxville)

Am J Obstet Gynecol 210:352.e1-352.e4, 2014

Objective.—The objective of the study was to analyze a large number of patients receiving vancomycin chemoprophylaxis and evaluate the maternal and neonatal cord blood levels at the time of delivery.

Study Design.—Every mother who entered labor with a positive group B streptococcal culture and a high-risk penicillin allergy with resistance to clindamycin or unknown sensitivity was consented to participate in the study. In the initial phase of the study, patients received the standard intravenous dose of 1 g every 12 hours. Based on the results, this was changed to a dosing of 15 mg/kg every 12 hours in the second phase and then further modified to 20 mg/kg every 8 hours in the third phase. Maternal and cord blood vancomycin levels were obtained at delivery and evaluated.

Results.—A total of 55 patients consented to participate in the study, with 31 in phase I, 12 in phase II, and 12 in phase III. For the standard-dosing phase I group, only 32% of maternal and 9% of cord blood samples were therapeutic at delivery. For phase II, 50% of maternal and 33% of cord blood values were therapeutic; however, in phase III, 83% of mothers and neonates had therapeutic levels at the time of delivery.

Conclusion.—With standard dosing, only 9% of neonates have therapeutic vancomycin levels at delivery. By using a regimen of 20 mg/kg intravenous every 8 hours (maximum individual dose 2 g), the newborn therapeutic level increases above 80%. The pharmacological pattern shows that transplacental passage occurs with fetal levels equaling maternal levels, but transplacental transport is somewhat slow in both directions.

► For intrapartum antibiotic prophylaxis against neonatal early-onset group B streptococcal (GBS) sepsis in infants born to women with a history of anaphylaxis, angioedema, respiratory distress, or urticaria after administration of a penicillin or cephalosporin, current Centers for Disease Control (CDC) guidelines recommend treatment with vancomycin unless the GBS isolated from antepartum screening for colonization has shown susceptibility to clindamycin or erythromycin. Increasing rates of resistance to those agents in recent years has correspondingly led to increased use of vancomycin in this setting. Very little is known about the extent or kinetics of transplacental passage of vancomycin, however. This work provides important data to address that knowledge gap. These authors report that the recommended dose of 1 g every 12 hours failed to produce therapeutic serum levels ($\geq$10 μg/mL) at birth in 68% of the mothers and 91% of the infants. They went on to determine that a regimen using doses of 20 mg/kg every 8 hours consistently produced therapeutic serum levels in both mothers and babies (83% for both groups). No subjects had measured levels greater than 40 μg/mL, the presumed upper limit of the therapeutic range. Based on these observations, the authors recommend consideration of that higher, more frequent dosing regimen for this indication, with the objective of minimizing development of or selection for resistant organisms. Although that represents responsible antibiotic stewardship, it is important to note that cord blood levels exceeding the recognized minimal inhibitory concentration for GBS (1 μg/mL) were achieved in 56 of 57 infants in this study, so use of the CDC-recommended dosing should not raise concerns about the potential efficacy of prophylaxis. The sole exception was an infant who was delivered before infusion of the first vancomycin dose could be completed, for whom the cord blood vancomycin level was below the limit of detection. Data on the minimal interval required to achieve a cord blood level greater than 1 μg/mL are not provided. Until that information becomes available, it will be important to heed the recommendation of these authors that "if delivery occurs shortly after a vancomycin infusion is begun, the neonate may not have coverage and this should probably be relayed to the pediatric care providers," but the significance of that information may be difficult for the latter providers to determine. These data do provide valuable reassurance that vancomycin reliably, albeit slowly, crosses the placenta and can provide important protection against GBS infection in this circumstance.

W. E. Benitz, MD

14 Postnatal Growth and Development/ Follow-up

Alterations in Brain Structure and Neurodevelopmental Outcome in Preterm Infants Hospitalized in Different Neonatal Intensive Care Unit Environments

Pineda RG, Neil J, Dierker D, et al (Washington Univ School of Medicine, St Louis, MO)

J Pediatr 164:52-60, 2014

Objective.—To evaluate associations between neonatal intensive care unit (NICU) room type (open ward and private room) and medical outcomes; neurobehavior, electrophysiology, and brain structure at hospital discharge; and developmental outcomes at 2 years of age.

Study Design.—In this prospective longitudinal cohort study, we enrolled 136 preterm infants born <30 weeks gestation from an urban, 75-bed level III NICU from 2007-2010. Upon admission, each participant was assigned to a bedspace in an open ward or private room within the same hospital, based on space and staffing availability, where they remained for the duration of hospitalization. The primary outcome was developmental performance at 2 years of age (n = 86 infants returned for testing, which was 83% of survivors) measured using the Bayley Scales of Infant and Toddler Development, 3rd Edition. Secondary outcomes were: (1) medical factors throughout the hospitalization; (2) neurobehavior; and (3) cerebral injury and maturation (determined by magnetic resonance imaging and electroencephalography).

Results.—At term equivalent age, infants in private rooms were characterized by a diminution of normal hemispheric asymmetry and a trend toward having lower amplitude integrated electroencephalography cerebral maturation scores ($P = .02$; $\beta = -0.52$ [CI −0.95, −0.10]). At age 2 years, infants from private rooms had lower language scores ($P = .006$; $\beta = -8.3$ [CI −14.2, −2.4]) and a trend toward lower motor scores ($P = .02$; $\beta = -6.3$ [CI −11.7, −0.99]), which persisted after adjustment for potential confounders.

Conclusion.—These findings raise concerns that highlight the need for further research into the potential adverse effects of different amounts of sensory exposure in the NICU environment.

▶ Recently, there has been a concerted effort to minimize infant stress in neonatal intensive care units (NICUs) by monitoring and eliminating excessive environmental light and noise and promoting the use of developmental care practices. A logical extension of this effort is the current trend of remodeling or building NICU space to create small private rooms in which both ambient light and noise are modified and families are afforded a more private setting for interactions with their infants. The results of the above exploratory study call into question the wisdom of focusing solely on decreasing excessive sensory experiences, such as sound and light. In fact, infants allocated to private NICU rooms had lower scores on developmental testing than infants cared for on open NICU wards. One plausible explanation is that the decrease in sensory experiences associated with private rooms was further decreased by infrequent family visitation, holding, and interactions with infants, which was the case in the study NICU.

As the authors state in the discussion section, the theory supporting the positive aspects of sound abatement and sensory minimization was conceived before the advent of NICU single rooms. It may be that we have gone too far in our efforts to minimize sensory stimuli and have reduced sensory experiences to levels that are detrimental to infant development.

L. A. Papile, MD

Comparison of Bayley-2 and Bayley-3 scores at 18 months in term infants following neonatal encephalopathy and therapeutic hypothermia

Jary S, Whitelaw A, Walløe L, et al (Univ of Bristol, UK; Univ of Oslo, Norway)
Dev Med Child Neurol 55:1053-1059, 2013

Aim.—Neuroprotection trials for neonatal encephalopathy use moderate or severe disability as an outcome, with the Bayley Scales of Infant Development, Second Edition (Bayley-2) Index scores of <70 as part of the criteria. The Bayley Scales of Infant and Toddler, 3rd Development, Third Edition (Bayley-3) have superseded Bayley-2 and yield higher than expected scores in typically developing and high-risk infants. The aim of this study, therefore, was to compare Bayley-2 scores and Bayley-3 scores in term-born infants surviving neonatal encephalopathy treated with hypothermia.

Method.—Sixty-one term-born infants (37 males, 24 females; median gestational age at birth 40 wks, range 36–42 wks; median birthweight 3280 g, range 2295–5050) following neonatal encephalopathy and hypothermia had contemporaneous assessment at 18 months using the Bayley-2 and Bayley-3.

Results.—The median Bayley-3 Cognitive Composite score was 7 points higher than the median Bayley-2 Mental Developmental Index (MDI) score and the median Bayley-3 Motor Composite score was 18 points higher than the median Bayley-2 Psychomotor Developmental Index (PDI) score. Ten children had a Bayley-2 MDI of <70; only three children had Bayley-3 combined Cognitive/Language scores of <70. Eleven children had Bayley-2 PDI scores of <70 and four had modified Bayley-3 Motor Composite scores of <70. Applying regression equations to Bayley-3 scores adjusted rates of severe delay to similar proportions found using Bayley-2 scores.

Interpretation.—Fewer children were classified with severe delay using the Bayley-3 than the Bayley-2, which prohibits direct comparison of scores. Increased Bayley-3 cut-off thresholds for classifying severe disability are recommended when comparing studies in this clinical group using Bayley-2 scores.

► The Bayley Scales of Infant Development (BSID) were revised in 2006. The revision included a separation of the original Mental Developmental Index (MDI) into distinct cognitive, receptive, and language scales and the Psychomotor Developmental Index (PDI) into fine and gross motor scales. This observational study adds to a growing body of literature demonstrating that the 2006 version BSID (BSID-III) yields higher scores on both the motor and developmental indices, making it difficult to compare outcome studies that used the previous version (BSID-II) with those using the BSID-III. The question that arises is whether the BSID-II underestimates or the BSID-III overestimates development. Both might be true.

A recent metaanalysis reported that sensitivity of the BSID-II MDI and PDI are low with higher specificity, indicating a high proportion of children in whom development improved over time.[1] Conversely, studies evaluating the BSID-III and using term control groups as a reference population report a mean score in each domain above 100 (cognitive development around 105, language development around 109, and motor development around 107).[2] With reported standard deviations of 10 to 15 points, the cutoff thresholds for identifying children with moderated delay on the BSID-III would be 80 to 90 instead of the cutoff threshold of 70 on the BSID-II. A conversion table for BSID-II MDI and PDI scores to BSID-III composite cognitive/language and motor scores that uses data from published studies is available as a supplemental table (SI) to the article.

L. A. Papile, MD

References

1. Luttikhuizen dos Santos ES, de Kieviet JF, Konigs M, van Elburg RM, Oosterlaan J. Predictive value of the Bayley scales of infants development of very preterm/very low birth weight children: meta-analysis. *Early Hum Dev.* 2013;89:487-496.
2. Anderson PJ, De Luca CR, Hutchinson E, Roberts G, Doyle LW; Victorian Infant Collaborative Group. Underestimation of developmental delay by the new Bayley-III scale. *Arch Pediatr Adolesc Med.* 2010;164:352-356.

Performance of the Parent Report of Children's Abilities–Revised (PARCA-R) versus the Bayley Scales of Infant Development III

Martin AJ, Darlow BA, Salt A, et al (Univ of Sydney, Australia; Univ of Otago, Christchurch, New Zealand; Ormond Street Hosp for Children, London, UK)
Arch Dis Child 98:955-958, 2013

Background.—The Parent Report of Children's Abilities-Revised (PARCA-R) assesses cognitive and language development at 24 months. It was validated against the Mental Development Index of the Bayley Scales of Infant Development II (BSID II), but this has now been superseded by BSID III.

Objective.—To compare the PARCA-R against the BSID III.

Methods.—PARCA-R and BSID III assessments scheduled at 24 months of age (corrected for prematurity) were completed in 204 infants with suspected or proven neonatal sepsis in the International Neonatal Immunotherapy Study. Associations between the scales were measured and the predictive accuracy of the PARCA-R for moderate cognitive delay and moderate language delay was assessed using Receiver Operating Characteristic (ROC) analysis.

Results.—Median birthweight was 911 g, median gestational age at birth was 27 weeks and 100 (49.0%) were girls. 4.4% and 8.4% met standard BSID III criteria for cognitive delay and language delay, respectively. These rates increased to 19.6% and 12.6% when an independent sample of normal term infants were used as the reference group suggesting standard BSID III reference norms may tend to underestimate delay. The Spearman correlation between PARCA-R and BSID scales were 0.43 for cognition and 0.71 for language. The PARCA-R successfully predicted cases of cognitive delay and language delay with the area under the ROC curves ranging from 0.83 to 0.97 depending on reference norms used.

Conclusions.—The results support the PARCA-R as a practical tool for the identification of appreciable cognitive and language delay at 24 months among critically ill premature and extremely low birthweight neonates.

▶ Traditionally, formal neurodevelopmental appraisals performed by trained assessors are used to monitor high-risk neonatal populations and for collecting outcome data on select populations enrolled in clinical trials. However, the model is expensive, reimbursement is often lacking, and it requires families to travel to the testing site.

In this report, the authors explored the strength of association between the Parent Report of Children's Abilities (PARCA-R), a parent-completed questionnaire developed to evaluate language and cognitive ability, and the Bayley Scales of Infant Development III (BSID-III) cognitive and language scales. The strength of association between the PARCA-R and BSID-III cognitive and language scales were quantified using Spearman correlation coefficients and a receiver-operator characteristics curve was constructed to evaluate the ability of the

PARCA-R to predict moderate or severe delay on the BSID-III cognitive and language scales. Prediction of an individual child's BSID III scores from the PAC + RCA-R was relatively imprecise. However, the PARCA-R performed well in predicting cases of moderate or severe language delay and moderate and severe cognitive delay. Although the PARCA-R has been used in several international clinical trials,[1] it is doubtful, given the information in this article, that the instrument will gain acceptance as a new criterion approach to developmental assessment.

L. A. Papile, MD

Reference

1. Brocklehurst P, Farrell B, King A, et al. Treatment of neonatal sepsis with intravenous immune globulin. *N Engl J Med.* 2011;365:1201-1211.

Effect of primary language on developmental testing in children born extremely preterm

Lowe JR, Nolen TL, Vohr B, et al (Univ of New Mexico School of Medicine, Albuquerque; RTI International, Durham, NC; Brown Univ School of Medicine, Providence, RI; et al)

Acta Paediatr 102:896-900, 2013

Aim.—The aim of this study was to better understand the impact of non-English language spoken in the home on measures of cognition, language and behaviour in toddlers born extremely preterm.

Methods.—Eight hundred and fifty children born at <28 weeks of gestational ages were studied. 427 male and 423 female participants from three racial/ethnic groups (White, Black and Hispanic) were evaluated at 18–22 months adjusted for age using the Bayley Scales of Infant Development third edition and the Brief Infant Toddler Social Emotional Assessment (BITSEA). Children whose primary language was Spanish (n = 98) were compared with children whose primary language was English (n = 752), using multivariable regression adjusted for medical and psychosocial factors.

Results.—Cognitive scores were similar between groups; however, receptive, expressive and composite language scores were lower for children whose primary language was Spanish. These differences remained significant after adjustment for medical and socio-economic factors. Spanish-speaking children scored worse on the BITSEA competence and problem scores using univariate analysis, but not after adjustment for medical and socio-economic factors.

Conclusion.—Our finding that preterm children whose primary language was Spanish had similar cognitive but lower language scores than those whose primary language was English suggests that using English language-based testing tools may introduce bias against non-English-speaking children born preterm.

▶ The Bayley Scales of Infant Development (BSID) were developed and standardized in English. Because there is no published non-English-based standardized test for the age group encompassed by the BSID, it is frequently translated and administered in the child's language by either a bilingual certified examiner or a certified examiner with an interpreter. In the above observational study, the authors explored the relationship between primary language spoken in the home and BSID scores in the areas of cognition and language.

The study cohort was born at less than or equal to 28 weeks' gestational age at 1 of the 16 centers participating National Institute of Child Health and Human Development Neonatal Research Network and underwent developmental assessment between 18 and 22 months' corrected age. Because the cohort of children with a primary language other than English or Spanish was small (7%), only children in English-speaking homes (n = 752) and in Spanish-speaking homes (n = 98) were included in the analyses. The mean and median cognitive scores were similar for the English-speaking and Spanish-speaking children (90 and 90 vs 90 and 88.3); however the difference in receptive and expressive language scores was significantly lower in the Spanish-speaking children, even when adjusted for numerous medical and socioeconomic factors.

This study highlights the potential hazard of translating a test standardized in English into another language to conduct neurodevelopmental testing. The authors speculate that the language scale of the BSID is altered when administered in a language other than English because of differences in translation, the varying dialects spoken and language structure. An additional explanation is that exposure to 2 languages may have contributed to overall language delays. At least 1 published study has shown that bilingual children born at term perform less well on language portions of neuropsychological assessments at school age but not on tests of attention and executive function.[1]

L. A. Papile, MD

Reference

1. Garratt LC, Kelly TP. To what extent does bilingualism affect children's performance on the NEPSY? *Child Neuropsychol.* 2008;14:71-81.

Predictive value of the amplitude integrated EEG in infants with hypoxic ischaemic encephalopathy: data from a randomised trial of therapeutic hypothermia

Azzopardi D, on behalf of the TOBY study group (Hammersmith Hosp, London, UK)

Arch Dis Child Fetal Neonatal Ed 99:F80-F82, 2014

The amplitude integrated EEG (aEEG) is reputed to be one of the best predictors of neurological outcome following hypoxic ischaemic encephalopathy in term newborns and was used to select infants into trials of neuroprotection with hypothermia, but its predictive value and the effect of moderate hypothermia on the aEEG have not previously been examined in a randomised study. The positive predictive value (PPV) of the aEEG recorded within 6 h of birth for death or disability at 18 months of age was determined in 314 infants born after 35 weeks gestation who were randomised to receive standard care with or without cooling for 72 h. The aEEG was classified according to voltage and by pattern. The PPV of a severely abnormal aEEG assessed by the voltage and pattern methods was 0.63 and 0.59 respectively in non-cooled infants and 0.55 and 0.51 in cooled infants ($p > 0.05$). Although the differences in PPV between cooled and non-cooled groups were not significant, they are consistent with observational studies showing a lower PPV in infants treated with hypothermia, probably due to a neuroprotective effect of cooling.

▶ The amplitude integrated electroencephalogram (aEEG) is reputed to be one of the best predictors of neurological outcome following hypoxic-ischemic encephalopathy (HIE) in term infants.[1] Additional observational studies showed that the predictive value of aEEG for adverse neurodevelopmental outcome was reduced in infants with HIE who were treated with therapeutic hypothermia compared with noncooled infants.[2]

In this report, the authors analyzed the aEEG data available from the TOBY randomized clinical of therapeutic hypothermia for neonatal encephalopathy. The inclusion criteria for the trial required the presence of an abnormal aEEG and clinical criteria of HIE. The aEEG was recorded for at least 30 minutes within 6 hours of birth before randomization and before initiation of whole-body cooling. aEEG records of an adequate quality were available for 314 of 325 participants in the trial; 158 in the standard care only arm and 158 in the standard care with cooling arm. Data regarding death or neurodevelopmental disability were available for each of the 314 infants. Positive predictive value was calculated for abnormal aEEG voltage and pattern including moderate or severe depression, discontinuous normal voltage, continuous low voltage, flat trace and burst, and also pattern combinations.

The finding that the predictive value for adverse outcome at 18 months of age of the aEEG recorded within 6 hours of birth is lower than previously reported suggests that caution is needed when using early aEEG findings to counsel families about the likely outcome of their encephalopathic infants.

L. A. Papile, MD

References

1. van Laerhoven H, de Haan TR, Offringa M, Post B, van der Lee JH. Prognostic tests in term neonates with hypoxic-ischemic encephalopathy. *Pediatrics*. 2013; 131:88-99.
2. Shankaran S, Pappas A, McDonald SA, et al. Predictive value of an early amplitude integrated electroencephalogram and neurologic examination. *Pediatrics*. 2011;128:e112-e120.

Antenatal steroid exposure and outcomes of very premature infants: a regional cohort study

Wong D, for the NICUS Network (Australian Natl Univ Med School, Canberra, Australian Capital Territory, Australia)

Arch Dis Child Fetal Neonatal Ed 99:F12-F20, 2014

Objective.—To compare mortality, short-term morbidity and long-term neurodevelopmental outcomes of <29 week premature infants with antenatal steroid exposure (none, incomplete and complete).

Patients and Methods.—Multicentre retrospective cohort study, within a geographically defined area in Australia served by a network of 10 neonatal intensive care units (NICUs), of infants <29 weeks gestational age, admitted to NICUs between 1998 and 2004. Outcome measures included hospital survival, perinatal complications and functional disability at 2–3 years follow-up.

Results.—2549 neonates were included; 319 (12.5%) received no exposure to steroids. Hospital mortality (OR 0.59, 95% CI 0.45 to 0.76, $p < 0.001$, intraventricular haemorrhage (IVH) (OR 0.58, 95% CI 0.42 to 0.81, $p = 0.001$) and necrotising entercolitis (NEC) (OR 0.62, 95% CI 0.42 to 0.91, $p = 0.018$) was less likely in infants with any steroid exposure. Any steroid exposure was associated with less need for surfactant (OR 0.41, 95% CI 0.30 to 0.57, $p < 0.001$) and mechanical ventilation (OR 0.30, 95% CI 0.17 to 0.52, $p < 0.001$). Subgroup analyses demonstrated differences in outcomes only with complete steroid coverage and not with incomplete coverage. Survival benefit and reduction in the incidence of severe IVH was evident from 24 to 28 weeks. Long-term neurodevelopmental data available for 1473 survivors showed no significant difference in outcomes with steroid exposure after multivariate analysis.

Conclusions.—Exposure to a complete course of antenatal steroids is associated with higher infant survival rates, lower rates of severe IVH and NEC compared to an incomplete course or no exposure. Any exposure to steroids reduces the risk of moderate cerebral palsy, however, long-term neurodevelopmental outcome may not be affected by steroid exposure.

▶ Published studies comparing mortality and perinatal morbidity according to antenatal steroid (ANS) exposure showed that ANSs confer survival benefit and reduce perinatal morbidity for infants born at gestational ages of 23 to 26 weeks only when a full course is administered. In this study, the authors assessed the impact of any ANS exposure on neurodevelopmental outcome in early childhood, as well as on mortality and perinatal morbidity, among a cohort of extremely preterm infants.

The data analyzed was abstracted from the Neonatal Intensive Care Units Data Collection, an ongoing prospective audit of infants admitted to 10 NICUs in a geographically defined region of Australia, and the Neonatal Intensive Care Units Follow-up Data Collection, an ongoing audit of admitted infants at 2 to

3 years corrected for prematurity. Of the 1970 infants less than 29 weeks of gestational age eligible for follow-up, data were available for 1473 (74.8%).

The abstract summary emphasizes the significant reduction in mortality and perinatal morbidity between the cohort exposed to any ANS and that not exposed. However, because extremely preterm birth frequently occurs before a complete course of ANS can be administered, the subgroup analysis comparing incomplete ANS exposure to no ANS exposure may be more clinically relevant. In that analysis, a partial course of ANS was not associated with a reduction in either mortality or the occurrence of major medical morbidities such as intraventricular hemorrhage or necrotizing enterocolitis from 24 to 28 weeks, a result similar to that noted in previous published studies. However, in contrast to previous reports, ANS exposure did not result in less developmental delay. The lack of benefit regarding neurodevelopmental outcome with ANS exposure suggests that at extremely low gestational ages, the beneficial effects of ANS are insufficient to counter the detrimental influence of prematurity and its attendant medical morbidities on subsequent neurodevelopment.

L. A. Papile, MD

Characteristics of extremely low-birth-weight infant survivors with unimpaired outcomes at 30 months of age

Kumar P, NICHD Neonatal Research Network (Northwestern Univ Feinberg School of Medicine, Chicago, IL; et al)

J Perinatol 33:800-805, 2013

Objective.—To evaluate characteristics of unimpaired outcome in extremely low-birth-weight (ELBW) survivors.

Study Design.—ELBW infants ($n = 714$) with 30 months' assessments were analyzed. Logistic regression was used to develop a model for the binary outcome of unimpaired versus impaired outcome.

Result.—Thirty-three percent of infants had an unimpaired outcome. Seventeen percent of ELBW survivors had a Bayley II Mental Developmental Index score of ≥101 and 2% had a score of ≥116. Female gender, use of antenatal steroids (ANS), maternal education ≥high school and the absence of major neonatal morbidities were independent predictors of unimpaired outcome. The likelihood of an unimpaired outcome in the presence of major neonatal morbidities was higher in infants exposed to ANS.

Conclusion.—The majority of unimpaired ELBW survivors had cognitive scores shifted toward the lower end of the normal distribution. Exposure to ANS was associated with higher likelihood of an unimpaired outcome in infants with major neonatal morbidities.

► Although this study was a secondary analysis of the glutamine trial and included only 62% of infants enrolled in the trial, there are several interesting findings. The first relates to the distribution of the Mental Developmental Index (MDI) scores for the cohort who was classified as unimpaired (MDI and Psychomotor Developmental Index scores >85, normal neurological examination, vision, hearing, functional ability for swallowing, and infant was walking). Only 17% had an MDI score greater or equal to 100, whereas 50% of a normal term cohort would be expected to score greater or equal to 100. The implications of this shift downward are unknown but potentially may explain the academic difficulties that extremely low birth weight children face at school age.

The second finding relates to the impact of major medical morbidities on neurodevelopment. Previous studies have suggested that infants who had 1 or more major medical morbidities have a 2- to 3-fold increased risk of poor developmental outcome.[1] In the study reviewed here, the overall rate of moderate to severe impairment of 33% was similar to that in previous published reports; however, the adverse impact of the presence of 1 or more major medical morbidities was much less pronounced. Of note the neurodevelopmental assessments in this study were done at 30 months' corrected age, whereas in previous studies, the assessments were carried out at 18 months' corrected age.

L. A. Papile, MD

Reference

1. Schmidt B, Asztalos EV, Roberts RS, Robertson CM, Sauve RS, Whitfield MF. Impact of bronchopulmonary dysplasia, brain injury, and severe retinopathy on the outcome of extremely low-birth-weight infants at 18 months: results from the trial of indomethacin prophylaxis in preterms. *JAMA*. 2003;289:1124-1129.

Two-Year Outcomes of a Randomized Controlled Trial of Inhaled Nitric Oxide in Premature Infants

Durrmeyer X, for the European Union Nitric Oxide Study Group (Centre Hospitalier Intercommunal de Créteil, France; et al)
Pediatrics 132:e695-e703, 2013

Background and Objectives.—The European Union Nitric Oxide trial was designed to assess the potential benefits of inhaled nitric oxide (iNO) compared with placebo in infants with respiratory failure. This follow-up study evaluated respiratory, neurodevelopmental, and other outcomes for infants entered into the European Union Nitric Oxide trial to age 2 years.

Methods.—In a multicenter, randomized, double-blind study, preterm infants born at <29 weeks' gestation with moderate respiratory failure were allocated to receive iNO (5 ppm) or placebo for 7 to 21 days. Subjects underwent assessments at 1 and 2 years corrected for prematurity.

Results.—At 36 weeks' postmenstrual age, 696 of 792 infants were alive; 4 in the iNO arm subsequently died before age 2 years compared with 7 in the control arm. We evaluated 95% of the survivors at 12 months and 90% at 2 years. In the iNO arm, 244 of 363 (67.2%) infants had survived without disability at age 2 years compared with 270 of 374 (72.2%) who received placebo ($P = .094$). Mean (SD) cognitive composite scores (Bayley Scales of Infant and Toddler Development, third edition) were 94 (13) in the iNO group and 95 (14) in the placebo group; in the iNO group, 19% scored <85 and 9.5% developed cerebral palsy compared with 13.3% and 9%, respectively. There were no significant differences in hospitalizations overall or due to respiratory illness in use of home oxygen therapy or respiratory medications, in growth, or in other health outcomes.

Conclusions.—At 2 years of age, low-dose (5 ppm) iNO started early (<24 hours after birth) for a median of 20 days did not affect neurodevelopmental or other health outcomes.

▶ Animal models suggest that alveolar development might be maintained by inhaled nitric oxide (iNO) during mechanical ventilation, resulting in improvement in lung function.[1] It also has been suggested that iNO may be neuroprotective.[2] However, these beneficial effects have not been evident in clinical trials of iNO in very preterm infants. One of the aims of this secondary study to the European Union Nitric Oxide Trial was to evaluate neurodevelopment and respiratory health in early childhood to ascertain if iNO therapy in the neonatal period had a longer-term benefit on later outcome.

The lack of difference between the iNO and control cohorts concerning neurodevelopmental outcome is consistent with the observations of previous investigators. Yet the percentage of surviving infants noted to have no or minimal disability at the 2-year follow-up (80% iNO vs 83% placebo) is much higher than that reported in previous studies of iNO. This observation most likely can be attributed to the underestimation of the proportion of children with developmental delay with the latest iteration of the Bayley Scales of Infant Development (BSID-III) when compared with the previous version (BSID-II).

There also was no difference noted regarding pulmonary health. By 1 year of corrected age, approximately 25% of the iNO study cohort and their control counterparts were hospitalized at least once with a respiratory illness, and an additional 25% were hospitalized for other reasons. Although the rate of hospitalization for respiratory problems decreased in the second year compared with first year corrected age for both groups, it was still notable at 10% to 13%. Medications related to respiratory problems were used by approximately 10% in both groups. The study is ongoing with the next assessment scheduled at 7 years of age, an age at which time a more robust neurodevelopmental assessment, as well as pulmonary function studies, can be obtained.

L. A. Papile, MD

References

1. McCurnin DC, Pierce RA, Chang LY, et al. Inhaled NO improves early pulmonary function and modifies lung growth and elastin deposition in a baboon model of neonatal chronic lung disease. *Am J Physiol Lung Cell Mol Physiol.* 2005;288: L450-L459.
2. Pansiot J, Loron G, Olivier P, et al. Neuroprotective effect of inhaled nitric oxide on excitotoxic-induced brain damage in neonatal rat. *PLoS One.* 2010;5:e10916.

Need for Supplemental Oxygen at Discharge in Infants with Bronchopulmonary Dysplasia Is Not Associated with Worse Neurodevelopmental Outcomes at 3 Years Corrected Age

Lodha A, Sauvé R, Bhandari V, et al (Alberta Children's Hosp, Calgary, Canada; Yale Univ School of Medicine, New Haven, CT)

PLoS One 9:e90843, 2014

Objectives.—To determine if chronic oxygen dependency (discharge home on supplemental oxygen) in children with bronchopulmonary dysplasia (BPD; defined as requirement for supplemental O_2 at 36 weeks postmenstrual age) predicts neurodevelopmental disability rates and growth outcomes at 36 months corrected age (CA).

Study Design.—Longitudinal cohort study.

Setting.—Southern Alberta regional center located at high altitude.

Participants.—Preterm infants weighing ≤1250 grams with no BPD, BPD, and BPD with chronic oxygen dependency.

Main Outcome Measures.—Neurodevelopmental and growth outcomes.

Results.—Of 1563 preterm infants admitted from 1995–2007, 1212 survived. Complete follow-up data were available for 1030 (85%) children. Children in BPD and BPD with chronic oxygen dependency groups had significantly lower birth weights, gestational ages, prolonged mechanical ventilation and oxygen supplementation and received more postnatal steroids, compared to those without BPD. Children with BPD and BPD with chronic oxygen dependency were more likely to be below the 5th centile in weight and height compared to those without BPD but there was little difference between the BPD and BPD with chronic oxygen dependency groups. After controlling for confounding variables, children who had BPD and BPD with chronic oxygen dependency had higher odds of neurodevelopmental disability compared to those without BPD [OR (odds ratio) 1.9 (95% CI 1.1 to 3.5) and OR 1.8 (1.1 to 2.9), respectively], with no significant difference between BPD and BPD with chronic oxygen dependency [OR 0.9 (95% CI 0.6 to 1.5)].

Conclusions.—BPD and BPD with chronic oxygen dependency in children predicts abnormal neurodevelopmental outcomes at 36 months CA. However, the neurodevelopmental disability rates were not significantly higher in BPD with chronic oxygen dependency children compared to children with BPD only. Compared to those without BPD, growth is impaired in children with BPD and BPD with chronic oxygen dependency, but no difference between the latter two groups.

▶ In this study, the authors conclude that the risk of poor growth and neurodevelopmental disability in early childhood does not differ for infants with a severe form of chronic lung disease (CLD) compared with those with a milder form. Although this may be correct, the data presented are not convincing. The need for supplemental oxygen at the time of discharge to home was used as a surrogate for a severe form of CLD. To meet the criteria for home oxygen dependency, all that was needed was a dated hard copy of pulse oximetry results 48 hours before discharge showing room air oximetry ≤89%. From the data presented, it is not possible to ascertain what proportion of infants who met the criteria for home oxygen therapy truly had CLD sufficiently severe to require oxygen supplementation for a prolonged period of time. Additional studies using a more circumscribed definition of CLD are needed to clarify the relationship between BPD severity in preterm infants and neurodevelopmental disability.

L. A. Papile, MD

Neurodevelopmental outcomes of extremely low birth weight infants with spontaneous intestinal perforation or surgical necrotizing enterocolitis

Wadhawan R, for NICHD Neonatal Research Network (Women & Infants Hosp, Providence, RI; et al)

J Perinatol 34:64-70, 2014

Objective.—To determine if extremely low birth weight infants with surgical necrotizing enterocolitis have a higher risk of death or neurodevelopmental impairment and neurodevelopmental impairment among survivors (secondary outcome) at 18–22 months corrected age compared with infants with spontaneous intestinal perforation and infants without necrotizing enterocolitis or spontaneous intestinal perforation.

Study Design.—Retrospective analysis of the Neonatal Research Network very low birth weight registry, evaluating extremely low birth weight infants born between 2000 and 2005. The study infants were designated into three groups: (1) spontaneous intestinal perforation without necrotizing enterocolitis; (2) surgical necrotizing enterocolitis (Bell's stage III); and (3) neither spontaneous intestinal perforation nor necrotizing enterocolitis. Multivariate logistic regression analysis was performed to evaluate the association between the clinical group and death or neurodevelopmental impairment, controlling for multiple confounding factors including center.

Result.—Infants with surgical necrotizing enterocolitis had the highest rate of death before hospital discharge (53.5%) and death or neurodevelopmental impairment (82.3%) compared with infants in the spontaneous intestinal perforation group (39.1 and 79.3%) and no necrotizing enterocolitis/no spontaneous intestinal perforation group (22.1 and 53.3%; $P < 0.001$). Similar results were observed for neurodevelopmental impairment among survivors. On logistic regression analysis, both spontaneous intestinal perforation and surgical necrotizing enterocolitis were associated with increased risk of death or neurodevelopmental impairment (adjusted odds ratio 2.21, 95% confidence interval (CI): 1.5, 3.2 and adjusted OR 2.11, 95% CI: 1.5, 2.9, respectively) and neurodevelopmental impairment among survivors (adjusted OR 2.17, 95% CI: 1.4, 3.2 and adjusted OR 1.70, 95% CI: 1.2, 2.4, respectively).

Conclusion.—Spontaneous intestinal perforation and surgical necrotizing enterocolitis are associated with a similar increase in the risk of death or neurodevelopmental impairment and neurodevelopmental impairment among extremely low birth weight survivors at 18–22 months corrected age.

▶ In this abstract, the investigators report the increased risks of death/neurodevelopmental impairment and neurodevelopmental impairment among survivors associated with spontaneous intestinal perforation (SIP) and surgical necrotizing enterocolitis (SurgNEC). The definition of neurodevelopmental impairment included the presence of 1 or more of the following: moderate or severe cerebral palsy, bilateral blindness, bilateral hearing loss requiring amplification, Bayley II mental developmental index (MDI), or psychomotor developmental index (PDI) <70. The following data from the article provide a more robust look at the global nature of the neurodevelopmental impairment:

	No NEC/No SIP (*N* = 5095)	SIP only (*N* = 140)	SurgNEC (*N* = 174)
MDI <70	30.4%	52.9%	50.6%
PDI <70	20.0%	49.6%	43.6%
Cerebral palsy	5.5%	17.0%	22.5%
Deaf	1.7%	4.8%	8.4%
Blind	0.6%	3.4%	5.2%

On the basis of previous published reports, the higher frequency of low Bayley II scores and cerebral palsy for infants with either SIP or SurgNEC is not unexpected; however, the almost 4-fold and 6 -fold increase in sensorineural impairment among ELBW infants with SIP and SurgNEC, respectively, is alarming and needs further exploration. The data illustrate the devastating consequences of these gastrointestinal conditions and the urgent need to find an antidote.

L. A. Papile, MD

Neonatal ECMO study of temperature (NEST): a randomized controlled trial

Field D, NEST Study Collaborative Group (Univ of Leicester, UK)

Pediatrics 132:e1247-e1256, 2013

Background.—Despite evidence to support the use of extracorporeal membrane oxygenation (ECMO) in defined groups of newborn infants, rates of impairment among survivors remain high. Therapeutic hypothermia has been shown to provide neuroprotection in mature infants exposed to perinatal asphyxia. We hypothesized that therapeutic hypothermia during ECMO would reduce the proportion of infants with brain injury, and thus later impairment.

Methods.—We conducted a randomized trial in the United Kingdom to compare ECMO with cooling (34°C for the first 48 to 72 hours) with standard ECMO (37°C). The primary outcome was the cognitive composite score of the Bayley Scales of Infant and Toddler Development, 3rd edition, at 2 years. Prespecified secondary outcomes included death, neonatal morbidity, and other neurodevelopmental and behavioral outcomes at 2 years.

Results.—A total of 111 infants were entered into the study, 14 died before 2 years of age (16% who received ECMO with cooling vs 9% who received ECMO alone). Two infants were lost to follow-up, and 8 were unable to complete the full range of tests. For 45 evaluated infants who received ECMO with cooling, mean cognitive scores at 2 years were 88.0 (SD: 16.2) compared with 90.6 (SD: 13.1) for 48 infants receiving ECMO only (difference in means: −2.6; 95% confidence interval: −8.7 to 3.4). The various secondary outcomes were not significantly different between the groups, but most favored ECMO without cooling.

Conclusions.—In newborn infants treated by ECMO, the use of mild hypothermia for the first 48 to 72 hours did not result in improved outcomes up to 2 years of age.

▶ The publication of randomized clinical trials demonstrating the efficacy of therapeutic hypothermia for the treatment of hypoxic/ischemic encephalopathy in term and near-term infants has prompted some clinicians to extend the use of this modality to more immature infants and also other conditions thought to be associated with hypoxic-ischemic brain injury. This trial illustrates the potential dangers of extrapolating existing research findings from one condition to another without appropriate evaluation.

The investigators hypothesized that therapeutic hypothermia initiated at the start of the extracorporeal membrane oxygenation (ECMO) run would mitigate brain injury likely to occur during the establishment of ECMO. However, the predominant pattern of brain injury noted after ECMO is white matter infarction with cortical involvement, suggesting that the injury likely results from a prolonged subacute rather than an acute insult. The disappointing results of this study would suggest that it is the underlying condition and/or the associated physiological changes rather than the use of ECMO that leads to an increased risk of later neurodevelopmental impairment.

L. A. Papile, MD

Late Outcomes of a Randomized Trial of High-Frequency Oscillation in Neonates

Zivanovic S, Peacock J, Alcazar-Paris M, et al (King's College London, UK; et al)

N Engl J Med 370:1121-1130, 2014

Background.—Results from an observational study involving neonates suggested that high-frequency oscillatory ventilation (HFOV), as compared with conventional ventilation, was associated with superior small-airway function at follow-up. Data from randomized trials are needed to confirm this finding.

Methods.—We studied 319 adolescents who had been born before 29 weeks of gestation and had been enrolled in a multicenter, randomized trial that compared HFOV with conventional ventilation immediately after birth. The trial involved 797 neonates, of whom 592 survived to hospital discharge. We compared follow-up data from adolescents who had been randomly assigned to HFOV with follow-up data from those who had been randomly assigned to conventional ventilation, with respect to lung function and respiratory health, health-related quality of life, and functional status, as assessed with the use of questionnaires completed when the participants were 11 to 14 years of age. The primary outcome was forced expiratory flow at 75% of the expired vital capacity (FEF75).

Results.—The HFOV group had superior results on a test of small-airway function (z score for FEF75, −0.97 with HFOV vs. −1.19 with conventional therapy; adjusted difference, 0.23 [95% confidence interval, 0.02 to 0.45]). There were significant differences in favor of HFOV in several other measures of respiratory function, including forced expiratory volume in 1 second, forced vital capacity, peak expiratory flow, diffusing capacity, and impulse-oscillometric findings. As compared with the conventional-therapy group, the HFOV group had significantly higher ratings from teachers in three of eight school subjects assessed, but there were no other significant differences in functional outcomes.

Conclusions.—In a randomized trial involving children who had been born extremely prematurely, those who had undergone HFOV, as compared with those who had received conventional ventilation, had superior lung function at 11 to 14 years of age, with no evidence of poorer functional outcomes. (Funded by the National Institute for Health Research Health Technology Assessment Programme and others.).

▶ The original clinical trial of high frequency oscillatory ventilation (HFOV) was conducted between August 1998 and January 2001. A review of the original article revealed that 92% of mothers received antenatal steroids, and approximately 91% of the babies enrolled were given a first dose of surfactant within 2 hours of birth. There was no difference in the primary outcome of death or chronic lung disease at 36 weeks' postmenstrual age between the HFOV and conventional ventilation cohorts.

Of the original 797 infants randomized in the trial, 592 survived until hospital discharge. For this report only 55% of surviving eligible children were evaluated, illustrating how difficult it is to obtain long-term outcome data for infants enrolled in neonatal trials. The primary reason for "lost to follow-up" was inability to contact the family (71%).

Children who were randomized to HFOV had superior lung function; however, the difference between the groups was modest at best and was not associated with any difference in the frequency of respiratory disorders, use of medication for chest problems, or hospital admission in the 12 months preceding the evaluation. Assessment of behavior and academic achievement by means of questionnaires indicated that almost 60% of the children were in mainstream school; however, more than half of these children were receiving learning support or help. An interesting finding that other investigators have noted is that the children rated their quality of life higher than did either their parents or their teachers.

L. A. Papile, MD

Long-term cognitive and neurological outcome of preterm infants with postnatally acquired CMV infection through breast milk

Goelz R, Meisner C, Bevot A, et al (Univ Children's Hosp, Tuebingen, Germany; Univ Hosp, Tuebingen, Germany)

Arch Dis Child Fetal Neonatal Ed 98:F430-F433, 2013

Introduction.—Long-term follow-up data on preterm infants with breast milk–acquired postnatal cytomegalovirus (CMV) infection are sparse.

Aim.—To systematically evaluate the long-term cognitive outcome and prevalence of cerebral palsy (CP) in patients after postnatal CMV infection.

Patients and Methods.—All surviving infants <1500 g born in our centre between 1 June 1995 and 1 June 2000, and with postnatal CMV infection acquired at up to 3 months of corrected age, were eligible for our study; this included neurological and neurocognitive assessment, using the Kaufman Assessment Battery for Children (K-ABC) at the age of >4 years. A blinded and controlled matched-pairs design was used with gestational age, gender and date of birth as matching criteria.

Results.—Of 50 eligible children, 42 (84%) could be tested. There was no difference in the prevalence of cerebral palsy. Following CMV infection during their hospital stay, infants had significantly lower results in the simultaneous processing scale of the K-ABC ($p = 0.029$) after correction for additional risk factors like socioeconomic status (SES). Results for the sequential and achievement scales were only slightly reduced ($p > 0.05$).

Conclusions.—It seems possible that breast milk-acquired CMV infection has a detrimental influence on cognitive development of preterm infants.

▶ Over the past several years, there has been an increasing emphasis on feeding extremely preterm infants mothers' milk. One of the risks of doing so is the transmission of cytomegalovirus (CMV). Although the technique of freeze-thaw and/or pasteurization of breast milk can decrease the risk of transmission, it does not entirely eliminate the risk. In this controlled matched-pairs observational study, the authors evaluated the cognitive and neurologic outcome in early childhood of preterm infants who acquired CMV by ingesting their mother's breast milk.

Congenital infection was excluded through a polymerase chain reaction (PCR)—negative and culture-negative urine sample and ear and throat samples collected within 3 days after birth. Postnatal CMV infection was proven by PCR-positive and culture-positive urine samples. Transfusions as a source of postnatal infection was excluded by the use of only CMV-negative and leukocyte-depleted packed red blood cells. All infants were examined for postnatally acquired CMV infection through biweekly surveillance during their neonatal intensive care unit (NICU) stay and at 3 months' corrected age.

Overall preterm children with postnatally acquired CMV scored lower on all 3 scales of the Kaufman Assessment Battery for Children; however, only the difference on the achievement scale was statistically, but not clinically, significant. The lowest scores were achieved by the cohort infected before NICU discharge. Cerebral palsy was noted in only 1 of the 84 children. The authors' conclusion that it is possible that breast-milk-acquired CMV had a detrimental influence seems somewhat pessimist, given the data presented.

L. A. Papile, MD

Neurodevelopmental outcome, psychological adjustment, and quality of life in adolescents with congenital heart disease

Schaefer C, von Rhein M, Knirsch W, et al (Univ Children's Hosp Zurich, Switzerland)

Dev Med Child Neurol 55:1143-1149, 2013

Aim.—The aim of this study was to examine neurodevelopment, psychological adjustment, and health-related quality of life (HRQoL) in adolescents after bypass surgery for congenital heart disease (CHD) during early childhood.

Method.—Fifty-nine adolescents (34 females, 25 males) with CHD were examined at a median age of 13 years 8 months (range 11 y 5 mo-16 y 11 mo). Outcome was assessed with the Wechsler Intelligence Scale for Children, (fourth edition); the Beery Test of Visual-Motor Integration; the Rey-Osterrieth Complex Figure Test; the Zurich Neuromotor Assessment; the Strengths and Difficulties Questionnaire; and the KIDSCREEN questionnaires. Results were compared with those of 40 age- and sex-matched healthy comparison individuals.

Results.—Outcome with regard to full-scale IQ, perceptual reasoning, and the working memory scale was poorer in patients with CHD than in the comparison group (all $p \leq 0.001$). Visual perception, visuomotor integration ($p \leq 0.001$), and executive functions (Rey figure copy: $p = 0.05$) were also affected. Patients with CHD also had lower scores on all motor domains ($p < 0.02$) except static balance. Psychological adjustment was affected only in the 'peer relationship' domain ($p = 0.05$). Quality of life was similar to that of typically developing peers.

Interpretation.—Adolescents with CHD may manifest persistent cognitive and motor impairments, while psychological adjustment and self-reported HRQoL are mostly typical. Thus, long-term neurodevelopmental evaluations are necessary to provide early educational and therapeutic support.

► This observational study adds to the growing body of evidence that minor neurologic dysfunction occurs more frequently than severe disabilities in children who were born very low birth weight.[1] Moreover, it demonstrates that the majority of minor neuromotor dysfunctions identified in early childhood are still present at 10 years of age, suggesting that they are the result of neonatal neurologic injury rather than maturational delay. Motor coordination problems have a number of important consequences for a child. For instance, they may be associated with neurocognitive deficits such as visuomotor or visuoperceptual impairments and with learning difficulties.[2] In addition, slow motor speed can affect fine motor and graphomotor function and therefore can have a significant impact on school performance.[3] Moreover, motor problems have been associated with behavioral difficulties and behavioral disorders such as attention-deficit/hyperactivity disorder, as well as impaired social skills that may affect general well-being of the children.[4]

L. A. Papile, MD

References

1. Latal B. Prediction of neurodevelopmental outcome after preterm birth. *Pediatr Neurol.* 2009;40:413-419.
2. Seitz J, Jenni OG, Molinari L, Caflisch J, Largo RH, Latal Hajnal B. Correlations between motor performance and cognitive functions in children born <1250 g at school age. *Neuropediatrics.* 2006;37:6-12.
3. Smits-Engelsman BC, Niemeijer AS, van Galen GP. Fine motor deficiencies in children diagnosed as DCD based on poor grapho-motor ability. *Hum Mov Sci.* 2001; 20:161-182.
4. Lingam R, Golding J, Jongmans MJ, Hunt LP, Ellis M, Emond A. The association between developmental coordination disorder and other developmental traits. *Pediatrics.* 2010;126:e1109-e1118.

Tracheostomy for Infants Requiring Prolonged Mechanical Ventilation: 10 Years' Experience

Overman AE, Liu M, Kurachek SC, et al (Children's Hosps and Clinics of Minnesota, Minneapolis; Children's Respiratory and Critical Care Specialists, Minneapolis, MN; et al)
Pediatrics 131:e1491-e1496, 2013

Background.—Despite advances in care of critically ill neonates, extended mechanical ventilation and tracheostomy are sometimes required. Few studies focus on complications and clinical outcomes. Our aim was to provide long-term outcomes for a cohort of infants who required tracheostomy.

Methods.—This study is a retrospective review of 165 infants born between January 1, 2000 and December 31, 2010 who required tracheostomy and ventilator support. Children with complex congenital heart disease were excluded.

Results.—Median gestational age was 27 weeks (range 22–43), and birth weight was 820 g (range 360–4860). The number of male (53.9%) and female (46.1%) infants was similar ($P = .312$). Infants were divided into 2 groups based on birth weight ≤1000 g (A) and >1000 g

(B). Group A: 87 (57.6%) infants; group B 64 (42.4%). Overall tracheostomy rate was 6.9% (87/1345) for group A versus 0.9% (64/6818) for B ($P < .001$). Group A had a longer time from intubation to positive pressure ventilation independence, 505 days (range 62–1287) vs 372 days (range 15–1270; $P = .011$). Infants who had >1 reason for tracheostomy comprised 78.8% of the sample; 69.1% of infants were discharged on ventilators. Birth weight did not affect time from tracheostomy to decannulation ($P = .323$). More group A infants were decannulated ($P = .023$). laryngotracheal reconstruction rate was 35.8%. Five-year survival was 89%. Group B had higher mortality ($P = .033$). 64.2% of infants had developmental delays; 74.2% had ≥2 comorbidities.

Conclusions.—Tracheostomy rates were higher for extremely low birth weight infants than previously reported rates for all infants. Decannulation rates and laryngotracheal reconstruction rates were consistent with previous studies. Survival rates were high, but developmental delay and comorbidities were frequent.

▶ There is surprisingly little information available regarding the long-term outcome of infants who undergo tracheostomy while in the neonatal intensive care unit (NICU). In this retrospective observational study, the authors provide a descriptive report of the long-term outcomes for a cohort of infants who were discharged from Children's Hospitals and Clinics of Minnesota after tracheostomy placement.

Of the 8163 infants admitted to the NICU, 151 (1.8%) required tracheostomy, a rate similar to that reported previously.[1,2] However, infants who weighed less that 1000 grams at birth (extremely low birth weight; ELBW) were nearly 8 times as likely to require a tracheostomy compared with their heavier counterparts (6.9% vs 0.9%). Among the ELBW cohort, the primary reason for tracheostomy was bronchopulmonary dysplasia (95.4%). In comparison, heavier infants underwent tracheostomy for a variety of reasons, the majority of which related to congenital cardiac, airway, or pulmonary anomalies. These data indicate that the primary reason for tracheostomy has shifted away from airway obstruction to prolonged ventilation over the past 20 years. The longer time between intubation and either tracheostomy placement or decannulation in the ELBW cohort most likely reflects institutional practice of delaying tracheostomy until an infant is near a corrected age of 40 weeks.

Surprisingly, almost half of the ELBW cohort required laryngotracheal reconstruction (47.1%), whereas the rate among the heavier cohort was 25%, despite a higher rate of congenital anomalies in the latter group. The most common reason for laryngotracheal reconstruction was subglottic stenosis (75.9%). Because of the retrospective nature of the study, the validity of the neurodevelopmental data presented is uncertain. Most likely, the rate of development impairment is higher than that reported.

L. A. Papile, MD

References

1. Sidman JD, Jaguan A, Couser RJ. Tracheotomy and decannulation rates in a level 3 neonatal intensive care unit: a 12-year study. *Laryngoscope*. 2006;116:136-139.
2. Pereira KD, MacGregor AR, McDuffie CM, Mitchell RB. Tracheostomy in preterm infants: current trends. *Arch Otolaryngol Head Neck Surg*. 2003;129: 1268-1271.

Postnatal corticosteroids and neurodevelopmental outcomes in extremely low birthweight or extremely preterm infants: 15-year experience in Victoria, Australia

Cheong JL, Victorian Infant Collaborative Study Group (Royal Women's Hosp, Parkville, Victoria, Australia; et al)

Arch Dis Child Fetal Neonatal Ed 98:F32-F36, 2013

Objective.—Postnatal corticosteroids (PCS) are used to prevent or treat bronchopulmonary dysplasia (BPD) in extremely low birthweight (ELBW; <1000 g) or extremely preterm (EPT; <28 weeks) infants. In the early 2000s, concerns were raised about increased risks of cerebral palsy (CP) in association with PCS, which may have affected prescribing of PCS, and influenced rates of BPD, mortality or long-term neurosensory morbidity. Our aim was to determine the changes over time in the rates of PCS use and 2-year outcomes in ELBW/EPT infants in Victoria, Australia.

Design.—All ELBW or EPT infants born in Victoria, Australia in three distinct eras (1991–92, 1997 and 2005) who were alive at 7 days were included. Rates of PCS use, rates of BPD (oxygen dependency at 36 weeks' corrected age), death before 2 years of age, CP and major disability (any of moderate/severe CP, developmental quotient <–2 SD, blindness or deafness) were contrasted between cohorts.

Results.—The rate of PCS use and the dose prescribed diminished significantly in 2005 compared with earlier eras, but the rate of BPD rose. Non-significant changes in the rates of mortality over time were mirrored by non-significant changes in the rates of CP or major disability. Combined outcomes of mortality with either major disability or CP were similar over the three eras.

Conclusions.—PCS use decreased in 2005 compared with earlier eras, and was accompanied by a rise in BPD, with no significant changes in mortality or neurological morbidity.

▶ This study is yet another retrospective analysis of the relationship of postnatal corticosteroids (PCS) and neurodevelopmental outcome in extremely preterm infants. The authors hypothesized that the rate of PCS use would fall, the rates of bronchopulmonary dysplasia (BPD) and mortality would rise, and the rate of neurodevelopmental disability in survivors would fall over the 3 eras.

The rate of PCS use fell from 34.8% in the first epoch to 22.7% in the third epoch, as did the duration of treatment (27 vs 13.5 days). In addition, the median dexamethasone equivalent dose of PCS decreased from 7.7 mg/kg to

2.0 mg/kg. However, data regarding the rates of BPD and major disability reported in the abstract are somewhat misleading because they only reflect the outcome of infants who survived the first week after birth. Because the diagnosis of BPD was not made until 36 weeks' adjusted age, the diagnosis precluded infants who died before that time. If the competing outcomes of death and BPD are considered, the rate for BPD or death was similar in the 3 epochs (62%, 52%, and 59%), and there was a steady decline in the rate of death or major disability (56%, 50%, and 47%). Thus, it would appear that a decline in the use of PCS did not adversely affect the rate of BPD or death but rather was associated with an improvement in survival and neurodevelopmental outcome.

L. A. Papile, MD

Motor skills at 23 years of age in young adults born preterm with very low birth weight

Husby IM, Skranes J, Olsen A, et al (Norwegian Univ of Science and Technology, Trondheim, Norway)
Early Hum Dev 89:747-754, 2013

Background.—Motor skills have previously not been reported in young adults born with very low birth weight (VLBW), although they are commonly reported in children and adolescents.

Aim.—To compare fine and gross motor skills in VLBW young adults with matched term-born controls, and to study longitudinal changes in the VLBW group.

Study Design.—A geographically based follow-up study of a VLBW group and a control group.

Subjects.—Thirty-six VLBW (birth weight $\leq$ 1500 g) young adults, including four participants with cerebral palsy (CP), and 37 matched controls (birth weight $\geq$ 10th centile) were examined at 14 and 23 years of age.

Outcome Measures.—Fine and gross motor skills were assessed using Grooved Pegboard test (GP), Trail Making Test-5 (TMT-5), Movement Assessment Battery for Children-2 (Movement ABC-2) and High-level Mobility Assessment Tool (HiMAT).

Results.—VLBW young adults were slower than controls on GP ($p = 0.026$) and TMT-5 ($p < 0.001$). Mean total Movement ABC-2 score was 69.7 ± 20.2 in the VLBW group compared with 74.1 ± 14.4 in the control group ($p = 0.017$). Differences were also seen in manual dexterity and balance. Additionally, HiMAT showed reduced balance and speed in gross motor skills in the VLBW group. The proportion of participants with motor problems did not change between age 14 and 23. After exclusion of participants with CP, scores were essentially the same.

Conclusion.—VLBW young adults had overall poorer fine and gross motor skills compared with controls. Reduced speed seemed to be an underlying problem. Longitudinal findings indicate that VLBW children have not outgrown their motor problems when entering adulthood.

▶ Numerous studies have documented the prevalence of poor fine and gross motor skills from childhood through adolescence among children who were born either very preterm or very low birth weight (VLBW) and did not have cerebral palsy. The most pronounced motor problems were related to balance and manual dexterity. This study extends this observation of poor fine and gross motor skills through adulthood. When compared with results obtained previously at 14 years of age, the proportion of VLBW subjects with motor problems did not change between the 2 time periods; however, the proportion with poor performance with the nondominant hand was increased. Of particular interest was the finding that the low scores on tests of gross and fine motor skills were caused by failure to complete timed tests, rather than accuracy, suggesting that the general problem relates to motor speed. Poor manual dexterity combined with reduced motor speed may have a negative influence on computer typing and writing skills, which, in turn, can interfere with academic achievement and work success. The authors speculate that the poor motor speed and poor motor skills observed may be caused primarily by reduced connectivity in motor networks. Correlation of magnetic resonance imaging and motor outcomes in a cohort of very preterm or VLBW children who do not have cerebral palsy may help clarify this.

L. A. Papile, MD

15 Ethics

23andMe and the FDA

Annas GJ, Elias S (Boston Univ School of Public Health, MA; Northwestern Univ, Chicago, IL)

N Engl J Med 370:985-988, 2014

Background.—The Food and Drug Administration (FDA) has not yet determined how to govern direct-to-consumer (DTC) genetic testing. However, companies such as 23andMe have offered products such as the Saliva Collection Kit and Personal Genome Service (PGS) to consumers. Such products rely on single-nucleotide polymorphism (SNP) technology to identify genetic markers associated with hundreds of specific diseases and conditions. The stated goal is to inform people about their health and how to improve it. The 23andM3 campaign was halted by the FDA until PGS receives marketing authorization, but regulations for products such as PGS remain unclear.

Issues.—The debate weighs the concepts of medical (or government) paternalism against individuals' right to information about themselves. Direct patient access to medical records and test results has already been granted in other areas. It is likely that within the foreseeable future, most health plans will provide for members to have their entire genomes sequenced and linked to their electronic health records, with software available to help them understand what the genome profiles say, perhaps including consultation with a physician or genetic counselor. Currently the FDA and the National Institute of Standards and Technology are developing reference materials to fill the massive data bank this access will require. However, unless genomic tests are validated, the information gathered may be misleading or wrong, which could create harm rather than good. Often family history tells as much about a person's health risks as SNP-based testing. The FDA is therefore not depriving people of useful information but rather requiring that companies show their products are safe and effective–fulfilling their role of traditional consumer protection.

Privacy issues also arise. A person's private DNA information must be protected from individuals who might use it without the person's consent or make it available to others who could misuse it. An example would be releasing the information to deny someone life or disability insurance. Companies suggest that the massive collection of genetic information can be used and sold for medical research and discoveries. However, DNA donors must retain the right to consent to such a use and to maintain their privacy rights, both of which can be difficult to regulate reliably.

Informed Consent Protocols.—The American College of Medical Genetics and Genomics (ACMG) recommends that when a physician orders a clinical sequencing test, the laboratory should also test for pathogenic (or likely pathogenic) mutations in 56 genes, related to 24 serious disorders. Patients cannot opt out of the reporting of these findings to the clinician, which amounts to the patient waiving rights to decide what tests will be performed and who will receive the results. 23andMe offered customers a chance to not find out about the results of specific tests. Before whole-genome screening is widely performed, a more sophisticated informed consent protocol is needed so that individuals retain the right not to have specific genes sequenced.

Conclusions.—A regulatory framework for whole-genome-n-sequencing platforms is needed to manage the privacy and informed consent issues that arise. The clinical interpretation of an individual's genome and the formulation of useful recommendations to the consumer are essential. Genetic tests should improve patient health by providing accurate, clinically useful data that can inform patient decisions. Interpretation by a clinical geneticist or genetic counselor is needed to guide the application of genetic test results to clinical situations.

▶ This powerful commentary on the risks and benefits of genetic screening and the role of the Food and Drug Administration (FDA) highlights some of the ethical dilemmas facing the perinatal community as the genome screening becomes cheaper and more accessible to the public. "Whole-genome screening, whether ordered by physicians or consumers, will require more sophisticated informed-consent protocols, and we believe that individuals should also retain the right not to have specific genes sequenced at all."[1] Also as noted by the authors, "It seems reasonable to predict for example, that in the next decade or sooner, a majority of health plans will make it easy for their members to have their entire genomes sequenced and linked to their electronic health records and will provide software to help people interrogate their own genomes, with or without the help of their physicians or a genetic counselor supplied by the health plan. This service will, of course, require a massive data bank of genome reference materials, and the FDA and the National Institute of Standards and Technology are collaborating on the development of reference materials.[2,3] Before genomic tests have been validated, however, genomic information can be misleading—or just plain wrong—and could cause more harm than good in health care settings. In most cases, family history is likely to be at least as informative about an individual's health risks as single nucleotide polymorphism–based testing like that used by 23andMe." There will be troubled times before this is all sorted out. Genetics and the understanding of the genome is advancing at breakneck speed. There is an urgent need to slow down, gather the information, and make rational and thoughtful decisions that "will first do no harm."

A. A. Fanaroff, MD, FRCPE

References

1. Wolf SM, Annas GJ, Elias S. Point-counterpoint: patient autonomy and incidental findings in clinical genomics. *Science*. 2013;340:1049-1050.
2. Collins FS, Hamburg MA. First FDA authorization for next-generation sequencer. *N Engl J Med*. 2013;369:2369-2371.
3. Glantz L, Roche P, Annas GJ. Rules for donations to tissue banks—what next? *N Engl J Med*. 2008;358:298-303.

Views of parents and health-care providers regarding parental presence at bedside rounds in a neonatal intensive care unit

Grzyb MJ, Coo H, Rühland L, et al (Queen's Univ, Kingston, Ontario, Canada)
J Perinatol 34:143-148, 2014

Objective.—To examine the views of parents and health-care providers regarding parental presence during neonatal intensive care rounds.

Study Design.—Cross-sectional survey of parents whose children were admitted to a tertiary-care neonatal intensive care unit ($n = 81$). Medical trainees ($n = 67$) and nurses ($n = 28$) were also surveyed.

Result.—The majority of parents reported that attending rounds reduced their anxiety and increased their confidence in the health-care team. Nurses were more likely than medical trainees to support parental presence at rounds ($P = 0.02$). About three-quarters of medical trainees and nurses thought discussion is inhibited and 69% of trainees felt teaching is decreased when parents attend rounds.

Conclusion.—Most parents who attended rounds found the experience beneficial, but medical trainees' views were mixed. The positive impact on parents, and the learning opportunities created in family-centered care and communication when parents are present on rounds, should be highlighted for trainees and other neonatal intensive care personnel.

► It has always been a challenge to accomplish clinical decision making, communication with parents, and teaching (while maintaining compliance with Health Insurance Portability and Accountability Act in an open ward setting) during neonatal intensive care unit (NICU) rounds. This article reported the results of a survey in which parents, medical trainees, and nurses expressed their attitudes about the presence of parents during rounds in the NICU. Not surprisingly, parents thought it to be quite beneficial and improved their overall satisfaction and confidence. Medical trainees (residents and senior medical students) were less positive, feeling that parental presence inhibited teaching, whereas nurses were supportive of the concept.

Anecdotally, this has also been my own observation. In the era of family-centered care, parents are encouraged to be integral members of the health care team and to participate in decision making. Their attendance during rounds is essential to accomplish this, as well as to be able to ask medical or nursing questions of the neonatal team. As the study shows, demonstration of multidiscipline care and problem solving inspires confidence and may enhance both patient safety and satisfaction.

Part of the art of communication in this setting is making it clear when a teaching point is being made, perhaps by making an effort to explain this to the parents beforehand, that the attending or fellow is trying to make a point or two that are unrelated to the parents' baby but might need to be considered in similar situations. No parent wants to hear that the differential diagnosis of glucose intolerance might include pancreatic carcinoma, so not discussing it on rounds may miss a teaching opportunity. Prefacing this by saying, "this doesn't apply to your baby, but it's something the younger doctors need to know" can accomplish both.

In our own institution, introduction of single-room care has altered the parent-health care team interactions. One or both parents are more likely to be present on rounds. Discussion is more open because of privacy, and our rounding group is a bit smaller (and less intimidating) than it used to be before we split the service. It hasn't solved the trainee situation entirely, and it is entirely possible that some of the trainee insecurity is an outgrowth of the truncated hours that they now spend in the NICU.

S. M. Donn, MD

Medical interventions for children with trisomy 13 and trisomy 18: what is the value of a short disabled life?

Janvier A, Watkins A (Sainte-Justine Hosp Univ of Montreal, Quebec, Canada; Mercy Hosp for Women, Heidelberg, Melbourne, Victoria, Australia)

Acta Paediatr 102:1112-1117, 2013

Children with trisomy 13 and trisomy 18 (T13 or T18) have low survival rates, and survivors have significant disabilities. Life saving interventions (LSIs) are generally not recommended by many healthcare providers (HCPs). After a diagnosis of T13 or T18, many parents chose termination of pregnancy or comfort care at birth, but others consider treatment to prolong the lives of their children. While LSIs may be effective at prolonging the life of some children, the quality of life of survivors and the possible burden on the family may be considered negatively by HCP, which may lead to conflicts with families. Resource allocation considerations are often invoked to withhold LSI for T13 or T18 even though they are seldom mentioned for older patients with comparable outcomes.

Conclusion.—We should strive to improve communication with parents by 1. Investigating these conditions further to be able to better inform parents and 2. Providing balanced information for families and personalised care for each child.

▶ This commentary by 2 neonatologists well known for their thoughtful writings on ethical issues in perinatal medicine apparently was inspired by a short article in the same journal issue, in which 3 health professionals describe experiences when their own babies were found to have trisomy 13 or 18. We can hope that they are not representative, but those short anecdotes leave no room for doubt that as providers of perinatal care, we are still failing mothers of babies with these conditions much too often. As these mothers report:

"We sought support and information to make the best decisions for our babies. Regrettably our carefully made, reasonable goals were met with opposition or disrespected, compounding our grief and diminishing the joy of the brief time we had with our children. The medical care we requested was not selfish, nor without benefit to our children. Unfortunately, we discovered that, for some healthcare professionals, the standards of 'respect' and 'shared decision-making' are trumped by a 'one-size-fits-all' approach for trisomy babies."[1]

In those instances, the common theme was denial of access to medical interventions, but the "one-size-fits-all" descriptor may apply equally to insistence on maximal medical interventions without respect to parents' wishes or thoughtful articulation of the specific benefits to be obtained for a particular child. The plea here is not for any unitary prescription for care of these babies but for a collaborative decision-making process that respects the individuality of each child and family. Both articles offer practical suggestions for pursuit of that objective. Barriers include several misapprehensions or incorrect assumptions that flavor thinking and discussions about these matters. First, there is a difference between what is permissible and what is mandated or prohibited. For example, the Neonatal Resuscitation Program advice that "noninitiation of resuscitation may be appropriate" is not the same as "resuscitation measures are never appropriate" for affected infants. Second, the observation that some children with trisomy 13 or 18 live comfortably for years must not be taken to indicate that this outcome can be achieved in all or most by aggressive medical interventions. Conversely, there is little information to guide selective medical interventions, because the assumption that they will be ineffective has precluded asking the question of whether they may be on occasion. Corrective heart surgery (for example) will do nothing to ameliorate intractable seizures or life-threatening episodes of central apnea but may enhance comfort or prolong life. Third, perspectives on utility and futility often differ greatly between parents and providers. Health care providers often profoundly underestimate the meaning that parents attach to these infants and how much love they feel for them, failing to appreciate the value of the time they may get to have with their babies. As a group of professionals, we clearly have much to learn about approaching these babies and their families with humility, compassion, balance, and commitment to individualized management. These two articles are essential reading for all who participate in their care.

W. E. Benitz, MD

Reference

1. Thiele P, Berg SF, Farlow B. More than a diagnosis. *Acta Paediatr.* 2013;102: 1127-1129.

End-of-life care in Toronto neonatal intensive care units: challenges for physician trainees

El Sayed MF, Chan M, McAllister M, et al (The Hosp for Sick Children, Toronto, Ontario, Canada)

Arch Dis Child Fetal Neonatal Ed 98:F528-F533, 2013

Background.—Physician trainees in neonatology can find it extremely challenging to care for patients from diverse linguistic and multicultural backgrounds. This challenge is particularly highlighted when difficult and ethically challenging end-of-life (EOL) decision-making with parents is required. While these interactions are an opportunity for growth and learning, they also have the potential to lead to misunderstanding and uncertainty and can add to trainees' insecurity, unpreparedness and stress when participating in such interactions.

Objectives.—To explore the challenges for trainees when EOL decisions are undertaken and to encourage them to reflect on how they might influence such decision-making.

Design and Interview.—An in-depth, semi-structured interview guide was developed: the interview questions address trainees' beliefs, attitudes, preferences and expectations regarding discussions of EOL neonatal care. Twelve interviews were completed and the audio records transcribed verbatim, after removal of identifying personal information.

Results.—Participants identified six domains of challenge in EOL care: withdrawal of life-sustaining treatment based on poor outcome, explaining 'no resuscitation options' to parents, clarifying 'do not resuscitate (DNR)' orders, empowering families with knowledge and shared decision-making, dealing with different cultures and managing personal internal conflict. Participants experienced the most difficulty during the initial stages of training and eventually reported good knowledge of the EOL care process. They had a sense of security and confidence working within a multidisciplinary care team, which includes experienced nursing staff as well as bereavement and palliative care coordinator within the neonatal intensive care unit.

Conclusions.—The challenges experienced by physician trainees when providing EOL care can serve as focal points for improving EOL educational programmes for neonatal fellowship training.

▶ This article summarizes the important challenges to fellows caring for seriously ill and dying neonates in Toronto. This important study effectively emphasizes the role of guided experience in helping physicians in training develop both skills and confidence. El Sayed and colleagues analyzed the detailed interviews of 12 senior-level fellows who expressed significant concerns regarding issues common to stressful areas of decision making and family support in neonatology practice.

The authors suggest that experience in end-of-life care helps promote confidence in these professionals' abilities to handle the practical, ethical, and emotional challenges involved in key areas: withholding and withdrawal of life-sustaining technologies, explaining and clarifying orders to limit escalation of care, and negotiating shared decision making. Each of these areas presented extra challenges when occurring in families from different cultures. The authors conclude that experience alone may not be enough. They propose that curricula be developed to help prepare trainees earlier in their professional development to alleviate provider stress and to achieve better outcomes for infants, families, and the professionals who care for them.

Promising models of such curricula are being tested and disseminated, although important downstream outcomes resulting from such training (family satisfaction, relief of infant suffering) are yet to be effectively shown. Online resources can be very helpful and continue to be downloaded, adapted, and implemented.

- The Initiative for Pediatric Palliative Care has an online end-of-life curriculum available at www.ippcweb.org
- The End-of-Life Nursing Education Consortium provides resources directed at nurses but can be used effectively for multidisciplinary learning. Web site is www.aacn.nche.edu/elnec/
- The Center to Advance Palliative Care provides tools and training tips on its Web site www.capc.org
- Workshops in End-of-Life Care for Professionals in Children's Hospitals is an open-source program available on a University of Michigan Web site. End-of-life training using this site's learning objectives, curricula, videos, and handouts has been a part of the Pediatric Academic Society's annual meeting "required curriculum for fellows" since 2012. These resources are available at www.open.umich.edu/education/med/resources/palliative-care/2010

As curricula, training models, and care pathways continue to be developed, implemented, and tested, Dr El Sayed's study adds weight to the importance of these initiatives.

K. Pituch, MD

Lack of physician-patient communication as a key factor associated with malpractice litigation in neonatal brachial plexus palsy

Domino J, McGovern C, Chang KWC, et al (Wayne State Univ, Detroit, MI; Univ of Michigan, Ann Arbor)

J Neursurg Pediatr 13:238-242, 2014

Object.—Perinatal disorders are prone to malpractice litigation. Neonatal brachial plexus palsy (NBPP) results from stretching the nerves in the perinatal period and may lead to paresis or paralysis and sensory loss in the affected arm. Little is known about the key factors associated with malpractice litigation by families of patients with NBPP and whether these factors reflect the practice environment or are inherent to the condition. In this study, the authors documented the percentage of families of

NBPP patients at a specialty center that had filed a malpractice suit and described the key factors associated with that pursuit of legal action.

Methods.—The families/caregivers of 51 patients with NBPP who had presented to the University of Michigan Interdisciplinary Brachial Plexus Program participated in this study. A qualitative research design was applied using both a questionnaire to examine psychosocial factors and a dynamic tool to measure health outcomes from the patient perspective via parent proxy (Patient-Reported Outcomes Measurement Information System [PROMIS] assessment instruments). Statistical analysis included the Fisher exact test, chi-square test, and Student t-test. The study protocol was approved by the University of Michigan institutional review board.

Results.—Forty-seven percent of the families pursued malpractice litigation. In comparing patient families that had pursued legal action with those that had not, significant differences were revealed in the perception that the sustained birth injury was unnecessary ($p = 0.002$), the information received in the perinatal period was inadequate ($p = 0.003$), family concerns were ignored in the perinatal period ($p = 0.005$), and family concerns were not adequately addressed ($p < 0.001$). Sixty-six percent of the families received external advice to pursue legal action. The PROMIS survey revealed significant group differences in depressive symptoms ($p = 0.008$), fatigue ($p = 0.02$), pain ($p = 0.01$), and anger ($p = 0.004$). In contrast, the extent of NBPP was not associated with malpractice litigation ($p = 0.18$). Age, sex, and race were not significantly different between litigation and nonlitigation groups.

Conclusions.—Physician-controllable factors, such as communication in the perinatal period, are associated with malpractice litigation in NBPP. The perceived level of global disability may affect the pursuit of malpractice litigation, whereas the isolated extent of nerve root involvement and/or upper extremity dysfunction are not significant factors in pursuing litigation. Identifying and ameliorating these factors within the practice environment may decrease the animosity between families and health care providers and improve overall outcome for patients with NBPP.

▶ The single biggest problem in communication is the illusion that it has taken place.

—George Bernard Shaw

Communication is at the heart of the physician-patient relationship. Yet when an adverse outcome occurs, physicians often find it very difficult to have an honest conversation with the family. Families are understandably concerned, often angry, and want answers that may be difficult to provide. Clinicians may be embarrassed or ashamed, or feel inadequately trained and prepared to have such conversations. Additionally, they often fear a lawsuit.

Yet, there is both an ethical and legal obligation to be honest with parents. Honesty and integrity form the basis for the American Medical Association Code of Medical Ethics and are at the heart of professionalism. Legally, the Joint Commission has mandated open disclosure of unanticipated outcomes during patient care,[1] and in Pennsylvania hospitals are required to notify parents of minors in writing within 7 days of a serious event.[2]

In this article, Domino et al showed that "a breakdown in physician-patient appears to be a key factor associated with the pursuit of malpractice litigation by families of children with NBPP [Neonatal Brachial Plexus Palsy]." The study site is a specialty referral center for neonatal brachial plexus palsy. Thus, all study patients have the same basic condition, and the authors are then able to compare those families who filed a malpractice lawsuit with those who did not. This is a unique perspective compared with most malpractice literature that only looks at families who have already filed a lawsuit.

Interestingly, the degree of injury did not correlate with the decision to pursue litigation. Rather, a perception by the family that they did not receive adequate information in the perinatal period or that their concerns were ignored were significantly associated with a decision to file a lawsuit. The study takes place at a single center and with 51 patients is relatively small. By directly addressing families' concerns and helping them to understand their child's injuries, however, a physician will not only be fulfilling their ethical and legal professional obligations but may very well be decreasing the risk of being named in a malpractice lawsuit.

J. M. Fanaroff, MD, JD

References

1. Joint Commission on Accreditation of Healthcare Organizations, Standard RI.1.2.2. Accessed July 1, 2001.
2. Pa. Stat. Ann. Tit. 40 §1303.308.

Facing Persistent Challenges in Pediatric Decision-Making: New Hastings Center Guidelines

Berlinger N, Barfield R, Fleischman AR (The Hastings Ctr, Garrison, NY; Duke Univ, Durham, NC; Albert Einstein College of Medicine, Bronx, NY)
Pediatrics 132:789-791, 2013

Background.—Compared to 2.5 million total deaths, the 50,000 deaths of pediatric patients in the United States may seem insignificant but they have a significant impact on both the families and the clinicians involved. Challenges facing pediatric clinicians include a significant lack of knowledge about ethical and legal issues, concerns of conscience when providing end-of-life care, and tension among team members about how to provide appropriate care. Relevant issues related to ethics guidelines were discussed.

Best Interests.—The role of surrogate decision-maker can be psychologically stressful for clinicians in any end-of-life situation, but with a patient too young to have formed values it is especially difficult. Parents and guardians may help to inform clinicians' decisions. Even very young children can have strongly expressed preferences about what they like or don't like, especially when their lives have been spent dealing with chronic illness and medical interventions. Continually discussing patient preferences helps all parties understand who the child is and how he or she could be helped or hurt by a proposed course of action. The discussion must include the impact of treatment on the child's experiences of living. Electronic media, which are often a primary means for communication for young patients, offer decision-making tools that may engage them and help clarify preferences. The setting must also be patient-centered and respectful of the child and the effects of treatment. Seeing things from the patient's perspective may be especially important with older children or adolescents, but the clinician must also be mindful that a patient may be unable to understand all the consequences of a choice. Parents must also be helped to cope with the reality of a child's worsening condition. Patience, time, and strong communication skills are essential. Clinicians may also seek out ethics professionals or family social workers on the health care team.

Preventing Suffering.—Both curative and palliative medicine approaches are used for pediatric patients from diagnosis onward. Palliative medicine and nursing provide optimal support for pain and symptom management. Professionals can confidently promise to provide expert management of the child's pain and symptoms, even if the prognosis is uncertain. Palliative modalities should be explained in terms of their benefits for the child, reassuring parents that the child will always be cared for. The child's access to pain and symptom relief should not depend on an individual physician's willingness to collaborate with palliative care colleagues or subjective judgment about when these individuals should be included in the care plan.

Teamwork Issues.—During handoff procedures, new team members should be informed of all previously documented decisions and preferences and prepared to support them. Teams must also be given the opportunity to discuss concerns or differences in perceptions or values. If left unaddressed, these differences can sabotage the care plan.

Conclusions.—The newborn intensive care unit (NICU) is often an end-of-life setting, since over half of all pediatric deaths occur in the first year of life. Good NICU care includes the use of life-saving and life-sustaining technologies as well as end-of-life interventions. Family-centered approaches should prioritize family preferences and values in making decisions involving premature infants. Among the practical steps clinician educators can take to support professional and family caregivers are modeling good care, sharing information about care innovations, and integrating reflection about caring for children into clinical tasks. It is often difficult for parents to forgo curative interventions even when a child is near the end of life. New and innovative health policies, including hospice services, may promote better care in these situations. The Physician Orders for Life-Sustaining Treatment model helps in documenting patient preferences as portable medical orders and may be used for chronically ill children who are cared for primarily at home. Pediatric clinicians may have difficulty talking about hospice or forgoing life-sustaining treatment for pediatric patients. Moral distress is common, but the continuing integration of palliative care and expertise in communication into pediatric settings may help. Health care professionals who care for seriously ill children and their families may need opportunities to reflect on the personal experience of dealing with these issues and handling the intensive emotions that arise with the loss of a pediatric patient.

▶ As someone who frequently provides end-of-life care to neonates and often answers the phone when calls to ethics committee come in about dying children in our hospital, I am often reminded of how hard it is for many of us to care for these kids. Across the pediatric subspecialties, many of us will find ourselves caring for children with devastating and tragic illnesses, acute and chronic, that burden and shorten their lives. Regardless of our comfort and experience in looking after these patients (and their parents), we all find ourselves embroiled in those cases that weigh us down, give us gray hairs, and wonder how on earth we're going to help these people. This article gives us exactly what we need when it comes to embracing our responsibilities as compassionate and competent providers of end-of-life care to infants, children, and adolescents. It is laid out in such a simple and straightforward manner that one might miss that these issues are complicated and distressing—it's nice to get a reminder that we're all capable of doing this well, if we just take the time and effort to think critically about the issues.

What I like about this article is that it empowers us to tackle these tough cases, to face our own fears and biases, and to work to improve the systems and institutions that deliver end-of-life care to dying children. The burden is on us to understand the ethics, context, and procedural roadblocks such that we can recognize and meet the needs of pediatric patients at the end of their lives. The article also addresses some issues that don't seem to get as much press these days. With all due respect to great strides we've made in recognizing the role of parents, siblings, and extended families in the care of sick children, the authors take a rather brave position in affirming the importance of individual patients' interests and preferences, which sometimes seem to get lost in the oft-invoked "family-centered care" model. The authors also tackle dicey issues such as long-standing tensions between intensive care providers and palliative care teams, the complications of the shift-based health care model and accompanying handoffs, and the importance of recognizing and managing moral distress. Leave it all on the field, but don't forget to rehydrate.

N. Laventhal, MD, MA

Is Treatment Futile for an Extremely Premature Infant With Giant Omphalocele?

Feltman D, Stokes T, Kett J, et al (Evanston Hosp, IL; Walter Reed Med Ctr, Bethesda, MD; Seattle Children's Hosp, WA; et al)
Pediatrics 133:123-128, 2014

Doctors have no ethical obligation to provide futile treatment. This has been true since the time of Hippocrates who warned physicians not to treat patients who were "overmastered by their disease." This principle remains valid today but, as the Society for Critical Care Medicine notes, it is difficult to identify treatment as absolutely futile in all but a few clinical situations. Far more common, they note, are "treatments that are extremely unlikely to be beneficial, are extremely costly, or are of uncertain benefit." These, they say, "may be considered inappropriate and hence inadvisable, but should not be labeled futile." So what should doctors do when they have a case that seems close to the futility threshold but does not, perhaps, quite cross it? In such cases, is it appropriate to make unilateral decisions to withhold life-sustaining treatment even if the family objects? Or should treatment be provided knowing that it might cause pain and suffering to an infant with no likelihood of benefit? To address these questions, we present a case of an extremely premature infant with a giant omphalocele and ask 3 neonatologists, Dr Dalia Feltman of Evanston Hospital, Dr Theophil Stokes of the Walter Reed Medical Center, and Dr Jennifer Kett, a neonatologist and fellow in bioethics at Seattle Children's Hospital, to comment.

► In Greek mythology, Sisyphus was a man doomed to spend eternity rolling a boulder up a hill, at which point it would roll down again, and he would have to start all over again. To some this may be the definition of futility, a concept that has been "debated in the medical community with a vehemence that few philosophical concepts elicit."[1]

This article uses an "ethics rounds" format to discuss whether intervention should be provided for a 25-week preemie with a giant omphalocele. The parents, aware and prepared for the giant omphalocele but with no previous counseling regarding extreme prematurity, become angry and upset when told that resuscitation in this situation would be "futile." They demand treatment and threaten to call a lawyer. What should the neonatologist do in this situation?

The 3 commentators all bring a different perspective and approach to the same difficult and tragic situation. Would aggressively treating this infant violate the Hippocratic injunction not to do so to patients who are "overmastered by their disease?"[2] Or is this case, as the authors elegantly state, close to the futility threshold without quite crossing the line, in which case it may be "reasonable to support the family's strong desire to attempt resuscitation." There may be no single right answer to these difficult ethical dilemmas. One absolute, however, is to always listen to the parents, determine their level of understanding of the situation and their desires, and ultimately maintain a humane, compassionate, and patient-centered approach to these families at all times.

J. M. Fanaroff, MD, JD

References

1. Helft PR, Siegler M, Lantos J. The rise and fall of the futility movement. *N Engl J Med.* 2000;343:293-296.
2. *Oath of Hippocrates.* Scientific Papers: Physiology, Medicine, Surgery, Geology. Harvard Classics, vol 38. Boston, MA: P.F. Collier and Son; 1910:3.

Ethical and legal aspects of noninvasive prenatal genetic diagnosis

Dickens BM (Univ of Toronto, Canada)

Int J Gynaecol Obstet 124:181-184, 2014

The new technology that will allow genetic testing of a fetus within the first trimester of pregnancy by isolating cell-free fetal DNA (cffDNA) in the mother's blood raises a range of ethical and legal issues. Considered noninvasive, this test is safe and reliable, and may avoid alternative genetic testing by amniocentesis or chorionic villus sampling, which risks causing spontaneous abortion. Ethical and legal issues of cffDNA testing will become more acute if testing expands to fetal whole-genome sequencing. Critical issues include the state of the science or diagnostic art; the appropriateness of offering the test; the implications of denying the test when it is available and appropriate; disclosure and counseling following test results; and management of patients' choices on acquiring test results. A challenge will be providing patients with appropriate counseling based on up-to-date genetic knowledge, and accommodating informed patients' legal choices.

▶ Cassandra is one of the more tragic figures in Greek mythology. The powerful deity Apollo, enamored by her beauty, gave her the power to see the future. When she spurned his advances, however, he made her powerless to change it. Is genetic testing of fetuses and neonates analogous to a Cassandra situation? Newborn screening has been the focus of a vigorous moral debate in the past several years as programs have expanded significantly without clear evidence of benefit and a multitude of concerns that have led the President's Council on Bioethics to conclude that the benefits of screening may be "outweighed by the potential harms.[1] These harms range from the challenge of informed consent to fears of discriminatory Eugenics, where parents may screen embryos so that their child will have blue eyes.

The article by Dickens provides an overview of the myriad ethical and legal issues surrounding noninvasive prenatal genetic diagnosis, one of the newer forms of prenatal testing. Of course, genetic screening during pregnancies is not new. With cell-free fetal DNA (cffDNA) testing, however, the era of safe, inexpensive, whole-gene sequencing of a fetus may be rapidly approaching, with the consequent risk of "trivializing a procedure that might compel exceptionally difficult decisions to be made, with lifelong consequences." For example, parents are generally not allowed to test their children for Huntington disease, a lethal disorder that does not manifest until adulthood. Should such information be disclosed through cffDNA? As is often seen with new technologies, the article raises more questions than answers. But raising the questions is an important first step to ensure that, as President's Commission Chairman Edmund Pellegrino notes, "the future benefits of new techniques to expand our knowledge ... will be facilitated in an ethically sensitive way."[1]

J. M. Fanaroff, MD, JD

Reference

1. *The Changing Moral Focus of Newborn Screening*. Washington, DC: The President's Council on Bioethics; 2008.

Article Index

Chapter 1: The Fetus

Conservative management of antenatally diagnosed cystic lung malformations 1

Absent Fetal Nasal Bone: What Does it Mean for the Euploid Fetus? 2

Chapter 2: Epidemiology and Pregnancy Complications

The Effect of Real-Time Continuous Glucose Monitoring in Pregnant Women With Diabetes: A randomized controlled trial 5

Impact of ART on pregnancies in California: an analysis of maternity outcomes and insights into the added burden of neonatal intensive care 7

Amnioinfusion in very early preterm prelabor rupture of membranes (AMIPROM): pregnancy, neonatal and maternal outcomes in a randomized controlled pilot study 8

EXPRESS study shows significant regional differences in 1-year outcome of extremely preterm infants in Sweden 10

Outcomes of Infants Born at 22 and 23 Weeks' Gestation 12

Antecedents of Cerebral Palsy and Perinatal Death in Term and Late Preterm Singletons 14

Claims for compensation after alleged birth asphyxia: a nationwide study covering 15 years 15

Assisted reproductive technologies impair the expression and methylation of insulin-induced gene 1 and sterol regulatory element-binding factor 1 in the fetus and placenta 16

Chapter 3: Genetics and Teratology

DNA Sequencing versus Standard Prenatal Aneuploidy Screening 19

Minor Anomalies: Can They Predict Specific Major Defects? A Study Based on 23 Major and 14 Minor Anomalies in Over 25,000 Newborns with Birth Defects 21

Fetal DNA Methylation Associates with Early Spontaneous Preterm Birth and Gestational Age 22

Analysis of epigenetic changes in survivors of preterm birth reveals the effect of gestational age and evidence for a long term legacy 23

Neonatal Genome-Wide Methylation Patterns in Relation to Birth Weight in the Norwegian Mother and Child Cohort 25

Additional value of prenatal genomic array testing in fetuses with isolated structural ultrasound abnormalities and a normal karyotype: a systematic review of the literature 26

Anomalies associated with gastroschisis and omphalocele: Analysis of 2825 cases from the Texas Birth Defects Registry 27

Accuracy of Ultrasonography at 11–14 Weeks of Gestation for Detection of Fetal Structural Anomalies: A Systematic Review 29

Chapter 4: Labor and Delivery

Triggers of Spontaneous Preterm Delivery – Why Today? 31

Behavioural, educational and respiratory outcomes of antenatal betamethasone for term caesarean section (ASTECS trial) 32

The effect of obstetric practice change to reduce early term delivery on perinatal outcome 33

Immersion in Water During Labor and Delivery 34

Effect of Delayed vs Early Umbilical Cord Clamping on Iron Status and Neurodevelopment at Age 12 Months: A Randomized Clinical Trial 35

The effects of umbilical cord milking in extremely preterm infants: a randomized controlled trial 37

Rapid target allopurinol concentrations in the hypoxic fetus after maternal administration during labour 38

Vaginal delivery versus caesarean section in preterm breech delivery: a systematic review 40

Resuscitation intensity at birth is associated with changes in brain metabolic development in preterm neonates 41

Terminal Fetal Heart Decelerations and Neonatal Outcomes 43

Delay in intervention increases neonatal morbidity in births monitored with cardiotocography and ST-waveform analysis 45

The impact of introducing universal umbilical cord blood gas analysis and lactate measurement at delivery 46

Training Neonatal Cardiopulmonary Resuscitation: Can It Be Improved by Playing a Musical Prompt? A Pilot Study 48

Improving Delivery Room Management for Very Preterm Infants 49

Perinatal outcomes for extremely preterm babies in relation to place of birth in England: the EPICure 2 study 51

Selected perinatal outcomes associated with planned home births in the United States 52

Chapter 5: Infectious Disease and Immunology

Stratification of Risk of Early-Onset Sepsis in Newborns ≥34 Weeks' Gestation 55

Effect of Fluconazole Prophylaxis on Candidiasis and Mortality in Premature Infants: A Randomized Clinical Trial 57

Using vaginal Group B *Streptococcus* colonisation in women with preterm premature rupture of membranes to guide the decision for immediate delivery: a secondary analysis of the PPROMEXIL trials 59

Maternal Antibody at Delivery Protects Neonates From Early Onset Group B Streptococcal Disease 60

Impact of Perinatal Practices for Early-onset Group B Streptococcal Disease Prevention 61

The microbiota regulates neutrophil homeostasis and host resistance to *Escherichia coli* K1 sepsis in neonatal mice 63

Probiotic Effects on Late-onset Sepsis in Very Preterm Infants: A Randomized Controlled Trial 65

Toll-like receptor genetic variants are associated with gram-negative infections in VLBW infants 67

Neutrophil CD64 for Daily Surveillance of Systemic Infection and Necrotizing Enterocolitis in Preterm Infants 68

Concurrent Bloodstream Infections in Infants with Necrotizing Enterocolitis 71

Chapter 6: Cardiovascular System

A randomised placebo-controlled trial of early treatment of the patent ductus arteriosus 73

Comparison of Oral Paracetamol versus Ibuprofen in Premature Infants with Patent Ductus Arteriosus: A Randomized Controlled Trial 74

Oral Paracetamol versus Oral Ibuprofen in the Management of Patent Ductus Arteriosus in Preterm Infants: A Randomized Controlled Trial 76

Hypotension in Preterm Neonates: Low Blood Pressure Alone Does Not Affect Neurodevelopmental Outcome 77

Use of Antihypotensive Therapies in Extremely Preterm Infants 79

Targeted neonatal echocardiography (TnECHO) service in a Canadian neonatal intensive care unit: a 4-year experience 80

Pulse oximetry screening for critical congenital heart defects in newborn infants: Should it be routine? 81

Late Detection of Critical Congenital Heart Disease Among US Infants: Estimation of the Potential Impact of Proposed Universal Screening Using Pulse Oximetry 83

Cardiovascular function in children who had chronic lung disease of prematurity 86

Unilateral Vocal Fold Paralysis After Congenital Cardiothoracic Surgery: A Meta-analysis 87

Chapter 7: Respiratory Disorders

Effects of Targeting Higher vs Lower Arterial Oxygen Saturations on Death or Disability in Extremely Preterm Infants: A Randomized Clinical Trial 89

Respiratory Outcomes of the Surfactant Positive Pressure and Oximetry Randomized Trial (SUPPORT) 91

Oxygen Saturation and Outcomes in Preterm Infants 92

Oxygen Saturation and Outcomes in Preterm Infants 94

Temporal quantification of oxygen saturation ranges: an effort to reduce hyperoxia in the neonatal intensive care unit 95

Transcribed oxygen saturation vs oximeter recordings in very low birth weight infants 97

Reducing Unplanned Extubations in the NICU 98

Comparative effectiveness of surfactant preparations in premature infants 99

Surfactant Deficiency in Infants with Severe Acute Viral Bronchiolitis 101

A Randomized Controlled Trial of Two Nasal Continuous Positive Airway Pressure Levels after Extubation in Preterm Infants 102

Heliox for mechanically ventilated newborns with bronchopulmonary dysplasia 104

Impact of early surfactant and inhaled nitric oxide therapies on outcomes in term/late preterm neonates with moderate hypoxic respiratory failure 106

Tracheomegaly in Infants with Severe Congenital Diaphragmatic Hernia Treated with Fetal Endoluminal Tracheal Occlusion 107

Extracorporeal Life Support in Patients with Congenital Diaphragmatic Hernia: How Long Should We Treat? 108

Fetal growth restriction and pulmonary hypertension in premature infants with bronchopulmonary dysplasia 109

Variation in the Use of Diuretic Therapy for Infants With Bronchopulmonary Dysplasia 111

Death or Neurodevelopmental Impairment at 18 to 22 Months Corrected Age in a Randomized Trial of Early Dexamethasone to Prevent Death or Chronic Lung Disease in Extremely Low Birth Weight Infants 112

Association between Postnatal Dexamethasone for Treatment of Bronchopulmonary Dysplasia and Brain Volumes at Adolescence in Infants Born Very Preterm 114

Mesenchymal Stem Cells for Bronchopulmonary Dysplasia: Phase 1 Dose-Escalation Clinical Trial 115

Late Outcomes of a Randomized Trial of High-Frequency Oscillation in Neonates 116

Accurate Automated Apnea Analysis in Preterm Infants 118

Application of Transcutaneous Carbon Dioxide Tension Monitoring with Low Electrode Temperatures in Premature Infants in the Early Postnatal Period 119

Test–retest reliability of the infant car-seat challenge 120

Two-Year Outcomes of a Randomized Controlled Trial of Inhaled Nitric Oxide in Premature Infants 121

Chapter 8: Central Nervous System and Special Senses

Intraventricular Hemorrhage and Neurodevelopmental Outcomes in Extreme Preterm Infants 125

Risk Factors for Intraventricular Hemorrhage in Term Asphyxiated Newborns Treated With Hypothermia 127

Can neurophysiological assessment improve timing of intervention in posthaemorrhagic ventricular dilatation? 128

Cerebral desaturations in preterm infants: a crossover trial on influence of oxygen saturation target range 129

Neuroimaging in the Evaluation of Neonatal Encephalopathy 130

Neuroimaging in the Evaluation of Neonatal Encephalopathy 132

Xenon Ventilation During Therapeutic Hypothermia in Neonatal Encephalopathy: A Feasibility Study 133

Predictive value of the amplitude integrated EEG in infants with hypoxic ischaemic encephalopathy: data from a randomised trial of therapeutic hypothermia 134

Acute neonatal encephalopathy and seizures recurrence: A combined aEEG/EEG study 136

Factors Associated with Permanent Hearing Impairment in Infants Treated with Therapeutic Hypothermia 137

Anticonvulsant effect of xenon on neonatal asphyxial seizures 139

Moderate and Late Preterm Birth: Effect on Brain Size and Maturation at Term-Equivalent Age 140

Association between Postnatal Dexamethasone for Treatment of Bronchopulmonary Dysplasia and Brain Volumes at Adolescence in Infants Born Very Preterm 141

Association between Postnatal Dexamethasone for Treatment of Bronchopulmonary Dysplasia and Brain Volumes at Adolescence in Infants Born Very Preterm 142

Human milk feeding prevents retinopathy of prematurity (ROP) in preterm VLBW neonates 144

Ophthalmologic Outcome at 30 Months' Corrected Age of a Prospective Swedish Cohort of Children Born Before 27 Weeks of Gestation: The Extremely Preterm Infants in Sweden Study 146

Neonatal stroke: a review of the current evidence on epidemiology, pathogenesis, diagnostics and therapeutic options 148

Alterations in Brain Structure and Neurodevelopmental Outcome in Preterm Infants Hospitalized in Different Neonatal Intensive Care Unit Environments 149

Chapter 9: Gastrointestinal Health and Nutrition

Gut microbiota in preterm infants: assessment and relevance to health and disease 153

Intestinal epithelial cell apoptosis and loss of barrier function in the setting of altered microbiota with enteral nutrient deprivation 154

Three Main Factors Define Changes in Fecal Microbiota Associated With Feeding Modality in Infants 157

Milk oligosaccharide sialyl(α2,3)lactose activates intestinal CD11c$^+$ cells through TLR4 158

Effects of Different Complementary Feeding Regimens on Iron Status and Enteric Microbiota in Breastfed Infants 160

Fecal S100A12: Identifying Intestinal Distress in Very-Low-Birth-Weight Infants 161

Secretory antibodies in breast milk promote long-term intestinal homeostasis by regulating the gut microbiota and host gene expression 163

Epigenetic Effects of Human Breast Milk 165

A Pacifier-Activated Music Player With Mother's Voice Improves Oral Feeding in Preterm Infants 166

A Pacifier-Activated Music Player With Mother's Voice Improves Oral Feeding in Preterm Infants 168

Randomized Trial of Exclusive Human Milk versus Preterm Formula Diets in Extremely Premature Infants 169

Randomized Trial of Exclusive Human Milk versus Preterm Formula Diets in Extremely Premature Infants 171

Effect of Fortifiers and Additional Protein on the Osmolarity of Human Milk: Is It Still Safe for the Premature Infant? 173

Variability in human milk composition: benefit of individualized fortification in very-low-birth-weight infants 175

A standardized nutrition approach for very low birth weight neonates improves outcomes, reduces cost and is not associated with increased rates of necrotizing enterocolitis, sepsis or mortality 177

Cohort Study of Probiotics in a North American Neonatal Intensive Care Unit 179

Randomized controlled trial of prophylactic rectal stimulation and enemas on stooling patterns in extremely low birth weight infants 180

Epidemiology and Trends of Necrotizing Enterocolitis in Sweden: 1987–2009 182

Abnormal heart rate characteristics before clinical diagnosis of necrotizing enterocolitis 183

Association of cord blood digitalis-like factor and necrotizing enterocolitis 184

Brain Magnetic Resonance Imaging in Infants with Surgical Necrotizing Enterocolitis or Spontaneous Intestinal Perforation versus Medical Necrotizing Enterocolitis 185

Intestinal location of necrotizing enterocolitis among infants with congenital heart disease 187

Cronobacter: an emerging opportunistic pathogen associated with neonatal meningitis, sepsis and necrotizing enterocolitis 188

Usefulness of abdominal ultrasound in diagnosing necrotising enterocolitis 190

A prospective comparison of intestinal sonography and abdominal radiographs in a neonatal intensive care unit 191

Interleukin-8 predicts 60-day mortality in premature infants with necrotizing enterocolitis 193

Cytokine Levels in the Preterm Infant with Neonatal Intestinal Injury 195

Randomized Controlled Trial of Slow vs Rapid Enteral Feeding Advancements on the Clinical Outcomes of Preterm Infants With Birth Weight 750–1250 g 196

Enteral L-Arginine Supplementation for Prevention of Necrotizing Enterocolitis in Very Low Birth Weight Neonates: A Double-Blind Randomized Pilot Study of Efficacy and Safety 198

Growth and Fatty Acid Profiles of VLBW Infants Receiving a Multicomponent Lipid Emulsion From Birth 199

Safety and Efficacy of Early Parenteral Lipid and High-Dose Amino Acid Administration to Very Low Birth Weight Infants 202

Vitamin D status of early preterm infants and the effects of vitamin D intake during hospital stay 204

Chapter 10: Hematology and Bilirubin

A Randomized, Masked, Placebo-Controlled Study of Darbepoetin Alfa in Preterm Infants 205

Cognitive Outcomes of Preterm Infants Randomized to Darbepoetin, Erythropoietin, or Placebo 206

Association, among very-low-birthweight neonates, between red blood cell transfusions in the week after birth and severe intraventricular hemorrhage 208

The effect of hematocrit on the efficacy of phototherapy for neonatal jaundice 210

Causes of hemolysis in neonates with extreme hyperbilirubinemia 211

Unbound Free Fatty Acids from Preterm Infants Treated with Intralipid Decouples Unbound from Total Bilirubin Potentially Making Phototherapy Ineffective 212

Bilistick: A Low-Cost Point-of-Care System to Measure Total Plasma Bilirubin 214

Predischarge Screening for Severe Neonatal Hyperbilirubinemia Identifies Infants Who Need Phototherapy 215

Severe Neonatal Hyperbilirubinemia in the Netherlands 217

Iron supplementation in premature infants using the zinc protoporphyrin to heme ratio: short- and long-term outcomes 219

Chapter 11: Renal, Metabolism, and Endocrine Disorders

Neonatal Thyrotoxicosis 221

Dextrose gel for neonatal hypoglycaemia (the Sugar Babies Study): a randomised, double-blind, placebo-controlled trial 223

Early Hyperglycemia Is Associated With Poor Gross Motor Outcome in Asphyxiated Term Newborns 225

ACTH and cortisol cord plasma concentrations in preterm and term infants 226

Chapter 12: Miscellaneous

Randomized controlled trial of Family Nurture Intervention in the NICU: assessments of length of stay, feasibility and safety 229

Online support for parents of preterm infants: a qualitative and content analysis of Facebook 'preemie' groups 230

Neonatal intensive care unit handoffs: a pilot study on core elements and epidemiology of errors 232

Examining the effects of a targeted noise reduction program in a neonatal intensive care unit 233

Breastfeeding Keratosis: This Frictional Keratosis of Newborns May Mimic Thrush 234

Prediction of Neonatal Outcomes in Extremely Preterm Neonates 235

Utility of delayed surgical repair of neonatal brachial plexus palsy 238

A comparison of the infant car seat challenge and the polysomnogram at the time of hospital discharge 240

Increased Enamel Hypoplasia and Very Low Birthweight Infants 241

Compliance with the Baby-Friendly Hospital Initiative and impact on breastfeeding rates 242

Deaths and near deaths of healthy newborn infants while bed sharing on maternity wards 244

Chapter 13: Pharmacology

Effect of Fluconazole Prophylaxis on Candidiasis and Mortality in Premature Infants: A Randomized Clinical Trial 245

Prophylactic Indomethacin Worsens Short-Term Respiratory Outcomes in Extremely Low-Birth-Weight Infants 247

Characterization of the Population Pharmacokinetics of Ampicillin in Neonates Using an Opportunistic Study Design 249

Accuracy of the concentration of morphine infusions prepared for patients in a neonatal intensive care unit 250

Unlicensed and off-label drug use in an Irish neonatal intensive care unit: a prospective cohort study 252

Transplacental passage of vancomycin from mother to neonate 253

Chapter 14: Postnatal Growth and Development/Follow-up

Alterations in Brain Structure and Neurodevelopmental Outcome in Preterm Infants Hospitalized in Different Neonatal Intensive Care Unit Environments 255

Comparison of Bayley-2 and Bayley-3 scores at 18 months in term infants following neonatal encephalopathy and therapeutic hypothermia 256

Performance of the Parent Report of Children's Abilities–Revised (PARCA-R) versus the Bayley Scales of Infant Development III 258

Effect of primary language on developmental testing in children born extremely preterm 259

Predictive value of the amplitude integrated EEG in infants with hypoxic ischaemic encephalopathy: data from a randomised trial of therapeutic hypothermia 260

Antenatal steroid exposure and outcomes of very premature infants: a regional cohort study 262

Characteristics of extremely low-birth-weight infant survivors with unimpaired outcomes at 30 months of age 263

Two-Year Outcomes of a Randomized Controlled Trial of Inhaled Nitric Oxide in Premature Infants 264

Need for Supplemental Oxygen at Discharge in Infants with Bronchopulmonary Dysplasia Is Not Associated with Worse Neurodevelopmental Outcomes at 3 Years Corrected Age 266

Neurodevelopmental outcomes of extremely low birth weight infants with spontaneous intestinal perforation or surgical necrotizing enterocolitis 267

Neonatal ECMO study of temperature (NEST): a randomized controlled trial 268

Late Outcomes of a Randomized Trial of High-Frequency Oscillation in Neonates 269

Long-term cognitive and neurological outcome of preterm infants with postnatally acquired CMV infection through breast milk 271

Neurodevelopmental outcome, psychological adjustment, and quality of life in adolescents with congenital heart disease 272

Tracheostomy for Infants Requiring Prolonged Mechanical Ventilation: 10 Years' Experience 273

Postnatal corticosteroids and neurodevelopmental outcomes in extremely low birthweight or extremely preterm infants: 15-year experience in Victoria, Australia 275

Motor skills at 23 years of age in young adults born preterm with very low birth weight 276

Chapter 15: Ethics

23andMe and the FDA 279

Views of parents and health-care providers regarding parental presence at bedside rounds in a neonatal intensive care unit 281

Medical interventions for children with trisomy 13 and trisomy 18: what is the value of a short disabled life? 282

End-of-life care in Toronto neonatal intensive care units: challenges for physician trainees 284

Lack of physician-patient communication as a key factor associated with malpractice litigation in neonatal brachial plexus palsy 285

Facing Persistent Challenges in Pediatric Decision-Making: New Hastings Center Guidelines 287

Is Treatment Futile for an Extremely Premature Infant With Giant Omphalocele? 289

Ethical and legal aspects of noninvasive prenatal genetic diagnosis 291

Author Index

A

Aguado-Lorenzo V, 250
Aguilera M, 157
Ahle M, 182
Ahn SY, 115
Ailes E, 83
Al Yazidi G, 127
Albert JM, 241
Albrechtsen S, 45
Alcazar-Paris M, 269
Alderliesten T, 77
Aldrink J, 187
Ali ZS, 238
Allen P, 107
Andersen HU, 5
Anderson PJ, 140
Andersson D, 35
Andersson O, 35
Andersson RE, 182
Andreasen S, 15
Annas GJ, 279
Aubertin C, 233
Azzopardi D, 134, 139, 260

B

Backe B, 15
Badawi N, 14
Baer VL, 208
Bagnoli F, 226
Bakar D, 238
Baker CJ, 60
Banderali G, 165
Barberi S, 165
Barfield R, 287
Barnette AR, 130, 132
Barrett M, 154
Barrington KJ, 179
Barrowman N, 233
Batton B, 79
Baum CF, 242
Bean JF, 188
Beers K, 98
Benders MJ, 217
Benders MJNL, 148
Benjamin B, 27
Benjamin DK Jr, 57, 245
Benkoe T, 193
Bennett C, 51
Berardi A, 61
Bergenhenegouwen LA, 40
Berlinger N, 287
Berrington JE, 153
Bevot A, 271
Bhandari V, 266
Bhatia AM, 195
Bhutani VK, 210, 215
Bianchi DW, 19
Bisschop PH, 221
Bizzarro MJ, 71, 95
Blair E, 14
Blanco CL, 169, 171
Boeke CE, 31
Bohnhorst B, 190
Bolisetty S, 125
Bouquot J, 234
Brown-Lum M, 41
Bruno MEC, 163
Bührer C, 230
Burge DM, 1
Butler TJ, 177
Buzzella B, 102

C

Cahill AG, 43
Campaña H, 21
Carey VJ, 60
Carnielli VP, 199
Caughey AB, 43
Chan M, 284
Chang KWC, 285
Chang YS, 115
Chau V, 41
Chaudhuri D, 247
Check J, 109
Cheng YW, 52
Cheong JL, 141, 275
Cheong JLY, 114, 142
Cheung HM, 68
Chorna OD, 166, 168
Christensen RD, 205, 206, 208, 211
Cismowski MJ, 195
Claure N, 102
Coda Zabetta CD, 214
Conneely KN, 22
Coo H, 281
Cozzi C, 187
Cristofalo EA, 169, 171
Cruickshank MN, 23

D

Däbritz J, 161
Daneman A, 191
Dang D, 74
Darlow BA, 258
Davis NL, 120
Dawodu A, 204
de Halleux V, 175
de Wit MC, 26
DeMauro SB, 49
Demehri FR, 154
DeRienzo C, 232
Deshmukh HS, 63
Dickens BM, 291
Dierker D, 149, 255
Dingley J, 133
Doherty DA, 46
Dold SK, 48
Domellöf M, 35
Domino J, 285
Douglas E, 49
Doyle LW, 140
Draper ES, 51
Drott P, 182
Duerden EG, 41
D'Ugard C, 102
Dukhovny S, 2
Durrmeyer X, 121, 264

E

Ehrenkranz RA, 71
El Sayed MF, 284
El-Khuffash A, 80
Elias S, 279
Embleton ND, 153
Engel SM, 25
Erdeve O, 76
Escobar GJ, 55
Ewer AK, 81

F

Feltman D, 289
Field D, 268
Fiocchi I, 136
Fiori HH, 101
Fleischman AR, 287
Foell D, 161

Fommei C, 226
Fontana P, 136
Frantz AL, 163

G

Gadzinowski J, 104
Gallagher PG, 71
Garland JS, 67
Ge WJ, 235
Geng C, 241
Gill A, 73
Gill H, 137
Gliddon AE, 32
Goelz R, 271
Goldstein M, 7
Gomez-Llorente C, 157
Gotink MJ, 217
Gotteiner N, 109
Govaerts LCP, 26
Graves SW, 184
Greco C, 214
Gregory ML, 120
Groenendaal F, 148
Grow JL, 177
Grzyb MJ, 281
Gupta MK, 87

H

Hacker MR, 37
Harris DL, 223
Hartmann F, 101
Hausmann M, 158
Hawkins SS, 242
Hegyi T, 212
Hellström A, 146
Hennet T, 158
Herbozo C, 80
Hernández-Díaz S, 31
Hirata K, 119
Holmström GE, 146
Hopfner RJ, 129
Horbar JD, 130, 132
Horvath M, 232
Howard BC, 253
Hunter CJ, 188
Husby IM, 276

I

Ishii N, 12
Iskander IF, 214
Islam S, 108

J

Jacobs SE, 65
Jain A, 80
Janeczko M, 240
Janvier A, 179, 282
Jary S, 256
Jeffery M, 73
Joshi S, 86
Joubert BR, 25

K

Kaandorp JJ, 38
Källen K, 146
Kamath-Rayne BD, 205, 206
Kapetanakis A, 139
Karagol BS, 196
Karp K, 49
Kathiravan S, 212
Katz K, 95
Kays DW, 108
Kelm M, 48
Kessler J, 45
Kett J, 289
Kiat-Amnuay S, 234
Kieran EA, 252
Kilaru V, 22
King TL, 52
Klebermass-Schrehof K, 128
Kluckow M, 73
Knirsch W, 272
Konduri GG, 106
Kotecha S, 86
Krebs NF, 160
Kreissl A, 173
Kumar P, 263
Kurachek SC, 273
Kurakevich E, 158

L

Lababidi SL, 225
Lam HS, 68
Lambert DK, 208
Lamola AA, 210
Lavrijsen SW, 217
Le F, 16
Lee H, 118
Lemmers PMA, 77
Lenfestey R, 232
Lenhof S, 129
Lewis MM, 98
Li B, 247
Li FY, 95
Li YR, 238
Little SE, 33
Liu M, 273
Liu X, 109, 133, 137
Liu Y, 63
Lodha A, 266
Lou H, 16
Lowe JR, 259

M

Malo J, 179
Manzoni P, 144
March MI, 37
Marlow N, 51
Martin AJ, 258
Martin W, 8
Mastrangelo M, 136
McAllister M, 284
McBride MC, 225
McGovern C, 285
McIntyre S, 14
Meertens LJE, 40
Meinzen-Derr J, 185
Meisner C, 271
Menkiti OR, 63
Merhar SL, 185
Merkel L, 98
Merritt TA, 7
Metze B, 230
Miller SM, 219
Moczko J, 104
Monangi N, 204
Mondal T, 247
Mori A, 226
Moster D, 45
Mulrooney NP, 67

N

Navarro OM, 191
Neil J, 149, 255
Nelson S, 241
Newnham JP, 46
Ng C, 1
Nicol K, 187
Nishihara M, 119
Nolen TL, 259
Nussenzveig RH, 211

O

O'Callaghan N, 252
O'Donnell CPF, 252
Ohls RK, 205, 206
Øian P, 15
Okumus N, 196
Olsen A, 276
Oncel MY, 76
Onwuchuruba CN, 253
Oshima Y, 119
Oshlack A, 23
Overman AE, 273

P

Paget-Brown AO, 118
Parets SE, 22
Parson AW, 37
Peacock J, 269
Peterson C, 83
Philips R, 7
Pineda RG, 149, 255
Plaza-Diaz J, 157
Poletta FA, 21
Polycarpou E, 198
Pones M, 193
Poon TCW, 68
Prefumo F, 29
Puopolo KM, 33, 55

R

Ralls MW, 154
Ramos Garcia PC, 101
Ramos Y, 185
Reagan PB, 111
Reck C, 193
Rench MA, 60
Repa A, 173
Rhein L, 120
Richards DS, 108
Riehle-Colarusso T, 83
Rigo J, 175
Ringholm L, 5
Rittler M, 21
Roberts D, 8
Robertson NJ, 139
Robinson JN, 33
Roehl KA, 43
Rogier EW, 163
Romans AT, 31
Rona Z, 128
Rook D, 202
Rossi AC, 29
Rühland L, 281
Ruiz TL, 97
Rukholm G, 87

S

Sáenz de Pipaón Marcos M, 180
Salt A, 258
Salvador A, 240
Sampath V, 67
Sanjosé B, 180
Sauvé R, 266
Schaaf J, 40
Schaefer C, 272
Schanler RJ, 169, 171
Schmid MB, 129
Schmidt B, 89
Schmölzer GM, 48
Schutzman DL, 240
Secher AL, 5
Sellars M, 107
Serenius F, 10
Sherlock LG, 160
Shipp TD, 2
Signal M, 223
Silva CT, 191
Sink DW, 97
Skranes J, 276
Slaughter JC, 166, 168
Slaughter JL, 111, 204
Smit E, 137
Snowden JM, 52
Soll RF, 130, 132
Spies EE, 225
Srebniak MI, 26
Srour M, 127
Stahl GE, 212
Stanwell J, 1
Stark AR, 112
Stenger MR, 111
Stern AD, 242
Stevens TP, 91
Stewart CJ, 153
Stokes T, 289
Stoll BJ, 195
Stone ML, 183
Strychowsky JE, 87
Stutchfield PR, 32
Szczapa T, 104
Szekely LJ, 177

T

Tajik P, 59
Tatum PM, 183
Teresa Montes Bueno M, 180
Thach BT, 244
Theda C, 23
Thoren EM, 230
Tooley J, 133
Towers CV, 253
Trembath A, 99
Tremoulet A, 249
Trzaski JM, 97
Tsolia M, 198
Tunstell P, 250

V

van der Aa NE, 148
van der Ham DP, 59
van Haastert IC, 77
van Trotsenburg ASP, 221
Vause S, 8
Verduci E, 165
Vergales BD, 118
Vermeulen MJ, 199, 202
Vlaardingerbroek H, 199, 202
Vohr B, 259
von Rhein M, 272

W

Wadhawan R, 267
Waldhör T, 128
Walløe L, 256
Walsh JM, 140
Wang D, 74, 233
Wang L, 166, 168
Watkins A, 282
Weeks K, 250
Weitkamp J-H, 183
Welch MG, 229
Westcott J, 160
Weston PJ, 223

Whitaker R, 32
White CRH, 46
Whitelaw A, 256
Wi S, 55
Wilkins-Haug L, 2
Wilson DG, 86
Wilson GN, 27
Wintermark P, 127
Wirth S, 161
Wong D, 262
Wong RJ, 210
Wu MC, 25

Y

Yaish HM, 211
Yoo HS, 115
Yurttutan S, 76

Z

Zachaki S, 198
Zafarmand MH, 59
Zani A, 107
Zenciroglu A, 196
Zhang C, 74
Zheng Y, 16
Zivanovic S, 116, 269
Zwiauer V, 173

FSC
www.fsc.org
MIX
Papier | Fördert
gute Waldnutzung
FSC® C083411

Kolibri 360 GmbH
Ferdinand-Jühlke-Straße 7
99095 Erfurt, Deutschland
produktsicherheit@kolibri360.de